Anesthesiology Boards

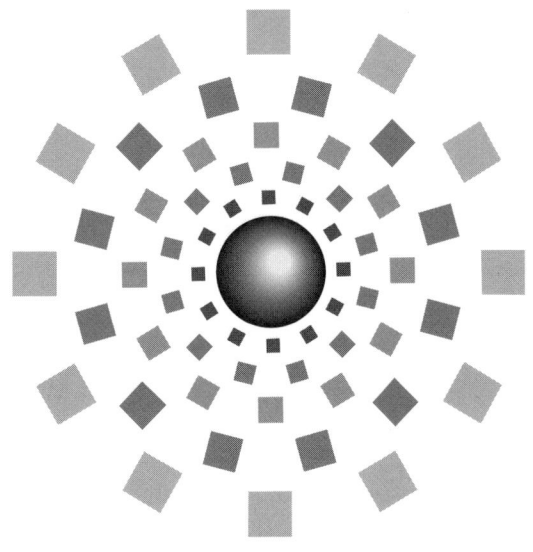

A Survival Guide

Michelle Starr, MD
Assistant Professor of Anesthesiology
Emory University School of Medicine

CHURCHILL LIVINGSTONE
An Imprint of Elsevier Science
New York   Edinburgh   London   Philadelphia

CHURCHILL LIVINGSTONE
An Imprint of Elsevier Science

The Curtis Center
Independence Square West
Philadelphia, Pennsylvania 19106

Library of Congress Cataloging-in-Publication Data

Starr, Michelle.
    Anesthesiology boards : a survival guide / Michelle Starr.
       p.   cm.
    ISBN 0-443-07619-7
    1. Anesthesia Terminology. 2. Anesthesiology Examinations, questions, etc. 3. Anesthesia Dictionaries. I. Title.
    [DNLM: 1. Anesthesiology Terminology—English. WO 215 S796a –2000]
    RD82.S73   2000
    617.9′6′014—dc21
    DNLM/DLC
                                       99-33417

ANESTHESIOLOGY BOARDS: A SURVIVAL GUIDE   ISBN 0-443-07619-7

Copyright © 2000 by Churchill Livingstone

All rights reserved. No part of this publication may be reproduced or transmitted in any form or by any means, electronic or mechanical, including photocopy, recording, or any information storage and retrieval system, without permission in writing from the publisher.

Churchill Livingstone® and the ™ are trademarks of Elsevier Science.

Printed in the United States of America

Last digit is the print number: 9 8 7 6 5 4

PREFACE

While studying for the written portion of the American Board of Anesthesiology examination, I, like many students of anesthesiology, adopted a keyword-oriented approach. It sounded good in theory . . . if I just looked up all the information pertaining to the keywords I'd missed on my in-training exams, then I'd be ready for the real thing! Reality came crashing down when I looked up that first keyword and realized that it was listed in FOURTEEN different places in one text! "Uh, oh . . . this could be harder than I thought!" is a nice way of saying what came to mind. Obviously, many of my peers felt the same way and chose instead to use the keyword-oriented review texts available at the time. Other residents chose to study by answering thousands upon thousands of practice questions, also available in review book form. For me, neither approach was satisfactory. The keyword-oriented review texts were written in full-text format, just as the major anesthesia reference texts are. I, as many students, find it easier to memorize lists, and found myself having to take notes from the review texts, forced to create my own lists from which to study. The only way I found "question-and-answer" type review books helpful was to wade through them after reading a topic *elsewhere* and find the one or two questions they had regarding the said topic to see if I'd understood it. Cumbersome. Time-consuming. Not at all what I had in mind. Both approaches had merit, but how to make them work better?

As a result of my frustration, I created this book to try to achieve the best of both worlds. You'll notice that the book is thin . . . that's because I intentionally left out ALL THE STUFF THEY NEVER ASK YOU. I have compiled keyword-specific information and presented it in a bullet-list format (easier to memorize), accompanied by text for topics requiring greater explanation. Flowcharts are included to clarify physiologic pathways. Sections are brief, with narrow focus, and each section is followed by sample questions to reinforce the information presented. The length of sections and number of questions per section reflect the amount of attention the topic is given on the exam.

So . . . *how do you use this book*? You can either look up a specific keyword in the index and find the section(s) it's covered in, or you can look at the table of contents and find out which keywords are covered in which sections. Either way, you'll be presented with the years in which the topic appeared on the exam, so you can get an idea of the favorites of the examiners.

It is my hope that you find this book to be as "user-friendly" as I envisioned it to be and that it serves as a useful study tool. Good luck. Study hard. Call me when you pass. I'll be rooting for you.

Michelle Starr, MD

ACKNOWLEDGMENTS

My appreciation to Dr. Peter Sebel for planting the seed of the idea for this book . . . he saw my extensive notes created during my study efforts and commented: "You ought to try to get this published!" I'm glad I didn't realize then how much work it would be! My utmost appreciation to my secretary, Ms. Emily Hazelwood, for her diligence and efficiency during the preparation of this manuscript. (She's a whiz kid with a computer scanner!) My thanks to my many colleagues at Emory University School of Medicine and in particular at Grady Memorial Hospital, for never telling me to get lost when I shoved a newly typed section under their noses and said "Here. Read this and tell me what you think." Finally, my heartfelt thanks to my father, Terry Starr, without whose undying faith and support this dream would never have begun.

CONTENTS

SECTION 1
Inhalational Anesthesia

1 ■ Minimum Alveolar Concentration...3

KEYWORDS	TEST YEAR
MAC: definition	1994
MAC: factors affecting	1994, 1996, 1998×2
MAC and volatile anesthetic potency	1994×2

2 ■ Uptake and Distribution of Inhaled Anesthetics 5

KEYWORDS	TEST YEAR
Uptake and distribution of inhaled anesthetics	1993, 1994, 1998×2
Desflurane: rate of rise of F_A/F_I vs. N_2O	1996
Volatile agent uptake: effect of cardiac output	1993
Inspired anesthetic concentration: determinants	1994
Congenital heart disease: effect of intracardiac shunt on uptake	1993, 1994, 1996
Inhalational induction: child vs. adult	1995, 1998
Inhalational induction in infants	1993, 1998
Second gas effect	1993, 1998
Concentration effect	1993

3 ■ Pulmonary Effects of Inhalational Agents...................................9

KEYWORDS	TEST YEAR
Inhalational anesthesia: respiratory effects	1994, 1995, 1998
General anesthesia and pulmonary gas exchange	1995
Volatile agents: cardiopulmonary effects	1993, 1994, 1995
CO_2 response curve: anesthetic implications	1994
CO_2 response curve: drug effect	1994, 1998
Desflurane pharmacology	1995

4 ■ Cardiovascular Effects of Inhalational Agents.............................11

KEYWORDS	TEST YEAR
Volatile agents and nonischemic heart disease	1994
Volatile agents: cardiopulmonary effects	1993, 1994, 1995, 1998
Halothane: cardiovascular effects	1993, 1995

vii

viii   Contents

Halothane: ventilatory response to hypoxia	1993
Isoflurane effects: CBF and CMRO$_2$	1993, 1998
N$_2$O: cerebral effects	1995
Isoflurane effects: CBF and CMRO$_2$	1993
Desflurane pharmacology	1995

5 ■ Nitrous Oxide 13

KEYWORDS	TEST YEAR
N$_2$O and air in closed spaces	1993, 1996
N$_2$O: physical properties	1994
N$_2$O: cerebral effects	1995
N$_2$O and eye surgery	1996

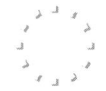

SECTION 2
Pulmonary Physiology

6 ■ Pulmonary Physiology 17

KEYWORDS	TEST YEAR
Pulmonary blood flow: distribution	1995
V/Q mismatch: factors affecting	1993, 1998×2
V/Q mismatch: effects	1995
Cardiac output and deadspace	1995
Effects: hypoventilation	1993
Work of breathing: factors affecting	1994
VD/VT: factors affecting	1996
Increased A-aDO$_2$: causes	1996, 1998
Lung compliance: anesthetic factors and disease	1996, 1998

7 ■ Apneic Oxygenation 20

KEYWORD	TEST YEAR
Apneic oxygenation	1993, 1994

8 ■ Oxyhemoglobin Curves, Oxygen Content, and Oxygen Delivery 21

KEYWORDS	TEST YEAR
O$_2$ delivery: determinants of	1995, 1998
O$_2$ transport, hematocrit and viscosity	1995
Altered p50 and tissue O$_2$ delivery	1995
Oxyhemoglobin shift: causes	1993, 1995, 1998
Fetal hemoglobin vs. adult	1993, 1995
Fetal hemoglobin	1995
Oxygen content: factors affecting	1994
Chronic anemia: compensatory mechanisms	1995
Maternal-fetal O$_2$ transport	1994

9 ■ Flow-Volume Loops 24

KEYWORDS	TEST YEAR
PFTs: flow-volume loop interpretation	1993, 1995
PFTs: in obstructive and restrictive disease	1994
Flow-volume loop in COPD	1996

10 ■ Pulmonary Function Tests and Disease States........................... 26

KEYWORDS	TEST YEAR
FRC and general anesthesia	1994, 1998
FRC: positional effects	1994, 1998
FRC: factors reducing	1996
Aging: effect on PFTs	1993
Morbid obesity: PFTs	1993, 1994
Pregnancy: PFTs during	1994
Hypoxic mechanisms in pregnancy	1993, 1994, 1995, 1996
Abdominal surgery: PFTs after	1993, 1994
Gas exchange after abdominal surgery	1993, 1998
Restrictive lung disease: pathophysiology	1995
Kyphoscoliosis: respiratory effects	1995
Pulmonary fibrosis: anesthetic considerations	1993
Myasthenia gravis: PFTs	1993, 1994

SECTION 3
Anesthesia and Disease States

11 ■ Chronic Obstructive Pulmonary Disease................................. 31

KEYWORDS	TEST YEAR
COPD: mechanical ventilation	1994, 1996
COPD: hemodynamic monitoring	1993
COPD: spinal anesthesia	1993, 1998
COPD: preoperative therapy	1996, 1998
COPD: PFTs in advanced disease	1996
Bronchitis: preoperative assessment	1993
Emphysema: chest X-ray	1993

12 ■ Adult Respiratory Distress Syndrome 34

KEYWORDS	TEST YEAR
ARDS: pathophysiology and treatment	1995, 1998
ARDS: CO_2 retention	1995
ARDS: mechanical ventilation	1993, 1995

13 ■ Asthma 37

KEYWORDS	TEST YEAR
Asthma: anesthetic considerations	1994
Intraoperative asthma: signs	1995
Intraoperative bronchospasm: diagnosis	1993
Asthma: management	1996, 1998

14 ■ Morbid Obesity 39

KEYWORDS	TEST YEAR
Morbid obesity: anesthetic implications	1993, 1995, 1998
Morbid obesity: pharmacokinetc considerations	1994
Morbid obesity: cardiovascular implications and complications	1994, 1998
Morbid obesity: PFTs	1993, 1994, 1996

15 ■ Cigarette Smoking 42

KEYWORDS	TEST YEAR
Cigarette smoking: pulmonary effects	1994
Preoperative smoking cessation	1993, 1998

16 ■ Carbon Monoxide Poisoning 43

KEYWORD	TEST YEAR
Carbon monoxide poisoning	1993×2, 1995, 1996, 1998×2

17 ■ Diabetes Mellitus 45

KEYWORDS	TEST YEAR
Hyperglycemia: preoperative management	1993
Hyperglycemia: perioperative management	1995, 1998
Chronic hyperglycemia: effects	1993
Acute perioperative hypoglycemia: signs	1994
Diabetic ketoacidosis	1995, 1996

18 ■ Thyroid Disease 47

KEYWORDS	TEST YEAR
Hyperthyroidism: perioperative concerns	1995, 1998
Hyperthyroidism: intraoperative management	1994
Hyperthyroidism: beta-blockers	1996
Hypothyroidism: anesthetic considerations	1993, 1998
Thyroid surgery: complications	1995
Thyroid surgery: airway obstruction following	1993, 1995
Hoarseness following thyroid surgery: causes	1994, 1996

19 ■ Pheochromocytoma 50

KEYWORDS	TEST YEAR
Pheochromocytoma: preoperative management	1994
Pheochromocytoma: management of hypotension after resection	1993, 1995

20 ■ Myasthenia Gravis 53

KEYWORDS	TEST YEAR
Myasthenia gravis	1995
Myasthenia gravis: PFTs	1993, 1994
Myasthenic crisis vs. cholinergic	1995
Acetylcholinesterase inhibitors: side effects	1995
Acetylcholinesterase inhibitors: muscarinic effects	1994

Contents xi

21 ■ Eaton–Lambert Syndrome (Myasthenic Syndrome).........................56

KEYWORD	TEST YEAR
Myasthenic syndrome: characteristics	1993, 1994, 1995

22 ■ Malignant Hyperthermia and Masseter Spasm............................58

KEYWORDS	TEST YEAR
Malignant hyperthermia history: anesthetic management	1994
Malignant hyperthermia: clinical signs	1993
Malignant hyperthermia: early diagnosis	1996
Malignant hyperthermia: testing susceptibility	1996
Masseter spasm: characteristics	1996
Dantrolene: pharmacology	1995, 1998
Succinylcholine: contraindications	1994
Succinylcholine: effects in Duchenne's	1995

23 ■ Neuroleptic Malignant Syndrome..62

KEYWORD	TEST YEAR
Neuroleptic malignant syndrome	1993

24 ■ Muscular Dystrophy..64

KEYWORDS	TEST YEAR
Muscular dystrophy: anesthetic implications	1994
Duchenne's: preoperative evaluation	1995
Duchenne's: succinylcholine effects	1995
Myotonic dystrophy: anesthetic implications	1995
Succinylcholine: contraindications	1994

25 ■ Parkinson's Disease..67

KEYWORDS	TEST YEAR
Parkinson's disease: anesthetic implications	1995, 1996
Parkinson's disease: drug interactions	1993

26 ■ Glaucoma...69

KEYWORDS	TEST YEAR
Glaucoma: drug interactions	1995, 1998
Closed angle glaucoma: anesthetic considerations	1996, 1998
Intraocular pressure: drugs affecting	1993
Eye surgery: regional vs. general	1994
Oculocardiac reflex: pathways	1994
Oculocardiac reflex: clinical implications	1993, 1994
Bradycardia during eye surgery	1995

27 ■ Transurethral Resection of the Prostate..................................71

KEYWORDS	TEST YEAR
TURP: complications	1994
TURP: coagulopathy	1993
TURP: hypervolemia	1993
TURP syndrome	1993, 1998

TURP: causes of agitation following	1995
TURP: causes of postoperative hypoxia	1995
TURP: effect of glycine during	1993, 1994, 1995, 1996
TURP: differential diagnosis of bladder perforation	1996
TURP: treatment of hyponatremia	1996
TURP: proximate nerve anatomy	1996

28 ■ Extracorporeal Shock Wave Lithotripsy 73

KEYWORDS	TEST YEAR
Lithotripsy and regional anesthesia: hemodynamic effects	1994
Lithotripsy: timing	1994

29 ■ Anesthetic Implications of Liver Disease 75

KEYWORDS	TEST YEAR
Hepatic blood flow: intraoperative determinants	1994, 1998
Liver disease: preoperative evaluation	1993, 1998×2
Liver function tests	1994
Liver disease: anesthetic implications	1995
Liver disease: anesthetic induction	1993
Thiopental and liver disease	1996
Muscle relaxants: liver disease	1993
Hypoxemia with severe liver disease	1993, 1995
Liver disease: intraoperative hypotension	1993
Coagulopathy in liver disease	1995
Acute ETOH intoxication: anesthetic implications	1993, 1995, 1996, 1998
Cirrhosis: cardiovascular abnormalities	1994
Cirrhosis: pharmacokinetic implications	1994
Cirrhosis and muscle relaxants	1995
Cirrhosis and liver function tests	1996, 1998
Postoperative hepatic dysfunction	1995, 1996, 1998

30 ■ Hepatitis B Infection 79

KEYWORDS	TEST YEAR
Hepatitis B testing: interpretation	1995
Hepatitis B: immmediate tx after exposure	1994

31 ■ Liver Transplant 80

KEYWORDS	TEST YEAR
Liver transplant: management	1994
Liver transplant: venovenous bypass during	1995

32 ■ Cocaine Intoxication 81

KEYWORDS	TEST YEAR
Acute cocaine intoxication: signs	1993, 1994
Cocaine intoxication: anesthetic implications	1995
Cocaine: treatment of hypertension after	1993

33 ■ Renal Disease...83

KEYWORDS	TEST YEAR
Muscle relaxants in renal failure	1993, 1994, 1995, 1998
Renal failure: pharmacokinetics	1993
Prerenal azotemia: diagnosis	1995, 1998×2
Prerenal oliguria	1993
Postoperative oliguria: causes	1995, 1998
Postoperative oliguria: diagnostic criteria	1994
Oliguria: interpretation of lab data	1993, 1995
Acute tubular necrosis: diagnostic criteria	1994, 1996
Electrolyte effects of renal failure	1996
Morphine: elimination in renal failure	1994, 1998
Fluoride toxicity	1993

34 ■ Human Immunodeficiency Virus...86

KEYWORDS	TEST YEAR
Inactivation of HIV	1994
HIV: management of contamination	1993

35 ■ Laparoscopy...87

KEYWORDS	TEST YEAR
Laparoscopy: complications	1995
Laparoscopy and gas embolism	1993
Laparoscopy: response to CO_2 insufflation	1993, 1998
Laparoscopy: pulmonary effects	1995

SECTION 4
Pediatric Anesthesia

36 ■ Respiratory Function: Infants versus Adults............................93

KEYWORDS	TEST YEAR
Infant vs. adult oxygenation	1993
Respiratory function: adult vs. child	1993
Neonatal hypoxemia: physiologic causes	1995
Neonatal respiratory failure	1993
Neonatal respiratory physiology	1996
Perioperative desaturation in neonates: mechanisms	1994
Neonates and postoperative apnea	1994, 1998

37 ■ Pediatric Fluid Management..96

KEYWORDS	TEST YEAR
Neonatal fluid management	1995, 1998
Pediatric fluid management	1993, 1996

38 ■ Pyloric Stenosis 98

KEYWORD	TEST YEAR
Pyloric stenosis: preoperative abnormalities	1993, 1994, 1998

39 ■ Tetralogy of Fallot 100

KEYWORDS	TEST YEAR
Tetralogy of Fallot: pathophysiology	1995, 1998
Tetralogy of Fallot: management of cyanosis	1993, 1994, 1995, 1996, 1998
Right to left shunt: management during anesthesia	1993

40 ■ Croup versus Epiglottitis 102

KEYWORD	TEST YEAR
Croup vs. epiglottitis	1993, 1995, 1998

41 ■ Diaphragmatic Hernia 104

KEYWORD	TEST YEAR
Diaphragmatic hernia: management	1993, 1994, 1995

42 ■ Omphalocele/Gastroschisis 106

KEYWORDS	TEST YEAR
Gastroschisis repair: anesthetic implications	1994
Omphalocele repair: complications	1995
Omphalocele: fluid therapy	1996

43 ■ Tracheoesophageal Fistula 108

KEYWORD	TEST YEAR
TE fistula: complications	1993, 1994, 1998

44 ■ Necrotizing Enterocolitis 110

KEYWORD	TEST YEAR
NEC: perioperative management	1994

45 ■ Pierre-Robin Syndrome 112

KEYWORD	TEST YEAR
Anesthetic implications	1994

46 ■ Infants Born to Myasthenic Women 114

KEYWORD	TEST YEAR
Infants born to myasthenic women: respiratory failure at delivery	1993

47 ■ Fetal and Neonatal Circulation 115

KEYWORDS	TEST YEAR
Factors causing persistent fetal circulation	1993, 1996, 1998×2
Fetal adaptation at birth	1993

48 ■ Neonatal Temperature Regulation 117

KEYWORDS	TEST YEAR
Neonatal temperature regulation	1995, 1998
Neonatal hypothermia: effects	1995
Preterm infants: hypothermia	1993
Intraoperative hypothermia in infants	1995
Neonatal vs. adult thermoregulation	1994, 1998

49 ■ Prematurity 119

KEYWORDS	TEST YEAR
Prematurity: anesthetic risks	1993
Retinopathy of prematurity	1995
Preterm infants: hypothermia	1993
Perioperative desaturation in neonates: mechanisms	1994
Neonates and postoperative apnea	1994
Preterm infants: hypothermia	1993

50 ■ Meconium Aspiration 121

KEYWORD	TEST YEAR
Resuscitation after meconium aspiration	1993, 1998

51 ■ Neonatal Resuscitation. 123

KEYWORDS	TEST YEAR
Neonatal resuscitation: maternal addiction	1994
Neonatal resuscitation	1995×4
Neonatal HCO_3^- therapy	1995
Magnesium toxicity: neonatal	1995
Fetal adaptation at birth	1993
Magnesium: neuromuscular effects	1995, 1996
Neonatal blood gas analysis	1998

SECTION 5
Obstetric Anesthesia

52 ■ Fetal Monitoring. 129

KEYWORDS	TEST YEAR
Fetal heart rate: monitoring	1993, 1996, 1998
Fetal monitoring	1993, 1998
Fetal heart rate decelerations: causes	1994
Fetal heart rate: drug effects	1993, 1996
Fetal distress: diagnosis	1994, 1998

53 ■ Physiologic Changes of Pregnancy 131

KEYWORDS	TEST YEAR
	1993, 1994, 1995, 1996
Hypoxic mechanisms in pregnancy	1993, 1998
Pregnancy: PFTs during	1994

54 ■ Utero-Placental Blood Flow 133

KEYWORDS	TEST YEAR
Uterine blood flow: determinants	1994, 1996
Uterine blood flow during labor	1995
Uteroplacental blood flow: physiology	1994, 1996
Uterine contractions: anesthetic effects	1993
Aortocaval compression: management	1995, 1996

55 ■ Placental Transfer of Drugs and Oxygen 135

KEYWORDS	TEST YEAR
Placental transfer: determinants	1993, 1995, 1998×2
Placental transfer: local anesthetics	1993, 1994
Placental transfer: relaxants	1996
Maternal-fetal O_2 transport	1994
Placental oxygen exchange	1993
Thiopental level: maternal-fetal	1995
Maternal-fetal levels of bupivicaine	1993, 1994
Fetal hemoglobin vs. adult	1993, 1995
Fetal hemoglobin	1995

56 ■ Labor Analgesia 137

KEYWORDS	TEST YEAR
First stage of labor: analgesia techniques	1994
Labor, fetal distress, and epidural	1994
Second stage of labor: dermatomes	1993, 1996

57 ■ Anesthesia for Cesarean Section 139

KEYWORDS	TEST YEAR
Anesthesia for C-section: neonatal effects	1995
General anesthesia for C-section: anesthetic considerations	1994
C-section: effects of low-dose halothane	1993
Pregnancy and volatile anesthetic induction	1994, 1996
Hypoxic mechanisms in pregnancy	1993

58 ■ Anesthesia for Breech Delivery 142

KEYWORD	TEST YEAR
Anesthesia for breech delivery	1994

59 ■ The Bleeding Parturient 144

KEYWORDS	TEST YEAR
Bleeding parturient: causes	1995, 1996
Placental abruption: management	1996

| Retained placenta: anesthesia for | 1993 |
| DIC in obstetric patients | 1994 |

60 ■ Pre-Eclampsia/Eclampsia 146

KEYWORDS	TEST YEAR
Pre-eclampsia: pathophysiology	1995
Pre-eclampsia: hemodynamic effects	1994
Pre-eclampsia and epidural anesthesia	1996
Magnesium: pharmacology	1996
Magnesium: neuromuscular effects	1995, 1996
Magnesium: drug interactions	1994
Magnesium: side effects	1993
Neonatal magnesium toxicity	1995
DIC in obstetric patients	1994
Succinylcholine and pre-eclampsia	1993

61 ■ Tocolytic Therapy 149

KEYWORDS	TEST YEAR
Tocolysis: effects and complications	1993, 1994, 1995, 1998
Tocolysis in preterm labor	1996

62 ■ Anesthesia for Nonobstetric Surgery during the First Trimester 151

KEYWORD	TEST YEAR
Anesthesia for first trimester	1994, 1995, 1998×2

SECTION 6
Regional Anesthesia and Pain Management

63 ■ Local Anesthetics 155

KEYWORDS	TEST YEAR
Local anesthetic: mechanism of action	1993
Local anesthetic: duration	1993
Local anesthetic: physicochemical properties	1994
Local anesthetic onset: pharmacologic manipulation	1994
Local anesthetic: alkalinization	1993, 1998
Local anesthetic: cardiotoxicity	1994, 1995
Local anesthetic: PABA allergy	1995, 1998
Intravascular administration: clinical implications	1994
Bupivicaine: toxicity	1993, 1998
Differential nerve sensitivity	1994, 1996
Methylparaben in local anesthetics	1998

64 ■ Spinal Anesthesia 161

KEYWORDS	TEST YEAR
Subarachnoid block: midline vs. paramedian anatomy	1994
Subarachnoid block: advantages of paramedian	1993, 1998

Subarachnoid block: physiologic effects of T4 level	1994
Subarachnoid block: cardiovascular effects	1995, 1998
Subarachnoid block: cardiovascular collapse and resuscitation	1994
Subarachnoid block: causes of hypotension during	1993, 1995, 1998
Subarachnoid block: mechanism of respiratory arrest during	1994
Subarachnoid block: dyspnea with high level	1994
Subarachnoid block: distribution of local anesthetic	1993, 1995, 1998
Subarachnoid block: local anesthetic: duration of action	1994
Subarachnoid block: duration of local anesthetic	1993
Subarachnoid block: recovery	1995
Subarachnoid block: differential neural sensitivity	1994, 1998
Subarachnoid block: causes of failed block	1995
Subarachnoid block: effects/signs of high level	1994, 1995
Subarachnoid block: nausea with high level	1995
Subarachnoid block: hypobaric spinal anesthesia	1995
Spinal headache	1993, 1994, 1996

65 ■ Epidural Anesthesia..166

KEYWORDS	TEST YEAR
Epidural space: anatomy	1996, 1998
Epidural anesthesia: duration	1994
Epidural anesthesia: effects of T8 level	1994
Epidural anesthesia: cardiorespiratory effects	1993×2
Epidural anesthesia: complications	1993×2, 1998×2
Epidural: management of retained catheter	1994
Epidural test dose failure	1993

66 ■ Pediatric Regional Anesthesia 170

KEYWORDS	TEST YEAR
Pediatric caudal anesthesia	1994, 1998
Pediatric caudal anesthesia: complications	1993
Pediatric postoperative pain management	1993

67 ■ Epidural and Intrathecal Opioids 173

KEYWORDS	TEST YEAR
Epidural opioids: site of action	1993
Epidural morphine: pharmacodynamics/pharmacokinetics	1993
Epidural opioids: rostral migration	1994
Epidural opioids: spread	1993
Epidural narcotics: respiratory depression	1993
Spinal opioids and ventilatory depression	1994

68 ■ Low Back Pain and Epidural Steroids 175

KEYWORDS	TEST YEAR
Epidural steroids: indications	1994, 1995, 1998
Epidural steroid: low back pain	1995
Low back pain: treatment	1993

Contents xix

69 ■ Sympathetically Mediated Pain Syndromes 177

KEYWORDS	TEST YEAR
Reflex sympathetic dystrophy: characteristics	1994, 1995, 1998
Reflex sympathetic dystrophy: early and late signs	1994, 1996×2, 1998
Reflex sympathetic dystrophy: management	1993, 1996, 1998
Causalgia: diagnosis	1993

70 ■ Stellate Ganglion Blockade 179

KEYWORDS	TEST YEAR
Stellate ganglion block: anatomy	1995, 1998
Stellate ganglion block: signs	1994
Stellate ganglion block: effects	1993
Stellate ganglion block: complications	1993, 1994

71 ■ Celiac Plexus Blockade 181

KEYWORDS	TEST YEAR
Celiac plexus block: physiology	1994, 1995, 1998
Celiac plexus block: anatomy	1994, 1996
Celiac plexus block: indications	1993, 1994
Celiac plexus block: complications	1995, 1996
Celiac plexus block: pancreatic cancer treatment	1994
Celiac plexus block: avoiding complications	1996

72 ■ Postherpetic Neuralgia 183

KEYWORD	TEST YEAR
Postherpetic neuralgia	1993, 1994, 1995

73 ■ Neurolytic Nerve Blocks 185

KEYWORDS	TEST YEAR
Chemical neurolysis: indications	1994, 1996
Intrathecal neurolytic block: techniques	1994
Neurolytic blocks: head and neck cancer	1994
Phenol vs. alcohol	1993, 1998

74 ■ Cervical Plexus Blockade 187

KEYWORDS	TEST YEAR
Superficial cervical plexus block: anatomy	1995
Deep cervical plexus block	1994
Cervical plexus block: complications	1996, 1998

75 ■ Brachial Plexus Anatomy and Blockade 189

KEYWORDS	TEST YEAR
Shoulder block interscalene block: anatomy	1994, 1998
Interscalene block: landmarks	1995
Interscalene block: complications	1993×2
Interscalene block and phrenic paralysis	1995
Brachial plexus block: onset characteristics	1994, 1996
Brachial plexus: anatomy	1993, 1998

xx Contents

Axillary block: anatomy	1994, 1998
Axillary block: diagnosis and treatment of inadequate block	1994, 1998
Axillary block: median nerve failure	1995
Axillary brachial plexus: anatomy	1994
Axillary block: factors affecting spread	1993
Anesthesia for upper arm vascular surgery	1995
Sensory innervation of the arm	1998

76 ■ Lower Extremity Nerve Blocks 193

KEYWORDS	TEST YEAR
Lower extremity blocks: anatomy	1993, 1994, 1995, 1998
Sciatic nerve: landmarks	1993
Femoral nerve block	1995
Nerves that must be blocked for knee surgery	1993, 1994, 1998
Ankle block: anatomy	1993×2, 1995×2, 1996, 1998

77 ■ Intravenous Regional Anesthesia 196

KEYWORDS	TEST YEAR
IV regional anesthesia: effects and duration	1994
IV regional anesthesia: technique	1994
IV regional anesthesia: termination of	1993
IV regional anesthesia: tourniquet management	1994

78 ■ Retrobulbar Block and Oculocardiac Reflex 198

KEYWORDS	TEST YEAR
Retrobulbar block: complications	1993, 1994, 1995, 1996, 1998
Retrobulbar block: apnea and	1993
Retrobulbar block: contraindications	1995
Retrobulbar block: effects	1996, 1998
Oculocardiac reflex: afferent and efferent pathways	1993
Oculocardiac reflex: causes	1993
Oculocardiac reflex: prevention and treatment	1993
Oculocardiac reflex: clinical implications	1993, 1994, 1998

SECTION 7
Cardiothoracic Anesthesia

79 ■ Coronary Blood Flow and Myocardial Oxygenation 203

KEYWORDS	TEST YEAR
Coronary blood flow: physiology	1993, 1996
Subendocardial blood flow	1993
Coronary steal: pathophysiology	1995
Myocardial oxygenation: determinants	1994
Myocardial O_2 supply: anesthetic effects	1994
Intraoperative myocardial ischemia: detection	1994, 1998
Treatment: postinduction hypotension in CAD	1993
Postoperative myocardial ischemia: treatment	1993

80 ■ Ventricular Function Curves 206

KEYWORDS	TEST YEAR
Frank Starling relationships	1993, 1996, 1998
Cardiac failure	1995
Acute LV failure: management	1996
Pressors and preload	1995, 1998
Intraoperative hypotension: therapeutic intervention	1993, 1995
CHF and myocardial O_2 consumption	1994, 1998

81 ■ Blood Pressure Monitoring 209

KEYWORDS	TEST YEAR
Blood pressure: viscosity	1995
Blood pressure measurement: effect of site	1993
Transducers: resonance/dampening effects	1994
Transducers: zeroing	1993×2, 1998, 1998×2
Arterial pressure monitoring: artifacts	1993, 1995
Arterial catheterization	1993

82 ■ Temperature Correction of Arterial Blood Gases 211

KEYWORDS	TEST YEAR
ABG interpretation during hypothermia	1994, 1998
Hypothermia and gas transport	1994

83 ■ Central Venous and Pulmonary Artery Catheters 213

KEYWORDS	TEST YEAR
CVP: venous waves	1994
CVP: accurate measurement	1996
Giant A waves: significance	1993, 1998
PAOP: interpretation	1993, 1996
PAOP: factors affecting accuracy	1996
PA catheter: and pulmonary hypertension	1993
Abnormal PAD:LVEDP gradient: causes	1994
PAOP and LV volume: pitfalls	1995
PA catheter: complications	1994

84 ■ Thermodilution Cardiac Output 216

KEYWORDS	TEST YEAR
Thermodilution CO: measurement errors	1993, 1994, 1996, 1998
Cardiac output thermodilution determination: valvular regurgitation	1995
Cardiovascular derived variables	1993, 1998
Cardiac output: effect of arteriovenous shunt	1996

85 ■ Mixed Venous Saturation 218

KEYWORDS	TEST YEAR
SvO_2: factors decreasing/increasing	1993, 1994, 1996, 1998
SvO_2: and high FiO_2	1996
O_2 supply and demand: assessment	1994, 1998
Pulmonary artery blood gas: interpretation	1994, 1998

86 ■ Cardiac Pacemakers 219

KEYWORDS	TEST YEAR
DVI pacer: perioperative inhibition	1994
DDD pacer function	1993, 1998
EKG: pacemaker	1994
Pacemakers: fixed vs. synchronous mode	1995
Pacemaker mode conversion	1994
Preoperative pacer insertion: indications	1994, 1996

87 ■ Cardiac Tamponade 222

KEYWORDS	TEST YEAR
Cardiac tamponade: diagnosis	1994, 1998
Cardiac tamponade: anesthetic management	1993
Tamponade: hemodynamic manipulation	1994

88 Mitral Stenosis 224

KEYWORDS	TEST YEAR
Mitral stenosis: pathophysiology	1994, 1998
Mitral stenosis: anesthetic management	1994
Mitral stenosis: signs and symptoms	1994
Acute intraoperative atrial fibrillation in mitral stenosis: treatment	1994
Mitral valve disease and tachycardia	1995

89 ■ Mitral Regurgitation 226

KEYWORDS	TEST YEAR
Mitral valve prolapse: anesthetic implications	1993, 1998
Mitral regurgitation: hemodynamic management	1995
Acute mitral regurgitation: management	1993, 1996

90 ■ Aortic Stenosis 228

KEYWORDS	TEST YEAR
Aortic stenosis: anesthetic considerations	1993
Aortic stenosis and spinal anesthesia	1996
Aortic stenosis and acute ischemia: management	1995, 1996

91 ■ Aortic Regurgitation 230

KEYWORDS	TEST YEAR
Aortic insufficiency: hemodynamics	1995, 1998
Aortic valve replacement: anesthetic management	1993
Acute aortic regurgitation: management	1996, 1998

92 ■ Idiopathic Hypertrophic Subaortic Stenosis 232

KEYWORDS	TEST YEAR
IHSS: intraoperative management	1993, 1995
Obstructive cardiomyopathy: drugs worsening	1994
IHSS: management of inhalational anesthesia	1996

93 ■ Thoracic and Abdominal Aneurysms 234

KEYWORDS	TEST YEAR
Aortic dissection: hypotensive treatment	1994, 1996
Thoracic aneurysm repair: paraplegia after	1995
Thoracic aneurysm repair: nerve injuries after	1996
AAA management: aortic declamping	1995
Renal preservation and aortic cross-clamping	1994
Aortic cross-clamp and myocardial ischemia	1996

94 ■ Heparin 237

KEYWORDS	TEST YEAR
Heparin: effects of preoperative administration	1993
Heparin resistance	1995
Heparin resistance: management	1996
Heparin: factors affecting duration	1993
Heparin-induced thrombocytopenia	1993, 1996
ACT: uses and limitations	1994, 1995, 1998

95 ■ Protamine and Other Things 239

KEYWORDS	TEST YEAR
Coumadin reversal for emergency surgery	1994, 1995, 1998
Reversal of fibrinolytics	1995
Protamine reaction and management	1993, 1994, 1995
Protamine: cardiovascular effects	1996

96 ■ Cardiopulmonary Bypass 241

KEYWORDS	TEST YEAR
CPB: flow and pressure determinants	1994
CPB: venous saturation during	1995
CPB: ABGs during	1993
CPB: causes of hypoxemia following bypass	1995
CPB: defibrillation after	1993
CABG: differential diagnosis for hypotension after	1993, 1998

97 ■ Intraaortic Balloon Pumps 243

KEYWORDS	TEST YEAR
IABP: hemodynamic effects	1995, 1998
IABP: limitations	1993

98 ■ Mediastinoscopy 245

KEYWORD	TEST YEAR
Mediastinoscopy: complications	1995

99 ■ Double-Lumen Tubes 247

KEYWORDS	TEST YEAR
Double-lumen tube: indications	1993
Double-lumen tube placement	1993, 1994
Double-lumen tubes: malposition	1996

100 ■ One-Lung Ventilation and Pneumonectomy 250

KEYWORDS	TEST YEAR
Lung resectability: criteria	1994
Lung resection and preoperative PFTs	1993, 1995, 1998
One-lung ventilation: anatomic considerations	1994
One-lung ventilation: PaO_2	1994
Hypoxia during one-lung ventilation: management	1993, 1995, 1998×2
Hypoxic pulmonary vasoconstriction during one-lung ventilation	1994
Hypoxic pulmonary vasoconstriction: drug effects	1996
Hypoxic pulmonary vasoconstriction: inhibition	1996

101 ■ Cardiopulmonary Resuscitation 253

KEYWORDS	TEST YEAR
ACLS: priorities for therapy	1995
Antegrade flow with chest compression	1994
ABGs during CPR: management	1994
HCO_3^- in cardiac arrest	1994, 1998
HCO_3^-: side effects	1993, 1998
Defibrillation: and thoracic impedence	1993
Sinus arrest: anesthetic implications	1994
Ventricular tachycardia: management	1993, 1994, 1996, 1998
SVT: management	1995, 1996, 1998
EMD: CPR	1993
EMD: causes	1996

SECTION 8
Transfusion Therapy

102 ■ Transfusion Therapy 261

KEYWORDS	TEST YEAR
Blood compatibility	1995, 1998
Type and screen	1994
Blood transfusion and typing	1993
Banked blood vs. cell saver	1994
Banked blood: characteristics and considerations	1993, 1996
Sodium citrate toxicity	1995
Citrate intoxication: predisposition	1994, 1998
Massive transfusion and coagulation	1994, 1998
Posttransfusion coagulopathy	1993

103 ■ Transfusion Reactions 265

KEYWORDS	TEST YEAR
Allergic transfusion reaction: management	1994
Diagnosis: transfusion reaction	1994
Hemolytic transfusion reaction: treatment	1994
Hemolytic transfusion reaction: tests for	1993, 1998
Transfusion reaction: causes	1996

104 ■ Blood Component Therapy 266

KEYWORDS	TEST YEAR
Massive transfusion and coagulation	1994
Posttransfusion coagulopathy	1993
Indications for platelet transfusion	1996
Platelet transfusion: thrombocytopenia	1993
FFP: indications	1993, 1994
DDAVP: perioperative indications for	1995
Prolonged bleeding time: preoperative therapy	1994
Prolonged PT	1996

105 ■ Intraoperative Fluid Therapy 268

KEYWORDS	TEST YEAR
Fluid resuscitation: distribution characteristics	1994
Colloid therapy: viral risks	1993
Colloid vs. crystalloid	1993
Hetastarch: pharmacology	1993
Dextran: side effects	1994

106 ■ Von Willebrand's Disease 271

KEYWORDS	TEST YEAR
Von Willebrand's disease rx	1995
Von Willebrand's disease: preoperative preparation	1996, 1998
Von Willebrand's disease: intraoperative tx	1993

107 ■ Hemophilia A and Hemophilia B (Christmas disease) 273

KEYWORD	TEST YEAR
Hemophilia A and emergency surgery	1995

108 ■ Sickle Cell Anemia 274

KEYWORDS	TEST YEAR
Sickle cell crisis: management	1994
Sickle cell anemia: neonatal considerations	1994
Sickle cell disease: anesthetic management	1998

SECTION 9
Neuroanesthesia

109 ■ Cerebral Blood Flow and Metabolism 279

KEYWORDS	TEST YEAR
CBF autoregulation: physiologic inferences	1994
CBF: autoregulation	1993×2, 1995, 1996
Cerebral perfusion pressure: determinants	1994, 1996, 1998
$CMRO_2$ and hypothermia	1995
Anesthetics and $CMRO_2$	1994, 1998
CBF: perioperative regulation	1995, 1998

110 ■ Closed Head Injury and Increased Intracranial Pressure 282

KEYWORDS	TEST YEAR
Glasgow coma scale: criteria	1994
Glasgow coma scale: use and limits	1994
Intracranial elastance	1995
Cerebral perfusion pressure: determinants	1994
Increased ICP: pharmocologic management	1993, 1994, 1996
Increased ICP: intraoperative management	1995×2, 1996×2
Head trauma: reduction of ICP	1993, 1998
Barbiturate coma: indications	1995
Barbiturates and cerebral protection	1993, 1996
Brain herniation: treatment	1994
Head trauma: anesthetic management	1993
Hypocarbia and cerebral perfusion	1994
Hypocarbia and brain swelling	1993
Hypotensive drugs and ICP	1994
Bradycardia during neurosurgery: causes	1995
Brain death: criteria	1994, 1996, 1998

111 ■ SIADH versus Diabetes Insipidus versus Fluoride Nephrotoxicity 286

KEYWORDS	TEST YEAR
Post traumatic diabetes insipidus	1994
Diabetes insipidus: diagnosis and treatment	1995, 1996, 1998
Diabetes insipidus vs. fluoride toxicity: differential diagnosis	1993
SIADH: treatment	1995
SIADH: diagnosis	1996
Fluoride toxicity	1993

112 ■ Cerebral Aneurysm Clipping 288

KEYWORDS	TEST YEAR
Cerebral aneurysm rupture at induction	1995
Aneurysm clipping: anesthetic management	1994
Cerebral vasospasm: treatment	1993, 1998
Cerebral vasospasm: characteristics	1996
Subarachnoid hemorrhage: signs of	1996

113 ■ Carotid Endarterectomy 291

KEYWORDS	TEST YEAR
CEA: ventilatory drive following	1994, 1996
CEA: carotid body denervation	1996
CEA: chemoreceptors after	1993
CEA: neurologic deficit following	1995
CEA: EEG interpretation	1994
CEA: physiologic effects of	1995

114 ■ Anesthetic Effects on EEG 293

KEYWORDS	TEST YEAR
EEG burst suppression: causes	1995, 1998
Anesthetic effects on EEG	1993, 1996
Cerebral ischemia detection	1995

115 ■ Sensory Evoked Potentials..295

KEYWORDS	TEST YEAR
SSEP: uses	1993
SSEP: pathways	1995
SSEP: moderating factors	1995
SSEP: anesthetic effects	1995, 1996
SSEP: spinal cord function	1995
SSEP: interpretation	1993, 1998×2
Auditory evoked response: anesthetic implications	1995

116 ■ Spinal Cord Transection..298

KEYWORDS	TEST YEAR
Acute spinal cord injury	1993, 1994, 1996
Spinal cord injury and succinylcholine	1993
Anesthesia and acute cervical cord injury	1995
Intubation after cervical trauma	1993
Autonomic hyperreflexia	1993, 1998
Autonomic hyperreflexia: bradycardia	1994
Autonomic hyperreflexia: prevention	1995×2
SAB: quadraplegia and	1994

117 ■ Electroconvulsive Therapy..302

KEYWORDS	TEST YEAR
ECT and hemodynamic management	1994
ECT: physiologic effects	1996, 1998
ECT: anesthetic considerations	1994
Seizure potential: anesthetic drugs	1993
Duration of seizure	1996

SECTION 10
Anesthesia Equipment

118 ■ Gas Cylinders..307

KEYWORDS	TEST YEAR
E cylinder: pressure, flow and volume	1994
Cylinders: pressures of gases	1993
Oxygen cylinder volume	1996
N_2O: physical properties	1994

119 ■ Oxygen Therapy..310

KEYWORDS	TEST YEAR
Oxygen delivery masks: characteristics	1994
FiO_2 with nasal prongs	1993

120 ■ Flowmeters 312

KEYWORDS	TEST YEAR
Physics: gas flow	1993
O_2 flowmeter leak	1994
O_2 flowmeter malfunction: consequences	1994
Flowmeter sequence	1993

121 ■ Vaporizers 315

KEYWORDS	TEST YEAR
Vaporizer output: determinants	1993
Vaporizer hazards	1996
Tipped vaporizer	1993
Vapor pressure: determinants	1994

122 ■ The Dreaded Copper Kettle 318

KEYWORD	TEST YEAR
Anesthetic vapor concentration: calculation of	1993

123 ■ The Desflurane Vaporizer 320

KEYWORD	TEST YEAR
Desflurane vaporizer: function	1995, 1996, 1998

124 ■ The Anesthesia Machine 322

KEYWORDS	TEST YEAR
Anesthesia machine check	1994
Machine check with no oxygen flow	1993, 1998
Anesthesia machine: check valves	1993, 1995
Machine design to prevent hypoxia	1994, 1998
Failsafe device in anesthesia machine	1993
Flow proportioning system	1996
Oxygen flush valve function	1995
Oxygen pressure safety devices	1994

125 ■ Mapleson Breathing Circuits 325

KEYWORDS	TEST YEAR
Pediatric circuits: fresh gas flow requirements	1993, 1994, 1996
Bain circuit	1994

126 ■ The Circle System 328

KEYWORDS	TEST YEAR
Circle system: deadspace	1993, 1995
Inspiratory valve malfunction: consequences	1994
Oxygen analyzer: function in the circuit	1993, 1996
Oxygen analyzer: malfunction	1996
CO_2 absorption in a circle system	1993, 1995
CO_2: causes of inspired	1994

127 ■ Closed-Circuit Anesthesia 331

KEYWORD	TEST YEAR
Closed-circuit anesthesia	1993

128 ■ CO_2 Absorbers 333

KEYWORDS	TEST YEAR
CO_2 absorption in a circle system	1993, 1995
Exhaustion of soda lime	1996
Byproducts of CO_2 absorption	1993, 1995, 1996, 1998

129 ■ Scavenging Systems 335

KEYWORD	TEST YEAR
Scavenging systems: features and types	1994, 1995

130 ■ Anesthesia Ventilators 337

KEYWORDS	TEST YEAR
Ventilatory disconnect: monitoring	1995, 1998
Ventilatory disconnect: detection	1996
Anesthesia ventilator: implications of bellows hole	1994
Anesthesia ventilator: mechanics	1993, 1998
Anesthesia ventilator: function	1993, 1994
Anesthesia ventilator: malfunction	1995

131 ■ Mechanical Ventilation 340

KEYWORDS	TEST YEAR
Pressure cycled ventilators	1993, 1995
Neonatal ventilation	1996
Compression volume: clinical implications	1994
Ventilators: factors affecting measured tidal volume	1993, 1998
Ventilators: factors affecting tidal volume	1995, 1998
Effect of flowrate on ventilation volume	1996
IMV: demand vs. continuous flow	1994
Spontaneous vs. control ventilation: effect on CO_2 gradient	1996
IMV vs. IPPV	1994
Positive pressure ventilation: physiologic effects	1995, 1996
Mechanical ventilation and increased VD/VT	1996
Mechanical ventilation: increased PIP	1993, 1996
Pressure support ventilation	1993, 1995
Barotrauma: sequelae	1995
PEEP: complications	1995
PEEP: cardiopulmonary effects	1994, 1996, 1998
PEEP: effect on right ventricle	1995
CPAP: induced lung changes	1995

132 ■ Perioperative Hypoxia 344

KEYWORDS	TEST YEAR
Intraoperative hypoxia: causes	1993, 1994, 1995, 1996
Hypoxia during emergence	1994
Early postoperative hypoxia: causes	1994
Diffusion hypoxia: principle	1993
Postoperative respiratory distress: causes	1994

133 ■ Intraoperative Hypercarbia and Hypocarbia 346

KEYWORDS	TEST YEAR
Intraoperative hypercarbia: effects	1993, 1996, 1998
Hypocarbia: physiologic effects	1994
Acute hypocarbia and arrhythmias	1993

134 ■ Pulse Oximetry 348

KEYWORDS	TEST YEAR
Pulse oximetry: artifacts	1993, 1996, 1998
SPO_2: causes of artifactual values	1995, 1996
SPO_2: causes of decreased	1994

135 ■ Capnography 350

KEYWORDS	TEST YEAR
Capnography: applications	1995
Capnography: differential diagnosis of abnormal waveforms	1993, 1996, 1998
Capnography and airway obstruction	1994
$ETCO_2$: factors affecting	1995, 1998
High $ETCO_2$: equipment causes	1994
Low $ETCO_2$: causes	1993
CO_2: causes of inspired	1994, 1998
Increased gradient $ETCO_2$/arterial CO_2: causes	1993, 1994, 1995, 1996, 1998
Venous air embolism: diagnosis	1993, 1994×2, 1996×2
Venous air embolism: end-tidal gases	1993

136 ■ Electrical Confusion in the Operating Room............................ 354

KEYWORDS	TEST YEAR
Electrical safety in the OR	1994
Burns and electrocautery units	1993, 1994, 1998
Line isolation monitor: function	1994
Line isolation monitor: alarm	1993
Leakage current: recommended level	1993
Microshock: causes	1996

SECTION 11
Airway Management

137 ■ The Infant Airway versus the Adult Airway 359

KEYWORDS	TEST YEAR
Infant airway: anatomy	1993, 1994, 1996
Airway: infant vs. adult	1993, 1996

138 ■ Functional Innervation of the Airway ... 361

KEYWORDS	TEST YEAR
Upper airway: innervation	1993, 1994, 1995, 1998
Innervation of the larynx	1995, 1996
Recurrent laryngeal nerve block: anatomy	1993
Recurrent laryngeal nerve block: effects	1995
Recurrrent laryngeal nerve resection: effects	1995, 1996
Recurrent laryngeal nerve paralysis: causes	1993
Superior laryngeal nerve	1993
Laryngeal function: local anesthesia and general anesthesia	1994

139 ■ Management of the Difficult Airway ... 363

KEYWORDS	TEST YEAR
Difficult airway: management	1995
Anesthesia for awake intubation	1994, 1996×2
Cricothyroidotomy: ventilatory implications	1994
Transtracheal jet ventilation technique	1993, 1995
Tracheal trauma: airway management	1994
Intubation after cervical trauma	1993
Nasotracheal intubation: complications	1993
Cricoid pressure: effects	1994
Endobronchial intubation: signs of	1995
Postoperative hoarseness: mechanisms	1994

140 ■ Laryngospasm ... 367

KEYWORDS	TEST YEAR
Laryngospasm: management	1995
Laryngospasm: consequences	1994
Laryngospasm: physiology	1996
Negative pressure pulmonary edema	1993

SECTION 12
Complications

141 ■ Airway Fire ... 371

KEYWORDS	TEST YEAR
Airway fire: management	1993, 1994, 1995, 1996
Laser airway fire: prevention	1993, 1995

142 ■ Pulmonary Aspiration of Gastric Contents ... 373

KEYWORDS	TEST YEAR
Perioperative aspiration: diagnosis	1996
Perioperative aspiration: management	1993, 1994
Metaclopramide: pharmacology	1993, 1994, 1996
Metaclopramide and cimetidine: GI effects	1995
H_2-blockers: drug interactions	1993

Extrapyramidal drug effects: treatment	1995
Drugs for gastric pH and emptying	1996
Lower esophageal sphincter: drug effects	1993
Aspiration prophylaxis: side effects	1994

143 ■ Methylmethacrylate 377

KEYWORD	TEST YEAR
Methylmethacrylate: hemodynamic effects	1993, 1994

144 ■ Tourniquet Troubles 378

KEYWORDS	TEST YEAR
Leg tourniquet pain: anesthetic implications	1994, 1998
Leg tourniquet pain: treatment	1996
Tourniquet release: physiologic effects	1993, 1994, 1996, 1998
Tourniquet release: hypotension	1998

145 ■ Deep Venous Thrombosis 380

KEYWORDS	TEST YEAR
DVT: perioperative	1995
DVT: prevention	1993

146 ■ Anaphylaxis 382

KEYWORDS	TEST YEAR
Latex allergy: anesthetic implications	1994, 1995, 1996, 1998
Anaphylaxis: management	1995, 1996, 1998
Anaphylactoid reaction: antibiotics	1993

147 ■ Intraoperative Hypothermia 384

KEYWORDS	TEST YEAR
GA and heat loss: mechanisms	1995, 1996
Heat loss in exposure: mechanisms	1994
Intraoperative hypothermia: prevention	1993
Moderate hypothermia: perioperative effects	1993, 1994, 1996, 1998
Profound hypothermia: effects	1995, 1996
Deliberate hypothermia: physiology	1993×2, 1994
Postoperative shivering: treatment	1993, 1994

148 ■ Perioperative Nerve Injury 386

KEYWORDS	TEST YEAR
Patient positioning: neurologic complications	1994, 1998
Perioperative nerve injuries: lower extremity positioning	1994, 1998
Lower extremity nerve injury: causes	1996
Positioning and peroneal nerve injury	1995, 1998
Nerve injuries: vaginal delivery	1993
Nerve injuries: forceps delivery	1996

149 ■ Venous Air Embolism..388

KEYWORDS	TEST YEAR
Venous air embolism: diagnosis and treatment	1993, 1994×2, 1996×2
Air embolus: end-tidal gases	1993
Air embolus: cardiopulmonary changes	1993
Sitting position: complications	1995
$ETCO_2$ and neurosurgery	1994, 1998
Laparoscopy and gas embolism	1993

150 ■ Fat Embolism..391

KEYWORD	TEST YEAR
Fat embolism: signs	1994, 1998

SECTION 13
Pharmacology

151 ■ Clonidine..395

KEYWORDS	TEST YEAR
Preoperative clonidine: anesthetic implications	1993, 1994
Antihypertensives: rebound hypertension	1994, 1998
Clonidine: side effects	1996

152 ■ Digitalis Toxicity..397

KEYWORDS	TEST YEAR
Digitalis toxicity: management of acute	1994, 1998
Digitalis toxicity: perioperative causes and treatment	1994, 1998

153 ■ Sodium Nitroprusside..399

KEYWORDS	TEST YEAR
Nitroprusside: pharmacology	1993
Nitroprusside toxicity: signs	1993, 1994
Cyanide toxicity	1995, 1998
Cyanide toxicity: treatment	1995

154 ■ Deliberate Hypotension..402

KEYWORDS	TEST YEAR
Nitroprusside: pharmacology	1993
Nitroprusside–propanolol interactions	1995
Nitroprusside vs. trimethaphan	1993
Nitroprusside: coronary steal	1994, 1995
Trimethephan: pharmacodynamics	1996
Nitroprusside vs. nitroglycerin: pharmacodynamics	1995

155 ■ Furosemide versus Mannitol 405

KEYWORDS	TEST YEAR
Furosemide: metabolic effects	1995
Mannitol vs. furosemide: cardiovascular effects	1994
Mannitol: pharmacology	1995, 1996, 1998
Mannitol: nondiuretic effects	1993

156 ■ Thiopental 407

KEYWORDS	TEST YEAR
Barbiturates: cerebral effects	1994, 1996
Barbiturates and cerebral protection	1993, 1996
Barbiturates: kinetics	1993, 1998
Thiopental and liver disease	1996
Thiopental: redistribution	1996

157 ■ Comparison of Thiopental and Methohexital 409

KEYWORDS	TEST YEAR
Thiopental: treatment of intraarterial injection	1996
Barbiturates: cerebral effects	1994, 1996
Barbiturates and cerebral protection	1993, 1996
Barbiturates: kinetics	1993

158 ■ Propofol 411

KEYWORDS	TEST YEAR
Propofol: pharmacodynamics	1994
Propofol: pharmacology	1993
Propofol: cardiovascular effects	1993, 1998

159 ■ Etomidate 413

KEYWORDS	TEST YEAR
Etomidate: comparative pharmacology	1994, 1998
Etomidate: side effects	1994, 1998
Etomidate: adrenal suppression	1993, 1996

160 ■ Ketamine 415

KEYWORDS	TEST YEAR
Ketamine: cardiovascular effects	1994
Ketamine: pharmacology	1993, 1994, 1996
Ketamine: adverse effects	1995

161 ■ Comparison of Physiologic Effects and Pharmacokinetics of Thiopental, Propofol, Etomidate, and Ketamine 417

KEYWORDS	TEST YEAR
Etomidate: comparative pharmacology	1994, 1998
Ketamine: pharmacology	1993, 1994, 1996
Propofol: pharmacology	1993
Propofol: cardiovascular effects	1993
Propofol: pharmacodynamics	1994

Barbiturates: cerebral effects	1994, 1996
Barbiturates and cerebral protection	1993, 1996
Barbiturates: kinetics	1993, 1998

162 ■ Benzodiazepines 419

KEYWORDS	TEST YEAR
Benzodiazepines: comparative pharmacology	1993, 1995, 1998
Midazolam vs. diazepam	1993
Midazolam vs. thiopental: pharmacology	1993
Benzodiazepines in the elderly	1995

163 ■ Flumazenil 421

KEYWORDS	TEST YEAR
Flumazenil: pharmacology	1994, 1998
Flumazenil: duration	1996

164 ■ Opioids 423

KEYWORDS	TEST YEAR
Morphine: site of action	1996
Opioids and muscle rigidity	1994, 1995
Opioids and histamine release	1996
Opioid side effects: treatment	1993, 1998
Opioids: treatment of opioid-induced biliary spasm	1995×2
Alfentanil: pharmacodynamics/pharmacokinetics	1993, 1995
Alfentanil vs. fentanyl: kinetics	1993
Fentanyl: pharmacokinetics	1993, 1996
Fentanyl: effect on heart rate	1996
Awareness and opioid anesthesia	1995
Morphine: elimination in renal failure	1994
Morphine: duration in renal disease	1995

165 ■ Mixed Narcotic Agonists/Antagonists 428

KEYWORDS	TEST YEAR
Naloxone: pharmacology	1994
Nalbuphine: pharmacology	1995
Opiate receptor antagonists	1993
Analgesia with narcotic agonists/antagonists	1994
Narcotic addict: premedication	1993

166 ■ Ketorolac 431

KEYWORDS	TEST YEAR
Ketorolac: contraindications	1994, 1998
Ketorolac: pharmacology	1993, 1995
Ketorolac vs. meperidine	1993

167 ■ Neuromuscular Relaxants 433

KEYWORDS	TEST YEAR
Nondepolarizing blockade: characteristics	1993
Nondepolarizing blockade: duration	1996

Nondepolarizing relaxants: pharmacodynamics	1994
Atracurium: factors affecting metabolism	1994
Atracurium: metabolism	1995
Atracurium and laudanosine	1993
Mivacurium duration of action: factors affecting	1996
Mivacurium: pharmacology	1996
Nondepolarizing blockers: dosing with diseases	1993
Nondepolarizing blockers: dosing with burns	1996
Nondepolarizing blockers: histamine release	1996
Hemiparesis: nondepolarizing muscle relaxants	1994
Muscle relaxants in renal failure	1993, 1994, 1995
Muscle relaxants in liver disease	1993
Cirrhosis and muscle relaxants	1995
Neuromuscular relaxation: differential muscle sensitivity	1994
Resistance to muscle paralysis	1995
Residual muscle blockade after GA	1995
Magnesium: drug interactions	1994
Magnesium: neuromuscular effects	1995, 1996, 1998
Neuromuscular blockade and antibiotics	1993
Relaxant pharmacology: neonate	1995
Vecuronium pharmacology: neonate	1996

168 ■ Reversal of Neuromuscular Blockade 437

KEYWORDS	TEST YEAR
Acetylcholinesterase: pharmacodynamics	1995, 1996
Neostigmine and relaxant metabolism	1994
Acetylcholinesterase inhibitors: muscarinic effects	1994
Reversal of NMR block: clinical influences	1993, 1994, 1998
Acetylcholinesterase inhibitors: side effects	1995, 1998
NMR reversal: atropine vs. glycopyrolate	1994, 1995
Glycopyrolate: effects	1995
Anticholinergic side effects: treatment	1993, 1995, 1996
Atropine and hyperthermia	1993
Atropine toxicity	1993
Central anticholinergic syndrome	1993
Central anticholinergic syndrome: treatment	1996
Extubation after NMR reversal: criteria	1994
Negative inspiratory force: intraoperative assessment	1994

169 ■ Succinylcholine 441

KEYWORDS	TEST YEAR
Succinylcholine: pharmacokinetics	1993
Phase II block	1993, 1995
Succinylcholine: contraindications	1994, 1998
Succinylcholine: effects in Duchenne's muscular dystrophy	1995
Succinylcholine and preeclampsia	1993
Succinylcholine and pseudocholinesterase deficiency	1993, 1998×2
Succinylcholine: hyperkalemia	1994, 1998
Succinylcholine after NMR reversal	1995
Succinylcholine: prolonged recovery	1996
Succinylcholine induced bradycardia	1998

170 ■ Pseudocholinesterase Deficiency 444

KEYWORDS	TEST YEAR
Pseudocholinesterase deficiency: diagnosis	1994, 1998×2
Pseudocholinesterase deficiency: clinical implications	1996
Pseudocholinesterase: pharmacology	1993
Plasma cholinesterase genotypes	1995
Dibucaine number: interpretation	1995, 1998
Succinylcholine and pseudocholinesterase deficiency	1993, 1998

171 ■ Droperidol 446

KEYWORDS	TEST YEAR
Antiemetics: pharmacology of	1995
Droperidol: side effects	1994, 1998
Droperidol: pharmacology	1993

172 ■ Monoamine Oxidase Inhibitors 448

KEYWORD	TEST YEAR
MAO inhibitors: anesthetic implications	1993, 1995, 1998

173 ■ Cyclosporine Toxicity 450

KEYWORD	TEST YEAR
Cyclosporine toxicity	1993, 1994

Keywords 451

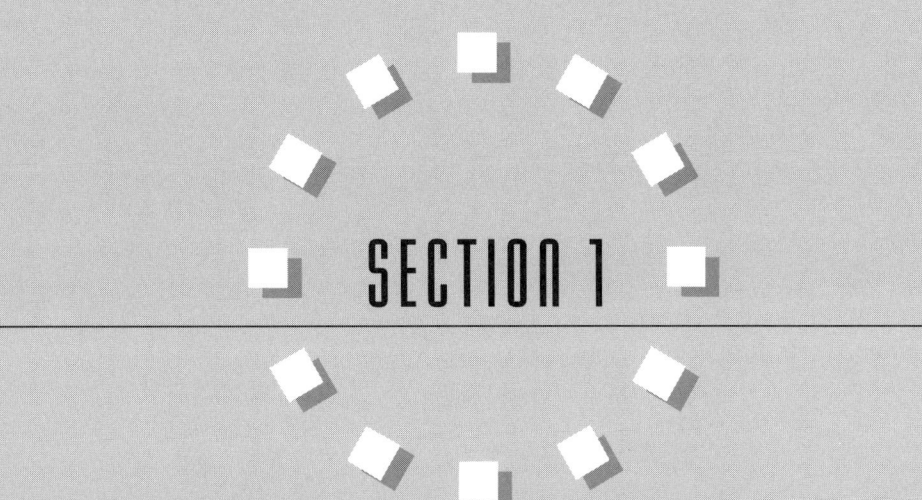

SECTION 1

Inhalational Anesthesia

CHAPTER 1

Minimum Alveolar Concentration

Definition of MAC: The minimum alveolar concentration (MAC) of a volatile anesthetic preventing movement in 50% of patients receiving a noxious stimulus (standardized as skin incision).[1]

What's the clinical significance of MAC?

It's the best measure of anesthetic potency available.

MAC and relative potency (% expired) of available agents

Halothane > isoflurane > enflurane > sevoflurane > desflurane > N_2O
0.75%   1.2%   1.4%   ~2%   ~6%   105%

Factors increasing MAC

1. Chronic alcohol abuse
2. Young age: highest MAC is at ~6 months old with a steady decline throughout life except for a blip during adolescence
3. Hyperthermia
4. Anything that promotes central neurotransmission: speed, cocaine, MAO inhibitors, L-Dopa

Factors decreasing MAC

1. Acute alcohol intoxication
2. Old age
3. Hypothermia
4. Barbiturates
5. Benzodiazepines
6. Narcotics
7. Ketamine
8. Local anesthetics
9. Pancuronium
10. Pregnancy
11. Acidosis and hypoxia, but NOT hyper-/hypocarbia

There are a lot more items that reduce MAC, and you can find exhaustive lists in any major anesthesia text, so I've listed only those that appear to be the favorites of the boards.

Sample questions: None . . . it's a pretty straightforward concept. Memorize, memorize, memorize.

Reference

1. Eger EI, II, Saidman LJ, Brandstater B. Minimum alveolar anesthetic concentration: a standard of anesthetic potency. Anesthesiology 26: 756, 1965.

CHAPTER 2

Uptake and Distribution of Inhaled Anesthetics

Anesthetic levels in the brain depend on anesthetic levels in the alveolus. Your goal is to rapidly achieve high alveolar concentrations (F_A), and thus, high brain levels. The main factor *you* can manipulate is the inspired concentration of anesthetic (F_I). It becomes obvious, then, that the speed of induction depends on the speed at which alveolar concentration approaches the inspired concentration (i.e.; the rate of rise of F_A/F_I).

Factors speeding the rate of rise of F_A/F_I

1. High gas inflow rates
2. High alveolar ventilation: especially important for highly soluble agents because the rate of rise of F_A/F_I is offset by rapid uptake of agent into the bloodstream. Insoluble agents are not taken up well by the blood, so their F_A/F_I rises fast, no matter what the alveolar ventilation is.
3. High concentration of inspired gas: especially important for a highly soluble gas, for reasons described above. High inspired concentrations also speed the rise of F_A/F_I by:
   A. Augmented alveolar ventilation: the uptake of gas from the alveolus creates a void that draws additional gas into the alveolus from the conducting airways.
   B. The concentration effect: You would expect that if half the *volume* of a gas is taken up from the lungs, then the *concentration* of the gas in the lungs would be halved, BUT IT'S NOT. This is because the *total volume* of the alveolus has been reduced. Thus, the new percent volume of the gas is somewhat *more* than half its original volume (i.e.; it's *concentrated* . . . see Figure 2–1).
   C. The second gas effect: The concentration effect *creates* the second gas effect. As uptake of one gas reduces alveolar volume, the concentration of a second alveolar gas increases because it's forced to reside in smaller alveolar volume. Since additional second gas is drawn into the alveolus during "augmented ventilation," the alveolar concentration remains increased, despite the return to original alveolar volume.
4. Anything that reduces uptake of agent.

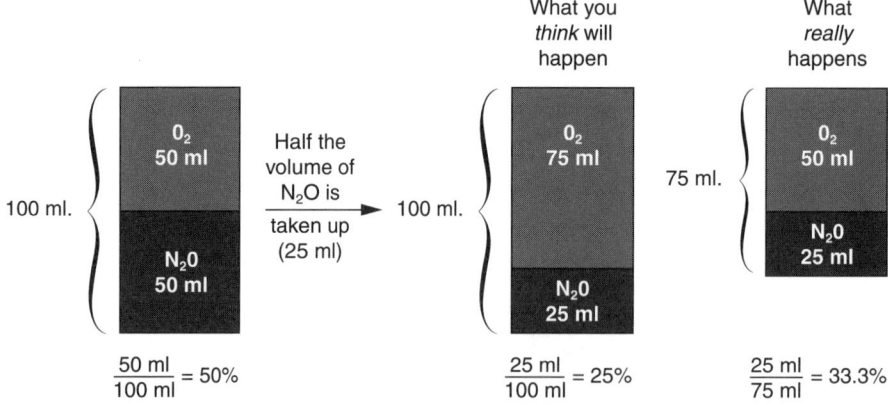

Figure 2–1.

Factors affecting uptake of inhaled agents

1. Solubility: quantified by blood:gas partition coefficient. (A blood:gas partition coefficient of 2 means that, at equilibrium, the amount of agent dissolved in blood is twice the amount in the gas phase.)
   A. High solubility = rapid entry into blood = slow induction because rise of F_A/F_I is slow.
   B. Relative solubilities: Hal > Enf > Iso > Sevo > N_2O > Des
   C. Note: Solubility increases as temperature decreases.
2. Cardiac output: High output = rapid removal of agent from alveolus = slow induction (slow rise F_A/F_I). Effect is more pronounced with highly soluble agents. (Same song . . . if an agent is insoluble, it doesn't matter how much you increase cardiac output, your output is still limited by how well the agent dissolves.) Effect is self-propagating:

   $\uparrow F_A \rightarrow$ myocardial depression $\rightarrow \downarrow CO \rightarrow \downarrow$ uptake $\rightarrow \uparrow\uparrow F_A$

   What if both cardiac output and ventilation are increased? No, they do not cancel each other out. The effect of cardiac output on F_A/F_I will be overshadowed by the rapid equilibration of the vessel-rich group (brain), and you'll have a more rapid induction of anesthesia.
3. Uptake by tissues: quantified by tissue:blood partition coefficient. Uptake by tissues is governed by the size of the tissue as well as the blood flow to the tissue. Thus, large tissues with low perfusion represent a slow filling reservoir for anesthetics.

   Relative tissue:blood coefficients: fat > muscle > brain ≈ liver ≈ kidney
4. Intracardiac shunting: A right-to-left shunt will slow induction because very little blood is available to take up the agent. (Induction is slow despite a rising alveolar concentration of agent.) On the other hand, left-to-right shunts have little effect on speed of induction, although they can reduce the effect of right-to-left shunts a bit.

Inhalational induction is faster in kids than in adults because

1. They have a smaller FRC.
2. They have proportionately more alveolar ventilation.
3. Their organs are better perfused. (Remember what we said about high cardiac output plus high alveolar ventilation?)
4. They send a disproportionately large amount of flow to the vessel-rich group of organs (the brain).

Sample questions

A = 1, 2, 3   B = 1, 3   C = 2, 4   D = 4 only   E = all are correct

1. A blood:gas partition coefficient of 1.5 means
   1. The concentration of agent is 1.5 times higher in the blood than in the alveoli
   2. The partial pressure of agent is 1.5 times higher in the blood than in the alveoli
   3. Each milliliter of blood holds 1.5 times as much agent as each milliliter of alveolar gas
   4. For a given amount of anesthetic agent, it takes 1.5 times as much blood to carry it than alveolar volume

2. A trauma patient is having an exploratory laparotomy. Blood pressure is 90/50 mmHg, pulse 135/min. During the first few minutes of mechanical ventilation and general anesthesia using halothane
   1. Alveolar partial pressure will be higher than expected
   2. More halothane is directed to the brain than to the kidneys
   3. Alveolar pressure will fall more following administration of dopamine than alveolar pressure of isoflurane would
   4. End-tidal carbon dioxide will be higher than expected

3. Inhalational induction in infants is faster than in adults because infants have
   1. A smaller percentage of body fat
   2. A disproportionate amount of blood flow to the vessel-rich group
   3. A smaller ratio of deadspace ventilation to alveolar ventilation
   4. Greater alveolar ventilation

4. Factors that slow the rate of rise of alveolar concentration of an anesthetic agent include
   1. Hypothermia
   2. High tissue:gas partition coefficient
   3. Tachycardia
   4. Hyperventilation

5.
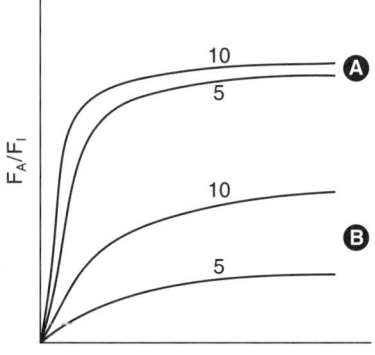

Figure 2–2.

True statements regarding Figure 2–2 include
1. Curve A represents an agent that is less soluble than curve B

2. A change in minute ventilation will affect the agent depicted by curve B more than curve A
3. Curve B represents an agent with a higher blood:gas partition coefficient
4. Curve A represents a more potent agent

6.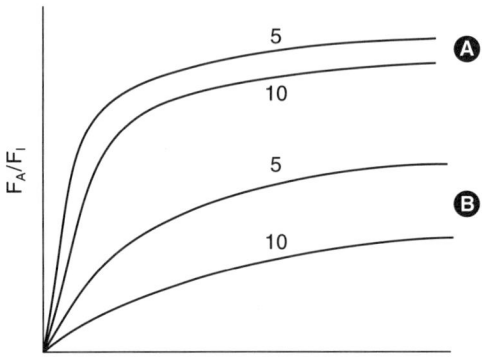

Figure 2–3.

True statements about Figure 2–3 include
1. Agent A is less soluble than agent B
2. The agent labeled B is less potent
3. The agent labeled A has a lower blood:gas partition coefficient
4. Shock will speed induction with agent B more than agent A

Answers: 1. B 2. B 3. C 4. A 5. A 6. B

CHAPTER 3

Pulmonary Effects of Inhalational Agents

(Other aspects are covered in the section Pulmonary Physiology)

All inhalational agents will produce

1. A dose-dependent increase in respiratory rate and decrease in tidal volume except isoflurane, which causes no further increase of respiratory rate beyond 1 MAC.
    A. Degree of increase in respiratory rate at one MAC: Nitrous > Hal > Des > Enf > Iso
2. Hypercarbia, except nitrous oxide.
    A. Degree of increase in $PaCO_2$ at 1 MAC: Enf > Des > Iso > Hal.
    B. $PaCO_2$ gradually returns to normal after several MAC hours.
3. A decreased ventilatory response to hypercarbia (i.e., for a given $PaCO_2$, the anesthetized patient responds with a smaller increase in minute ventilation than the nonanesthetized patient).
    A. Degree of respiratory depression at 1 MAC: Iso > Des > Enf > N_2O > Hal.
4. A decreased ventilatory response to hypoxemia, even at < 1 MAC. (Differs from CO_2 response . . . decreased responsiveness to hypercarbia is only seen at ≥ 1 MAC.)
5. Bronchodilation: halothane causes the greatest bronchial relaxation.
6. Inhibition of hypoxic pulmonary vasoconstriction.
7. Inhibition of intercostal muscle function (only seen with halothane).

Sample questions

A = 1, 2, 3   B = 1, 3   C = 2, 4   D = 4 only   E = all are correct

1. Compared to enflurane, isoflurane at 2 MAC causes
    1. More hypercarbia
    2. More tachypnea
    3. Similar tidal volume
    4. More impairment of intercostal muscle function

2. At 1 MAC, halothane increases the
    1. Respiratory rate
    2. Apneic threshold

3. PaCO$_2$
4. Pulmonary vascular resistance

3. Following general anesthesia with halothane, factors predisposing to postoperative hypercarbia include
   1. Chronic obstructive pulmonary disease
   2. Residual halothane
   3. Morphine
   4. Chronic anemia

Answers: 1. B   2. A   3. A

CHAPTER 4

Cardiovascular Effects of Inhalational Agents

● Table 4–1

Agent	Heart Rate	Systemic Vascular Resistance	MAP	Cardiac Output	Stroke Volume	Myocardial Contractility	Coronary Artery Resistance	Carotid Reflex
Halothane		↓	↓	↓	↓	↓↓	↓	↓↓
Enflurane	↑	↓	↓	↓	↓	↓	↓	↓
Isoflurane	↑	↓↓↓	↓		↓	↓	↓↓	↓
Desflurane		↓↓	↓		↓	↓	↓	↓
Sevoflurane		↓	↓		↓	↓	↓	↓
Nitrous	↑			↑		↓		

Key: ↑ = increased, ↓ = decreased, blank = no change. Note all these changes are at 1 MAC.

Highlights of this information (at 1 MAC)

1. Increase in heart rate: Greatest with isoflurane, but enflurane causes a dose-dependent tachycardia. Halothane decreases SA node automaticity and abolishes baroreceptor response.
2. Decrease in SVR: Greatest with isoflurane, least with halothane.
3. Decrease in MAP: Isoflurane and desflurane ↓ MAP via vasodilation and decreased SVR. Halothane and enflurane ↓ MAP via decreased myocardial contractility and CO.
4. Decreased CO: Enf > Hal >>> all the rest; nitrous actually increases CO when given alone.
5. Decreased contractility: Same distribution as decreased cardiac output.
6. Decreased coronary resistance: All agents increase coronary blood flow, but only isoflurane causes selective vasodilation in normal vessels, creating potential for "steal."

Additional points to ponder

Halothane: Sensitizes heart to catecholamines, supression of baroreceptor reflex will exacerbate hypotension caused by hypovolemia.
Enflurane: Lowers seizure threshold, causes dose-dependent tachycardia.
Nitrous: Causes sympathetic stimulation, thus increasing heart rate and cardiac output. Substitution of part of the anesthetic dose with nitrous while maintaining same total MAC will reduce the degree of hypotension seen with volatile agents. Same effect seen with cardiac output.

Effects of inhalational agents on renal function

1. ↓ renal vascular resistance (so renal blood flow is unchanged, despite a decreased MAP).
2. ↓ GFR.
3. ↓ urine output.

Effects of inhalational agents on cerebral function

1. Cerebral vasodilation, leading to ↑ CBF and ICP (Hal >> Enf > Iso, Sevo > N_2O).
2. ↓ cerebral metabolic rate (Iso > Enf > Hal > N_2O).

> **NOTE:** Hyperventilation and hypocarbia offset the vasodilation caused by all agents.

Sample questions

Single best answer

1. A 14-year-old male breathing spontaneously during inguinal hernia repair under general anesthesia with halothane, nitrous oxide, and oxygen develops a junctional rhythm of 60/min on EKG, blood pressure is 100/70 mmHg. The most appropriate action at this time is
   1. Administer atropine
   2. Administer epinephrine
   3. Discontinue halothane
   4. No action is required
   5. Discontinue nitrous oxide and hyperventilate with pure oxygen

2. A 3-year-old, 15-kg male undergoing hypospadius repair receives a field block by the surgeon with 7 ml 1% lidocaine with epinephrine 1:200,000. Spontaneous ventilation is maintained under general anesthesia with halothane, nitrous oxide, and oxygen. Shortly after incision, the EKG shows frequent premature ventricular contractions. The most appropriate action is
   1. Instruct the surgeon to switch to plain lidocaine
   2. Administer intravenous lidocaine 0.5 mg/kg until ectopic beats resolve
   3. Initiate positive pressure ventilation
   4. Deepen the halothane concentration
   5. Inform the surgeon that he has reached the toxic dose of lidocaine

   A = 1, 2, 3   B = 1, 3   C = 2, 4   D = 4 only   E = all are correct

3. Drugs that lower mean arterial pressure mainly by reducing systemic vascular resistance include
   1. Isoflurane
   2. Halothane
   3. Desflurane
   4. Enflurane

4. A dose-dependent reduction in cardiac output is seen with
   1. Isoflurane
   2. Halothane
   3. Desflurane
   4. Enflurane

Answers: **1.** 5   **2.** 3   **3.** B   **4.** C

CHAPTER 5

Nitrous Oxide

Rate of diffusion into air-filled space

$$N_2O \gg CO_2$$

Nitrous rapidly enters all gas-filled spaces. However, the effect of the nitrous depends on the compliance of the space it enters.

Effect of nitrous on noncompliant spaces

Causes a rapid increase in *pressure*. Examples of noncompliant spaces:

1. The middle ear: N_2O contraindicated for tympanoplasty.
2. Gas space created by pneumoencephalography.
3. Gas space created in eye by injection of sulfur hexafluoride or carbon octafluorine into vitreous during surgery for detached retina.

> **NOTE:** Risk of increased intraocular pressure following administration of N_2O exists for up to 4 weeks after intravitreal injection of opthalmologic gases.

Effect of nitrous on compliant spaces

Causes a rapid increase in *volume* with very little increase in pressure. Examples of compliant spaces:

1. Gas space created by pneumothorax.
2. Gas space created by pneumoperitoneum.
3. Bowel gas (most important in closed loops of bowel).
4. Air embolus.
5. Air-filled balloons: pulmonary artery catheter, endotracheal tube cuff.

Sample questions

A = 1, 2, 3   B = 1, 3   C = 2, 4   D = 4 only   E = all are correct

1. Diffusion of nitrous oxide into which of the following air-filled spaces will create an increased pressure?
   1. Middle ear
   2. Thorax
   3. Intraocular space
   4. Bowel

2. Nitrous oxide
   1. Will diffuse into air-filled spaces faster than air will diffuse out
   2. Has a higher blood:gas partition coefficient than air
   3. At equilibrium will exist at the same partial pressure in the alveoli and any air-filled space
   4. At equilibrium will exist at the same concentration in the alveoli and any air-filled space

Answers: 1. B   2. A

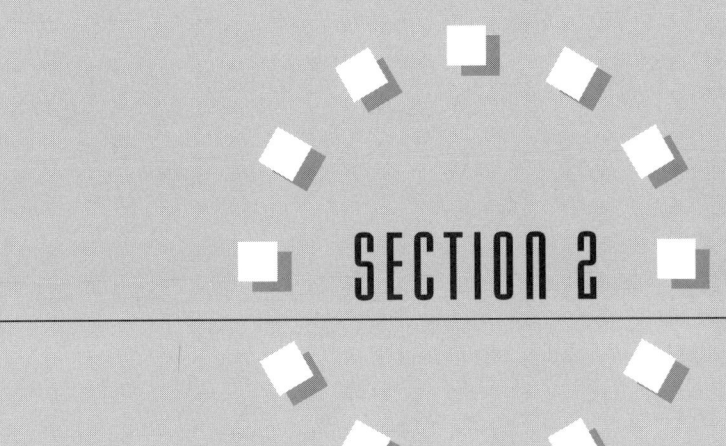

SECTION 2

Pulmonary Physiology

CHAPTER 6

Pulmonary Physiology

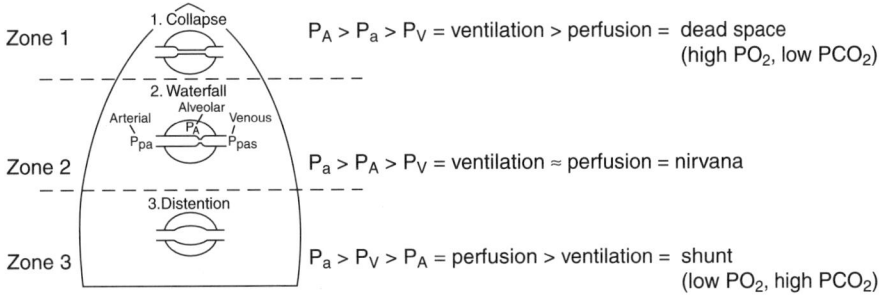

Figure 6–1. Modified from West JB, Dollery CT, Naimark A: Distribution of blood flow in isolated lung: relation to vascular and alveolar pressures. J Appl Phys 19: 723, 1964, with permission.

> **NOTE:** *Both* ventilation and perfusion are greatest at the base of the lung. However, gravity has a greater affect on blood (which is heavy) than on air (which is light), so perfusion exceeds ventilation at the base.

Factors affecting distribution of pulmonary blood flow

1. Gravity: biggest factor . . . blood runs downhill, so perfusion is best in *dependent* portion of lung, except when affected by:
2. Alveolar pressure: if $P_A > P_a$, blood is diverted to areas of lesser alveolar pressure, despite gravity.
3. Pulmonary vascular resistance: as PVR increases, pulmonary blood flow decreases, despite gravity.

Factors increasing pulmonary vascular resistance

1. Low cardiac output: less volume in vessel allows vessel to narrow, increasing resistance.
2. Hypoxia: causes hypoxic pulmonary vasoconstriction.
3. Hypercarbia: also causes reactive vasoconstriction.
4. Acidosis: ditto.

5. Any deviation from FRC: Volumes > FRC, distend alveoli and compress pulmonary arterioles.
Volumes < FRC, create hypoxia and pulmonary vasoconstriction.

Factors affecting distribution of ventilation

1. Gravity: biggest factor *during spontaneous ventilation* . . . the weight of the lung creates a relatively positive pleural pressure at the lung base, compressing basal alveoli more than apical. As the diaphragm falls and the rib cage expands during inspiration, basal alveoli undergo a greater change in volume per unit of pressure than apical alveoli (said another way: basal alveoli are more compliant, so air goes there). Thus, *even in positions other than upright*, spontaneous ventilation still goes to dependent portion of lung. *Exceptions:*
    A. Mechanical ventilation: compliance and resistance favor ventilation of nondependent areas.
    B. Anesthetized state: reduction of lung volumes due to hypoventilation makes nondependent areas more compliant than dependent areas.

So note: they'll ask you about ventilation in the lateral decubitus position:
   A. If the patient is breathing spontaneously, V_T goes to *dependent* lung.
   B. If anesthetized, but still breathing spontaneously, V_T goes to *nondependent* lung.
2. Compliance: meaning combined compliance of lung and chest wall.
3. Airway resistance: cross-sectional area of airways increases exponentially as you move distally, so resistance to flow is less.

Factors affecting work of breathing

1. Airway resistance: ↑ resistance = ↑ WOB (worsened by rapid, shallow breathing).
2. Compliance of lung or chest wall: ↓ compliance = ↑ WOB (worsened by slow, deep breaths).

Factors increasing dead space (i.e.; zone 1)

In general, anything that increases PVR or alveolar pressure.

1. PEEP/CPAP (↑ P_A).
2. Positive pressure ventilation (↑ P_A).
3. Bronchodilation (↑ anatomic dead space).
4. Low cardiac output (↑ PVR).
5. Pulmonary embolus (mechanically blocks perfusion).
6. Excessive ventilator tubing (↑ anatomic dead space . . . only at the Y-connector, remember?).

Factors increasing alveolar-arterial O_2 gradient

1. Smoking.
2. Advanced age.
3. Atelectasis (obesity, pregnancy, hypoventilation).
4. Chronic obstructive pulmonary disease.

Sample questions

A = 1, 2, 3   B = 1, 3   C = 2, 4   D = 4 only   E = all are correct

1. A reduction in cardiac output causes
   1. Increased pulmonary vascular resistance
   2. An increased ratio of deadspace to tidal volume
   3. An increased alveolar-arterial oxygen gradient
   4. An increase in arterial-alveolar carbon dioxide gradient

2. An asthmatic patient will have
   1. Decreased work of breathing if he takes slow, deep breaths
   2. Increased deadspace ventilation after receiving 0.4 mg intramuscular atropine
   3. Increased work of breathing with rapid shallow breaths
   4. Preferential distribution of tidal volume to the dependent lung during spontaneous ventilation in the lateral decubitus position

3. Distribution of ventilation in the anesthetized patient is
   1. Similar to what it is in the awake patient
   2. To the dependent portion of the lung if spontaneously breathing
   3. Altered due to cephalad migration of the diaphragm
   4. Altered by changes in lung compliance

4. Slow, deep inspiration will result in low work of breathing for the patient with
   1. Low total lung capacity and a high ratio of forced expiratory volume in 1 sec to vital capacity
   2. Low mid-expiratory flow rates
   3. Pulmonary fibrosis
   4. Significant pulmonary responsiveness to beta-adrenergic stimulation

Single best answer

5. Distribution of pulmonary blood flow is most dependent on
   1. Functional residual capacity
   2. Pulmonary vascular resistance
   3. Patient position
   4. Pulmonary compliance
   5. Spontaneous ventilation

Answers: 1. E   2. E   3. D   4. C   5. 3

CHAPTER 7

Apneic Oxygenation

What is it?

During apnea, the patient circuit is connected to a source of pure oxygen, creating a continuous column of oxygen from the y-connector to the alveolus. As oxygen is removed from the alveolus by pulmonary blood flow, oxygen in the circuit and conducting airways migrates into the alveolus, maintaining oxygenation.

Effectiveness is limited by

1. Increasing $PaCO_2$: rate of rise is 6 mmHg for the first minute, 3 mmHg each subsequent minute.
2. Starting $PaCO_2$: Duh. The higher you start, the faster you reach intolerable levels.
3. Incomplete denitrogenation: Because you reduce the volume of your "oxygen reservoir."
4. Low FRC: Again, because your reservoir volume is reduced.

How does a rising $PaCO_2$ limit oxygenation?

1. As the alveolus fills with CO_2, there's no space left in alveolus for oxygen to occupy.
2. Dysrythmias ensue.

Can I prevent hypercarbia without ventilating the patient?

Sure, by maintaining high flows of oxygen (about 1 L/kg/min).

Sample questions

None, because all they usually ask is for you to calculate the $PaCO_2$ after "x" minutes, if the starting $PaCO_2$ was "y."

CHAPTER 8

Oxyhemoglobin Curves, Oxygen Content, and Oxygen Delivery

Delivery of oxygen to the tissues is determined by

1. Cardiac output.
2. Total oxygen content of the blood.

} These two are the only variables the books ever talk about.

3. Type of hemoglobin: different species of Hb have different affinities for O_2, which affects release of O_2 to tissues . . . i.e.; O_2 delivery.

Determinants of oxygen content

O_2 only exists in the blood in two forms: dissolved or bound to hemoglobin, the greatest contribution being the bound Hb. This is expressed by that equation you've memorized a thousand times, but never really thought about:

$$O_2 \text{ content} = (.003 \times PaO_2) + (1.34 \times Hb \times SaO_2)$$

The amount of O_2 dissolved in blood at standard temperature and pressure (expressed in the first parentheses) depends on:

1. Atmospheric pressure: as P_{atm} increases, more O_2 is forced into solution (dissolved).
2. Solubility of oxygen: inversely related to temperature.
3. Partial pressure of oxygen in plasma (PaO_2).

} = .003

What's the significance of that number in the second parentheses? Each gram of Hb carries 1.34 ml O_2 *when fully saturated* (which is why we include the percent saturation in this calculation).

The oxyhemoglobin curve

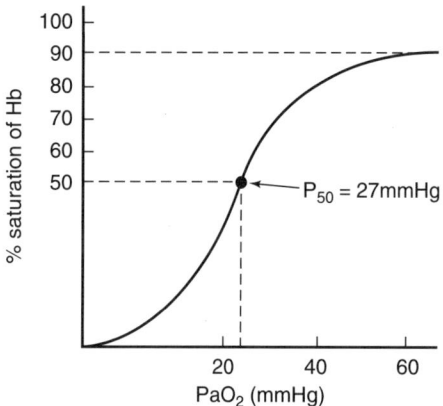

Figure 8–1.

Look at the curve and you'll see there's a quick-and-dirty way to estimate PaO_2 based on Hb saturation using the 40-50-60-70-80-90 rule:

If PaO_2 is: 40   50   60
Then saturation is: 70   80   90

Factors causing left shift (↑ affinity for O_2)	Factors causing right shift (↓ affinity for O_2)
1. ↓ H⁺ ion concentration (↑ pH)	1. ↑ H⁺ ion concentration
2. ↓ temperature	2. ↑ temperature
3. ↓ 2,3 DPG	3. ↑ 2,3 DPG (pregnancy, chronic anemia)
4. ↑ fetal hemoglobin	4. ↑ sickle hemoglobin
5. ↑ methemoglobin	
6. ↑ carboxyhemoglobin	

NOTE: Remember that high affinity for O_2 = decreased unloading of O_2 to the tissues and vice versa.

Betcha never thought about anemia and its effect on O_2 delivery, didja? Well, make sure you're familiar with the physiologic changes of anemia:

1. ↑ 2,3 DPG
2. ↑ P_{50}
3. ↑ cardiac output: via tachycardia if anemia is acute or low grade chronic. If chronic and severe, there's also an increase in stroke volume. Eventually, you reach a point where the oxygen demand for maintaining tachycardia outweighs the oxygen supplied by the tachycardia.
4. ↑ coronary artery blood flow: due to viscosity, cardiac output, and vasodilation.
5. ↑ oxygen extraction ratio: since less O_2 is delivered, tissues suck up all they can. Result: ↓ mixed venous O_2 content.
6. ↓ viscosity: reduces resistance to capillary flow and improves oxygen delivery to offset the effect of having fewer little red choo-choo trains.

Fine points about fetal hemoglobin

1. ↓ P_{50}
2. ↓ 2,3 DPG

3. Production stops at birth
4. ↑ levels found in sickle cell, β-thalassemia

Sample questions

A = 1, 2, 3   B = 1, 3   C = 2, 4   D = 4 only   E = all are correct

1. A patient with chronic anemia will have increased
   1. Cardiac output
   2. 2,3 DPG
   3. P_{50}
   4. Mixed venous oxygen saturation

2. A right shift of the oxyhemoglobin curve is expected in a patient with
   1. Intrauterine pregnancy at 36 weeks' gestation
   2. Asymptomatic sickle cell disease at 4 weeks of age
   3. Fever
   4. Uncorrected pyloric stenosis

3. Values required for calculation of arterial oxygen content include
   1. Cardiac output
   2. Amount of nonadult type hemoglobin present
   3. Hematocrit
   4. Percent saturation of hemoglobin

4. During repair of idiopathic scoliosis in a 20-year-old, reduction of blood loss is attempted using isovolemic hemodilution and deliberate hypotension with sodium nitroprusside. Blood pressure is 90/63 mmHg, pulse 105/min, hemoglobin 8.1 g/dL, PaO_2 95 on fiO_2 0.3, and mixed venous saturation is 63%. The most appropriate initial therapy is
   1. Institute positive end-expiratory pressure 10 cmH_2O
   2. Stop the sodium nitroprusside
   3. Administer methylene blue to reverse cyanide toxicity
   4. Transfuse with 2 units packed red blood cells
   5. Institute dopamine infusion at 7 µg/kg/min

Answers: 1. A   2. B   3. D   4. D

CHAPTER 9

Flow-Volume Loops

Clinical utility

Evaluation of presence and severity of airway obstruction.

Procedure

The patient performs a forced vital capacity maneuver followed by a forced inspiration to total lung capacity, and the spirograph plots the generated flows and achieved volumes.

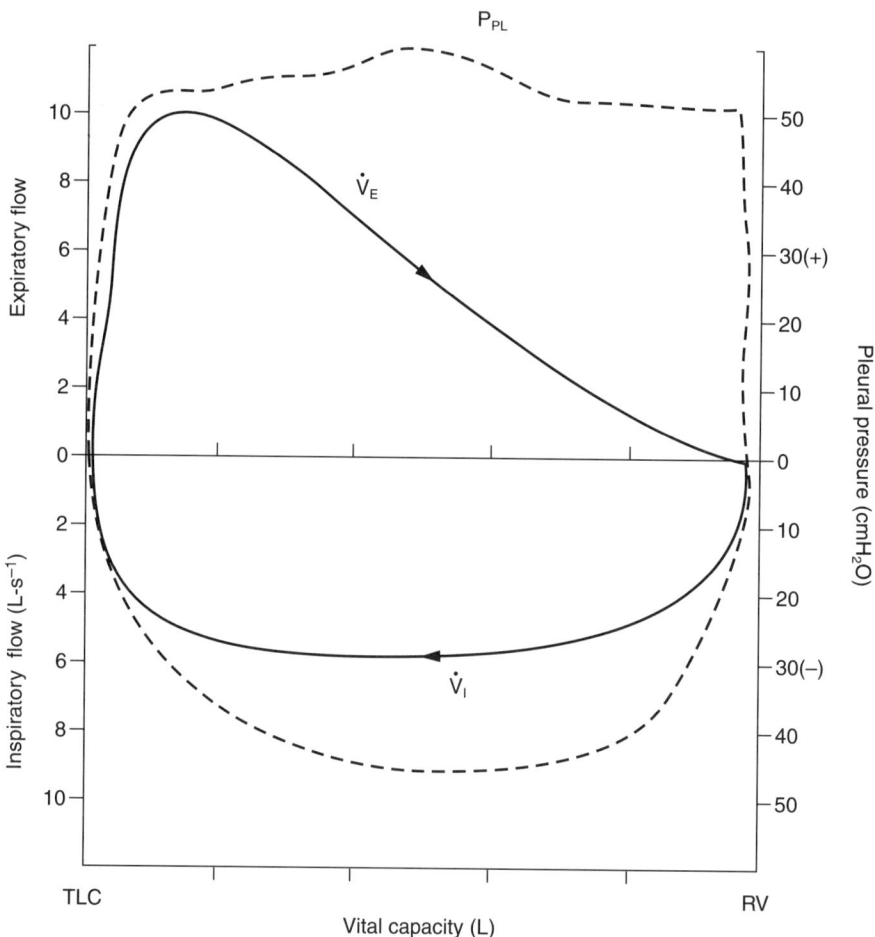

Figure 9–1. A typical flow-volume loop. From Miller RD, Cucchiara RF, Miller ED, Jr, Reves R, Roizen MF, Savarese JJ, eds. Anesthesia, ed 4. New York: Churchill Livingstone, 1994, p. 893. Reproduced with permission.

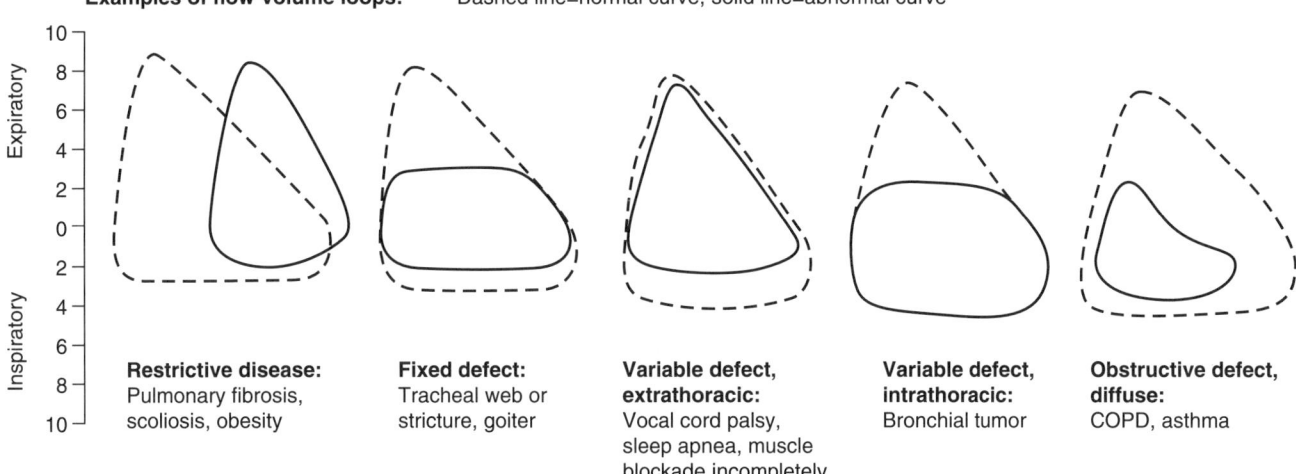

Figure 9–2.

> **NOTE:** Flow is proportional to pleural pressure (i.e., dependent on patient effort) throughout the entire curve, except during the last half of exhalation, where airway closure inhibits flow.

Types of airway obstruction

1. Diffuse disease: COPD, asthma, etc.
2. Upper airway obstruction
   A. Fixed. **Most common,** degree of flow impairment is unaffected by respiratory phase; thus, equal reductions of flow are seen in inspiration and expiration.
   B. Variable. *Intrathoracic:* negative pressure during inhalation stents open the airway; relative positive pressure during exhalation causes airway collapse and obstructs flow. *Extrathoracic:* intrathoracic pressure during inhalation is more negative than atmospheric pressure, causing upper airway collapse. Relatively positive intrathoracic pressure during exhalation forces air past obstruction, allowing normal flow.

Sample questions: None . . . you just need to be able to identify the various loops.

Chapter 10

Pulmonary Function Tests and Disease States

Abbreviations

TLC = total lung capacity
VC = vital capacity
FVC = forced vital capacity
FEV_1 = forced expiratory volume in 1 sec
IRV = inspiratory reserve volume
ERV = expiratory reserve volume
FRC = functional residual capacity ⎫ these two are not measurable
RV = residual volume ⎭ by simple spirometry

They expect you to know what volumes and capacities simple spirometry can measure.

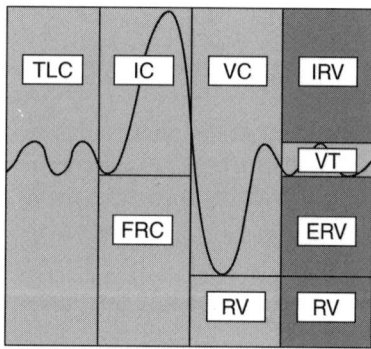

Figure 10–1. From Barash PG, Cullen BF, Stoelting RK. Clinical Anesthesia, ed 2. Philadelphia: Lippincott, 1992, p. 935. Reprinted with permission.

Normal spirometry parameters

● Table 10–1

Test	Male	Female
Total lung capacity (L)	6.5	5
Vital capacity (L)	5	4
Forced expiratory volume in 1 sec (FEV_1) (L)	4	3
% of forced vital capacity in 1 sec (L)	80	80
Functional residual capacity (L)	3.5	2

In general

Obstructive diseases reduce flows and FEV_1/FVC ratio, but volumes are unaffected. Restrictive diseases reduce volumes, but flows and FEV_1/FVC ratio remains 1.

- **Table 10–2**

Disease State	FEV_1	FVC	FEV_1/FVC
Obstructive (asthma, chronic bronchitis)	↓	normal	↓
Obstructive (emphysema)	↓↓	↓	↓
Restrictive (pulmonary fibrosis, kyphoscoliosis, obesity, pregnancy)	↓	↓	normal
Neuromuscular disease	↓	↓	normal

Other states that alter PFTs

1. Pregnancy: ↓ FRC, RV, ERV, but an ↑ IRV maintains normal TLC. V_T is also increased.
2. General anesthesia: ↓ FRC, V_T (tidal volume effect only seen in spontaneously breathing patient).
3. Elderly: ↑ FRC, RV, compliance, V_D, ↓ FEV_1 and response to hypoxia or hypercarbia.
4. Obesity: ↓ FRC, VC, IRV, ERV, but RV, closing capacity and flows are normal.

Other factors causing a reduction in FRC

1. Site of surgery: abdominal and thoracic procedures reduce FRC for several days postoperatively.
2. Position: when supine, diaphragm migrates cephalad.
3. Loss of muscle tone: thoracic muscles relax under anesthesia, decreasing opposition to elastic recoil.
4. Loss of "auto-PEEP": created by pursed-lip breathing in chronic lungers and by partially closing the glottis in children.

Sample questions

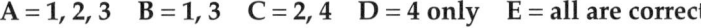

A = 1, 2, 3   B = 1, 3   C = 2, 4   D = 4 only   E = all are correct

1. A morbidly obese patient will demonstrate
   1. Less work of breathing with a respiratory pattern of rapid, shallow breaths
   2. An increased closing capacity
   3. A functional residual capacity less than closing capacity
   4. Reduced ratio of FEV_1 to FVC

2. The functional residual capacity is
   1. Increased in severe emphysema
   2. The combination of the expiratory reserve volume and the residual volume
   3. Increased in the elderly
   4. Increased with positive end-expiratory pressure

3. Changes in respiratory function in the elderly include
   1. Increased compliance
   2. Decreased arterial oxygen content

3. Decreased response to carbon dioxide
4. Increased alveolar oxygen content

4. Airway closure during normal tidal breathing occurs in
    1. Neonates
    2. Obesity
    3. Elderly
    4. Emphysema

Answers: 1. B   2. E   3. A   4. A

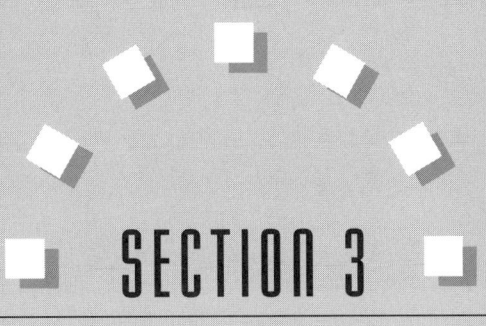

SECTION 3

Anesthesia and Disease States

CHAPTER 11

Chronic Obstructive Pulmonary Disease

Defect: Airway obstruction occurring during expiration but with normal inspiratory flow characteristics.

Two main categories

1. Chronic bronchitis
2. Emphysema

Factors contributing to obstruction

1. Increased secretions
2. Loss of lung parenchyma and its supportive action
3. Hypertrophy and spasm of bronchial smooth muscle

● Table 11–1

Clinical Parameter	Emphysema	Chronic Bronchitis
Structural defect	Loss of lung parenchyma	Hypertrophied glands Bronchospasm
$PaCO_2$	Normal	Elevated
PaO_2	Hypoxia *late* in clinical course	Hypoxia *early* in clinical course
Pulmonary function tests	↓ FEV_1/FVC ratio ↓ maximum voluntary ventilation ↑ RV/TLC ratio ↑ TLC, FRC, **RV** ↓ D_LCO (2° loss of diffusive surface area)	↓ FEV_1/FVC ratio ↓ maximum voluntary ventilation ↑ RV/TLC ratio ↑ TLC, FRC, **RV** D_LCO normal
Chest x-ray	Hyperlucent, flattened diaphragm Elongated heart shadow	Findings not pathognomonic
Incidence of cor pulmonale	Low	High (elevated pulmonary vascular resistance 2° hypercarbia/hypoxia)
Effect of bronchodilators	Not helpful	Helpful
Hematocrit	Normal	Elevated

Preoperative evaluation/preparation

1. ABG and pre/post-bronchodilator PFTs as indicated by history.
2. Pulmonary "tune-up": antibiotics, bronchodilators, chest physiotherapy.
3. Stop smoking (even temporary cessation will lower carboxyhemoglobin levels and improve oxygen delivery).
4. Expect need for mechanical ventilation if preop $PaCO_2 > 50$ mmHg and/or $FEV_1/FVC < 0.5$.

● Table 11-2

Anesthetic Management			
Regional		General	
Advantages	Disadvantages	Advantages	Disadvantages
1. Neuroaxial opioids may improve postop respiratory function	1. Limited by surgical site 2. Limited by level required (>T6 can impair ERV and ability to clear secretions) 3. Required sedation may compromise respiratory function	1. Volatile agents are bronchodilators	1. Agents inhibit hypoxic pulmonary vasoconstriction 2. Dries secretions 3. N_2O causes pulmonary vasoconstriction, limits F_IO_2, and increases bullae size (risk of pneumothorax)

Points to consider regarding mechanical ventilation of patients with COPD

1. Bronchospasm and secretions narrow the airways, creating turbulent flow and necessitating high peak airway pressures.
2. Airway obstruction and loss of elastic recoil necessitates long exhalation times.
3. Hypercarbia may be "normal" for patient, so don't try to completely correct it.
4. When extubating, remember that COPD patients may depend on hypoxic drive (high PaO_2 *suppresses* their drive).

In general, COPD patients will require

1. **Large tidal volumes** (10–15 mL/kg, may be better than PEEP because it improves oxygenation with less reduction on venous return to heart).
2. **Slow inspiratory rates** (reduces turbulence and level of peak inspiratory pressure required; therefore, less risk of pneumothorax).
3. **Low respiratory rates** (maximal expiratory time allows most complete CO_2 elimination, prevents air-trapping, and promotes venous return to the heart).

Sample questions

A = 1, 2, 3   B = 1, 3   C = 2,4   D = 4 only   E = all are correct

1. End-stage emphysema results in
    1. Diminished uptake of soluble anesthetic agents
    2. Decreased elastic recoil of the lung
    3. Increased deadspace ventilation
    4. Increased inspiratory reserve volume

2. In chronic obstructive pulmonary disease, it is common to have
    1. An increased alveolar–arterial PaO_2 gradient
    2. Elevated serum bicarbonate levels
    3. Prolonged elimination of soluble anesthetic agents
    4. A low PaO_2 that can be elevated by increasing the P_{AO_2}

Answers: 1. A   2. A

CHAPTER 12

Adult Respiratory Distress Syndrome

Pathophysiology

Inciting event → complement activation

Platelet aggregation   PMNs aggregate on pulmonary endothelium
↓   ↓
Pulmonary microemboli   Release inflammatory mediators
                                             ↓
                            Damage to alveolar-capillary membrane
                                             ↓
Leakage of plasma proteins, RBCs, WBCs, PMNs into alveoli and interstitium

Figure 12–1.

End results

1. Fluid and cell-filled alveoli leading to
   A. Decreased FRC.
   B. Increased right-to-left shunt.
   C. Hypoxemia refractory to increased F_iO_2.
   D. Increased secretions.
2. Fluid and cell-filled interstitium (noncardiogenic pulmonary edema) leading to
   A. Decreased lung compliance.
   B. Increased work of breathing.
   C. Diffuse bilateral infiltrates on chest x-ray.

Clinical progression

1. Early: tachypnea, ↓ PaO_2 and $PaCO_2$, ↑ work of breathing. If mild, may only need supplemental oxygen (usually able to adequately remove CO_2).
2. Late: tachypnea, ↓↓PaO_2, ↑ $PaCO_2$ (unable to keep up with oxygen demands, the patient "wears out").

Treatment of ARDS

1. Aggressive pulmonary toilet.
2. Antibiotics only if infective organism verified.
3. Steroids do not change outcome (~50% mortality, usually due to multiorgan system failure).
4. Meticulous fluid management (maintain cardiac output but avoid flooding lungs).
5. Supplemental oxygen, advance to mechanical ventilation as required.

Mechanical ventilation in ARDS

1. PEEP/CPAP essential for improving oxygenation (↑'s FRC and compliance, ↓'s shunt and deadspace).
2. Standard approach:
   A. **Large tidal volumes** (recruits alveoli).
   B. **High peak inspiratory pressures** (ensures delivery of adequate tidal volume).
   C. **Long inspiratory times or inverse I:E ratio** (maximizes time for oxygenation, and CO_2 removal usually not a problem).
3. Alternate approach: high-frequency jet ventilation (no difference in mortality).

CAVEAT: Beware that a volume ventilator will deliver the pre-set tidal volume no matter how much peak pressure is required to do so (high risk of barotrauma). You can minimize the risk of barotrauma by pressure limiting the ventilator (the remaining tidal volume "pops-off" beyond a certain peak pressure). The flipside of this is that as the lung compliance worsens the patient will receive less tidal volume.

Hemodynamic effects of PEEP

Increased alveolar pressure → pulmonary artery hypertension → RV afterload increase → ↑ CVP → ↓venous return → ↓ ventricular filling → systemic hypotension and decreased myocardial perfusion.

Common hemodynamic parameters in ARDS

1. CVP—high
2. PAP—high
3. PAOP—normal or low
4. LVEDV—normal or low

Sample questions

A = 1, 2, 3   B = 1, 3   C = 2, 4   D = 4 only   E = all are correct

1. A 70-kg female with adult respiratory distress syndrome is mechanically ventilated with a continuous-flow ventilator. Respiratory rate is 15/min, tidal volume is 600 mL, there is no preset pressure limit, and the inspiratory/expiratory ratio is 1:1. True statements regarding her ventilator settings include
   1. The maximum inspiratory flowrate delivered is 18 L/min
   2. Increasing the tidal volume would be the most appropriate first step to correct any hypercarbia
   3. The tidal volume received by the patient will decrease if the compliance of the ventilator circuit increases
   4. The delivered tidal volume will decrease as pulmonary compliance decreases

2. Expected findings obtained from a pulmonary artery catheter in a patient with adult respiratory distress syndrome being mechanically ventilated with 10 cm H_2O positive end-expiratory pressure include
   1. Elevated pulmonary artery pressure
   2. Elevated pulmonary artery occlusion pressure
   3. Elevated central venous pressure

4. Elevated left ventricular end-diastolic pressure

Single best answer

3. The most likely permanent sequelae of adult respiratory distress syndrome (besides death) is
   1. Proliferation of type I pneumocytes
   2. Decreased pulmonary compliance
   3. Aggregation of polymorphonuclear cells on the pulmonary endothelium
   4. Reduced diffusion capacity
   5. Chronic obstructive pulmonary disease

Answers: 1. A   2. B   3. 2

CHAPTER 13

Asthma

Defect: Hyperreactivity of airways causing reversible obstruction and chronic inflammation.

Symptoms

Wheezing/productive cough/dyspnea.

Pulmonary function tests

1. TLC normal
2. FRC increased (2° air trapping)
3. FEV_1, FEF_{25-75} decreased

Medications

1. Theophylline (aminophylline is I.V. form):
    Action: causes release of norepinephrine (direct β-agonist), inhibits phosphodiesterase-catalyzed breakdown of cAMP.
    Dose: load 5 mg/kg, maintenance infusion 0.5–1 mg/kg/hr
    Side effects: dysrythmias
    Caution: cimetidine increases plasma concentration to toxic levels; antagonizes barbiturate effect; crosses placenta
2. β-agonists (albuterol primarily)
    Action: direct-acting agonist
    Side effects: tachydysrythmias/hypokalemia
3. Anticholinergics (ipratroprium bromide): best for maintenance, not acute episode.
4. Corticosteroids (beclomethasone, triamcinolone): first-line drug.
5. Cromalyn sodium (mast cell stabilizer): first-line drug in children.

Anesthetic management

1. Regional if possible.
2. Establish deep plane of anesthesia prior to intubation (halothane best volatile bronchodilator, but sensitizes heart to catecholamines, and they're already on β-agonists).
3. Consider ketamine (prevents bronchoconstriction better than thiopental).
4. Avoid histamine-releasing drugs (atracurium, curare, thiopental, morphine).
5. Beware of reversal drugs (theoretical risk of precipitating spasm from cholinergic stimulation).

6. Mechanical ventilation (best achieved with humidified gas, low inspiratory flowrate, long exhalation).

Signs of intraoperative bronchospasm

1. Wheezing (or absent air exchange if spasm severe enough).
2. Excessive expiratory "up-sloping" on capnograph.
3. High peak inspiratory pressures.
4. Hypoxia/hypercarbia (if severe).
5. Prolonged exhalation time in spontaneously ventilating patient.

Differential diagnosis of intraoperative wheezing

1. Bronchospasm.
2. Reduced FRC (increases airway resistance and produces wheezing).
3. Light anesthesia (active expiratory efforts cause wheezing).
4. Endotracheal tube obstruction (kink, secretions, blood, overinflated cuff, bevel against tracheal wall).
5. Nasogastric tube in trachea.
6. Endobronchial intubation.
7. Rapid descent of a gravity-filled bellows (creates negative pressure in airway and "wheezing").
8. Zebras: pneumothorax, pulmonary embolus, pulmonary edema.

Sample question

Single best answer

1. Following rapid-sequence induction with 300 mg thiopental and 100 mg succinylcholine, a 60-kg patient on maintenance theophylline is noted to have a sharp upward slope on the carbon dioxide capnograph. Breath sounds are diminished bilaterally, but no wheezes are heard. Peak inspiratory pressures are 55 cmH$_2$O and the pulse oximeter reads 90% with f$_i$O$_2$ 1.0. Review of the chart reveals a theophylline level of 7.0 µg/mL. The most appropriate first step is
   1. Hand-ventilate with high concentration of volatile anesthetic
   2. Administer additional 120 mg thiopental intravenously
   3. Administer nondepolarizing neuromuscular blockade to improve ventilation
   4. Administer aminophylline 300 mg intravenously and initiate maintenance infusion
   5. Institute positive end-expiratory pressure 10 cmH$_2$O

Answers: 1. 1

Chapter 14

Morbid Obesity

Definition: Body weight ≥ two times the predicted ideal body weight

Cardiovascular system

1. ↑ blood volume
2. ↑ LVEDV
3. ↑ stroke volume
4. ↑ cardiac output
5. SVR normal
6. High incidence hypertension
7. High incidence dysrythmias

Schematic depiction of cardiovascular changes

Increased body mass
↓
Increased oxygen requirements
↓
Increased blood volume
↓
Increased LVEDV
↓
Increased stroke volume → LV hypertrophy → ↑ LVEDP → ↑ PAOP → Pulmonary hypertension
↓ ↓ ↓
Increased cardiac output   Eventual LV failure   Eventual RV failure

Figure 14–1.

Pulmonary system

Excess weight on chest and increased intraabdominal pressure produce a restrictive disorder. Resultant effects on PFTs:

1. ↓ total lung capacity
2. ↓ vital capacity
3. ↓ expiratory reserve volume
4. ↓ functional residual capacity
5. *Residual volume unchanged*
6. *Closing capacity unchanged*

> **Caveat:** Magnitude of changes is increased in the supine position and more so in Trendelenburg. FRC, in particular, is reduced by supine position and by induction of general anesthesia.

Why are they hypoxic at rest?

Tidal breathing occurs at lung volumes that are less than the closing volume. Thus, airway closure occurs during normal tidal breathing, leading to V/Q mismatch (shunting). Their FRC is also less than the closing volume. In addition, although they increase minute ventilation in an attempt to meet metabolic demands, their work of breathing consumes a disproportionate amount of oxygen, offsetting the benefits of increased minute ventilation.

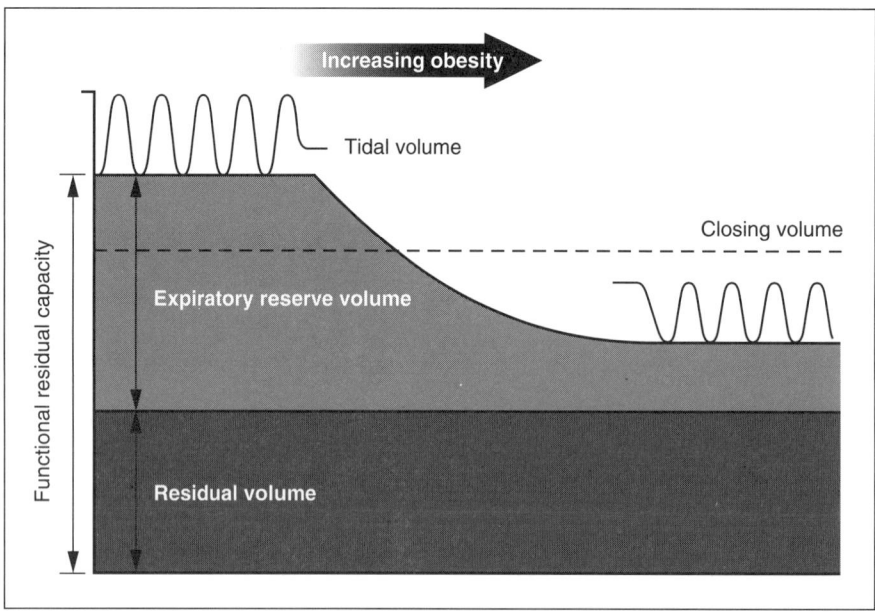

Figure 14–2. From Fox GS. Anaesthesia for intestinal short-circuiting in the morbidly obese with reference to the pathophysiology of gross obesity. Can Anaesth Soc J 22: 307, 1975, with permission.

Expected arterial blood gases

1. ↓ PaO_2, ↑ $A\text{-}aO_2$ gradient, normal $PaCO_2$, normal pH (and normal ventilatory response to carbon dioxide.
2. If patient has obese hypoventilation syndrome, **then** expect ↑ $PaCO_2$ and impaired response to CO_2.

Gastrointestinal/hepatic/renal changes

1. Gastric secretions have increased volume and acidity, but rate of emptying is not impaired.
2. Increased intraabdominal pressure increases risk of reflux and aspiration.
3. No increased incidence of hepatic/renal toxicity, but there is increased fluorination of volatile agents.

Pharmacokinetic considerations

1. Volume of distribution is increased for lipophilic drugs, so serum concentration is less than that seen with nonobese patients; however, terminal half-life is > expected since clearance is unchanged.
2. Increased biotransformation of volatile agents is seen, but doesn't cause delayed awakening.

Anesthetic management

1. Full stomach precautions (consider bicitra/H_2-blockers).
2. Potentially difficult/impossible intubation (consider awake laryngoscopy vs. fiberoptic).
3. General anesthesia preferred over regional (ensures ventilation/oxygenation, protects airway). Note: PEEP may be needed to prevent hypoxia, but beware of potential reduction of cardiac output.
4. Be prepared for high incidence of postop hypoxemia.

Sample questions

A = 1, 2, 3   B = 1, 3   C = 2, 4   D = 4 only   E = all are correct

1. Which of the following respiratory parameters is not decreased in morbid obesity?
   1. Total lung capacity
   2. Forced expiratory volume in 1 sec
   3. Expiratory reserve volume
   4. Forced vital capacity

2. True statements regarding pulmonary function in morbidly obese patients include
   1. The alveolar-arterial gradient is greater than in nonobese patients
   2. Even in the absence of obese hypoventilation syndrome, there is a decreased response to carbon dioxide
   3. Positive end-expiratory pressure may worsen oxygen delivery to the tissues
   4. Total thoracic compliance is increased

3. True statements regarding cardiac function in morbidly obese patients include
   1. Systemic vascular resistance is usually normal
   2. Systemic hypertension is common
   3. When related to body surface area, cardiac output is not increased
   4. Increased cardiac output is primarily a result of increased heart rate

4. Following administration of a single dose based on actual body weight in a morbidly obese patient
   1. Midazolam has a longer elimination half-life than in the nonobese patient
   2. Succinylcholine will demonstrate recovery time similar to those for the nonobese patient
   3. Vecuronium demonstrates prolonged time to twitch recovery
   4. Thiopental will not cause delayed emergence

5. Which ventilatory parameter undergoes the greatest change in morbidly obese patients?
   a. Inspiratory capacity
   b. Expiratory reserve volume
   c. Tidal volume
   d. Closing capacity
   e. Vital capacity

Answers: 1. C   2. B   3. A   4. E   5. B

CHAPTER 15

Cigarette Smoking

Physiologic effects of smoking

1. **Pulmonary effects** (besides the end result of COPD):
    A. Increased sputum production, airway reactivity, and carboxyhemoglobin.
    B. Decreased ciliary motility, FVC, and FEF_{25-75}.
2. **Cardiovascular** (besides the end result of cardiovascular disease): ↑ hematocrit (due to chronic tissue hypoxia), ↑ blood viscosity (due to high Hct), tachycardia (nicotinic effect).

Effects of preoperative smoking cessation

1. Effects seen within 12 to 48 hours
    A. ↓ carboxyhemoglobin (thus, more O_2-carrying capacity)
    B. Right shift of oxyhemoglobin curve (improved O_2 delivery to tissues)
    C. ↓ pulse
    D. ↑ mucociliary function (increased clearance of secretions)
    E. ↑ secretions ⎫
    F. ↑ airway reactivity ⎬ undesirable effects
2. Effects not seen until 8 weeks after cessation:
    A. ↓ secretions
    B. ↓ airway reactivity
    C. ↓ incidence of pulmonary complications

Sample question

A = 1, 2, 3   B = 1, 3   C = 2, 4   D = 4 only   E = all are correct

1. A 45-year-old with a 60-pack-year smoking history is scheduled for repair of an incarcerated inguinal hernia tomorrow. Abstinence from smoking for the next 24 hours will
    1. Improve oxygen delivery to the tissues
    2. Increase the P_{50}
    3. Increase the likelihood of bronchospasm
    4. Significantly reduce the chance of postoperative pulmonary complications

Answer: **1.** A

CHAPTER 16

Carbon Monoxide Poisoning

Clinical problem: Tissue hypoxia

Mechanism of hypoxia

1. Diminished O_2-carrying capacity because carbon monoxide binds hemoglobin with an affinity 200 times that of oxygen.
2. Decreased O_2 unloading to tissues due to a left shift of the oxyhemoglobin curve.

Signs and symptoms

1. Altered mental status (irritability, seizures, coma)
2. Headache, blurred vision
3. Nausea/vomiting
4. Angina
5. Cherry-red skin and mucous membranes
6. Respiratory failure (note that patient will not be tachypneic unless metabolic acidosis is present because the carotid bodies respond to the *normal* PaO_2)
7. Metabolic acidosis
8. Death

Diagnosis

1. Low arterial oxygen saturation in the presence of a normal PaO_2
2. Elevated measured carboxyhemoglobin (which can cause falsely high pulse oximeter reading)

Treatment

1. Administer 100% oxygen—displaces carbon monoxide from hemoglobin and speeds removal from body
2. Hyperbaric oxygen therapy if available (thought to decrease neurologic sequelae)

Sample question

A = 1, 2, 3   B = 1, 3   C = 2, 4   D = 4 only   E = all are correct

1. In carbon monoxide poisoning
   1. The degree of cyanosis is directly related to the amount of carboxyhemoglobin.

2. The pulse oximeter will read falsely low.
3. The PaO$_2$ decreases in proportion to the rise in carboxyhemoglobin.
4. Calculation of the arterial oxygen saturation based on the PaO$_2$ yields a falsely high value.

Answer: 1. D

CHAPTER 17

Diabetes Mellitus

Manifests as

1. Microvascular disease: retinopathy (blindness)
   nephropathy (renal failure)
2. Microvascular disease: coronary artery disease (myocardial infarction)
   cerebrovascular disease (stroke)
   peripheral vascular disease (claudication)
3. Neuropathy: autonomic (gastroparesis, resting tachycardia, hypotension)
   peripheral (foot ulcers)

Management

Besides the obvious complications that accompany the above problems, what they want you to know for the boards is the practical management of the three most common situations with diabetics:

1. **Hyperglycemia**
   A. Frequent glucose measurements (regardless of how you choose to administer insulin).
   B. Sliding scale or continuous infusion of regular insulin ~0.5–2 units/hr, both are equally acceptable.
   C. IV fluids to compensate for osmotic diuresis
   D. Consider monitoring ketones
2. **Hypoglycemia:** patients are tachycardic, hypertensive, diaphoretic, light-headed, eyes tearing
   A. D_{50} infusion .01–.02 mL/kg/min or bolus D_{50}.
   B. Frequent glucose checks.
   C. Withhold scheduled doses of β-blockers until hypoglycemia is corrected.
3. **Diabetic ketoacidosis:** precipitated by infection, stress; presents with nausea, vomiting, osmotic diuresis, and dehydration
   A. Aggressive rehydration with NaCl and supplemental K^+ (total body K^+ depleted due to attempts to correct acidosis, as acidosis improves, K^+ shifts back into cells and serum levels fall).
   B. Regular insulin infusion ~1–5 units/hr (titrate, continue until urine clear of ketones).
   C. Add dextrose to fluids when glucose <300 mg/dL.

D. Monitor and replace if necessary: magnesium, phosphate, sodium, potassium.
E. RARELY need to give HCO_3^-, acidosis improves as perfusion (hydration) improves.

Sample questions

Single best answer

1. A 60-year-old man with insulin-dependent diabetes and hypertension is undergoing repair of an inguinal hernia under general anesthesia with nitrous oxide and isoflurane 1.4%. He did not take his morning dose of propanalol and took only half of his morning insulin dose preoperatively. His preoperative glucose level was 150 mg/dL. During ligation of the hernia sack, he becomes diaphoretic, blood pressure is 160/100 mmHg, pulse is 105/min, and he is tearing. The most appropriate action at this time is
   1. Administer propanolol 1 mg intravenously
   2. Increase the isoflurane concentration
   3. Instruct the surgeon to reduce traction on the hernia sack
   4. Administer 25 mL dextrose 50% intravenous bolus and check serum glucose levels
   5. Administer 2 units regular insulin and check serum glucose level

2. A 14-year-old, 55-kg insulin-dependent diabetic is scheduled for emergency appendectomy. She has vomited several times today and her vital signs include temperature 38.5°C, pulse 110/min, blood pressure 125/70 mmHg, serum sodium 126 mEq/L, potassium 3.5 mEq/L, glucose 625 mg/dL, HCO_3^- 7.7 mEq/L. After administering antipyretics, antibiotics, and insulin, the most appropriate first therapeutic maneuver is to administer
   1. Intravenous 0.9% sodium chloride 2000 mL rapidly
   2. Intravenous 3% sodium chloride 1000 mL rapidly
   3. Intravenous sodium bicarbonate 16 mEq
   4. Intravenous sodium chloride 0.9% 3000 mL with 40 mEq potassium added
   5. Delay the procedure until her sodium is normalized

A = 1, 2, 3   B = 1, 3   C = 2, 4   D = 4 only   E = all are correct

3. True statements regarding the above patient include
   1. If blood transfusion is required, the level of dextrose in CPD preserved blood will significantly increase her glucose level
   2. Her serum sodium is actually much lower than indicated by the laboratory
   3. Her serum potassium will rise in response to fluid resuscitation with 0.9% sodium chloride
   4. As her fluid deficits are replaced, her pH will normalize

Answers: 1. 4   2. 4   3. D

CHAPTER 18

Thyroid Disease

Most common cause: Grave's disease

Signs and symptoms

1. Goiter: can cause external airway compression, leads to tracheal malacia.
2. Chronic hypermetabolic state
   A. Hyperdynamic circulation:
      —Tachycardia/tachydysrythmias
      —Increased cardiac output (with angina, high output failure)
      —Upregulation of β-receptors
   B. Heat intolerance
   C. Weight loss
   D. Adrenal cortical hyperplasia (increased cortisol requirement)
3. Skeletal muscle weakness: well known association with myasthenia gravis

Therapy

1. Propylthiouracil ⎫
2. Methimazole   ⎬ inhibit incorporation of iodine into tyrosine
3. β-blockers: prevents effects of excess sympathetic stimulation
4. Radioactive iodine
5. Subtotal thyroidectomy

Preoperatively

1. Render patient euthyroid!!!
   A. PTU/methimazole: takes 6–8 weeks
   B. propanolol: takes 7–14 days
   C. if surgery is emergent: IV propanolol boluses 0.5 mg, titrate to HR < 90
      OR: IV esmolol infusion, titrate to HR < 90
2. Avoid anticholinergics (may produce tachycardia).
3. Evaluate airway for compression and laryngeal nerve involvement.
4. Continue all antithyroid therapy.

Anesthetic management

1. Avoid sympathetic stimulants
   A. Induction/maintenance: avoid ketamine and pancuronium
   B. Reversal: gylycopyrolate is less chronotropic than atropine

2. Suppress responses to stimulation via β-blockers, narcotics, and agents.
3. Monitor for signs of thyroid storm.
4. Hypotension: treat with phenylephrine: action not dependent on catecholamine release.

> **PEARL:** MAC is not increased, but greater depth may be needed to ablate sympathetic responses.

Postoperative complications

1. Respiratory distress due to:
    A. Airway obstruction
       —Recurrent laryngeal nerve damage ⎫ immediately postop
       —Tracheomalacia ⎭
       —Hematoma with tracheal compression (early postop period)
    B. Hypocalcemia 2° to hypoparathyroidism (24–72 hr postop)
2. Hyperthyroidism recurrence
3. Hypothyroidism

Thyroid Storm

Due to sudden, excessive release of thyroid hormones; usually seen 6 to 18 hr postop, but can be intraop; looks like malignant hyperthermia.

1. **Signs/symptoms**
    A. ↑ temperature
    B. ↑ pulse
    C. High-output congestive heart failure
    D. Dehydration
    E. Shock
2. Management
    A. Cool the patient:
       —Cold IV fluids
       —Remove drapes
       —Cooling blankets
    B. β-blockers: continuous infusion of esmolol or bolus propanolol
    C. Cortisol: 100–200 mg IV
    D. PTU: 500 mg IV
    E. Sodium iodide: 1 g IV
    F. Pressors and inotropes as needed

Sample questions

A = 1, 2, 3   B = 1, 3   C = 2, 4   D = 4   E = all are correct

1. A patient develops respiratory distress in the PACU following a subtotal thyroidectomy. She has inspiratory stridor and suprasternal retractions. Her dressing has a scant amount of blood on it. Probable causes for her distress include
    1. Bilateral recurrent laryngeal nerve damage
    2. Hematoma
    3. Tracheomalacia
    4. Hypocalcemia

2. During subtotal thyroidectomy, a patient becomes hypotensive and does not respond to fluid administration. Appropriate measures at this time include
   1. Hydrocortisone 200 mg IV
   2. Placement of a PA catheter
   3. Phenylephrine 100 mcg IV
   4. Begin cooling efforts to treat thyroid storm

Answers: 1. A   2. B

CHAPTER 19

Pheochromocytoma

Defect: A catecholamine-secreting tumor, usually in the adrenal medulla or in the chromaffin tissue of the paravertebral sympathetic chains. Also called "the 10% tumor," because 10% are malignant, 10% are extraadrenal, and 10% are bilateral.

Patient population

1. 30–50 years old (but $1/3$ are in kids, males > females).
2. Can be part of MEN IIa, MEN IIb, or von Hippel-Landau syndrome.

Diagnosis

1. 24-hour urine collection and measurement of:
    A. Free norepinephrine—arguably the most sensitive
    B. Vanillylmandelic acid
    C. Normetanephrines
    D. Metanephrines
    E. Epinephrine
2. Clonidine suppression test: 0.3 mg PO of clonidine will decrease serum catecholamine levels in a patient with essential hypertension, but not in a patient with pheochromocytoma.

> **NOTE:** Normotension in the face of increased serum catecholamines indicates downregulation of adrenergic receptors.

3. CT scan to localize tumor.

Presentation

1. Paroxysmal hypertension and palpitations with associated diaphoresis, headache, and tremulousness
2. Weight loss
3. Hyperglycemia (alpha stimulation causes glycogenolysis and inhibits insulin release)
4. Decreased intravascular volume with resultant orthostatic hypotension and anemia
5. Cardiomyopathy and congestive heart failure (rare)

Preoperative preparation

1. Initiate alpha blockade (inhibits vasoconstriction, helps reestablish intravascular volume, prevents hypertension during tumor manipulation).
   Alpha-blocking agents:
   A. Phenoxybenzamine—drug of choice, given PO
      Prazosin (PO)
      Phentolamine (IV, rapid onset)
      Labetolol—runs risk of predominant β-blockade
2. Initiate β-blockade if tachycardia or dysrythymias persist.
3. Serial hematocrit measurements—indicative of normalization of intravascular volume.
4. ECHO if cardiomyopathy suspected.
5. Serial glucose measurements (α-blockade should correct hyperglycemia).

Anesthetic management

There are three distinct periods of high risk.

1. **Induction/laryngoscopy**
   A. Premedicate with benzodiazepines or scopalamine.
   B. Continue α- and β-blockade.
   C. Standard induction agents (avoid ketamine).
   D. Deepen with volatile agents (not halothane, because it sensitizes myocardium to catecholamines).
   E. Avoid relaxants that release histamine (curare) or are vagolytic (pancuronium).
   F. Administer lidocaine or fentanyl to blunt response to laryngoscopy.
   G. Nitroprusside infusion immediately available.
2. **Intraoperative tumor manipulation**
   A. Invasive blood pressure monitoring required
   B. Nitroprusside or nitroglycerin infusion immediately available
   C. Lidocaine for dysrythymias
3. **Ligation of venous drainage of tumor.** Severe hypotension possible. Treat with immediate infusion of crystalloid or colloid, decreased anesthetic depth, and have phenylephrine or norepinephrine infusion available.

Sample questions

A = 1, 2, 3   B = 1, 3   C = 2, 4   D = 4 only   E = all are correct

1. True statements regarding the initiation of β-blockade prior to α-blockade in a patient with pheochromocytoma include
   1. It is necessary to prevent reflex tachycardia caused by α-blockade.
   2. It helps control concomitant hyperglycemia.
   3. It may make α-blockade unnecessary.
   4. The risk of congestive heart failure is increased.

2. Treatment of persistent hypotension following removal of a pheochromocytoma includes
   1. Rapid infusion of crystalloid solution
   2. Reducing the concentration of volatile agent
   3. Phenylephrine infusion starting at 1.0 µg/kg/min
   4. Hydrocortisone 100 mg IV

19 ■ Pheochromocytoma

Single best answer

3. In the case of an unsuspected pheochromocytoma and the acute intraoperative onset of hypertension and arrythymias, the best choice of pharmacologic therapy would be
   1. Labetolol
   2. Propanolol
   3. Prazosin
   4. Phenoxybenzamine
   5. Phentolamine

Answers: 1. D   2. E   3. 5

CHAPTER 20

Myasthenia Gravis

Lesion: Autoimmune disorder with IgG antibodies against nicotinic cholinergic receptors

Clinical manifestations

1. Extraocular muscle weakness: diplopia, ptosis
2. Pharyngeal/laryngeal (bulbar) weakness: dysphagia, dysarthria, inability to manage secretions
3. Skeletal muscle weakness: worsens with activity
4. Increased risk of gastric aspiration

Common coexisting diseases

Most have an autoimmune etiology.

1. Thymoma
2. Hypo-/hyperthyroid
3. Lupus
4. Pernicious anemia
5. Idiopathic thrombocytopenia purpura
6. Sjögrens, scleroderma
7. Rheumatoid arthritis

Symptoms may be exacerbated by

1. Infection
2. Electrolyte disorders (hypocalcemia, hypokalemia)
3. Pregnancy
4. Surgery
5. *Drugs:* aminoglycosides, calcium channel blockers, quinidine, procainamide, lithium

Treatment

1. Anticholinesterases
   A. Increase the amount of acetylcholine available to bind the limited number of receptors.
   B. **BEWARE:** too much anticholinesterase also produces weakness ⇒ *cholinergic crisis*
   C. Diagnosis made by giving Edrophonium:
      —If it's myasthenic crisis, weakness improves

—If it's cholinergic crisis, weakness worsens *and* you get muscarinic side effects (salivation, miosis, bradycardia)
2. Steroids: interfere with production of IgG
3. Plasmapheresis (severe MG)
4. Thymectomy

How do they respond to neuromuscular relaxants?

- Table 20-1

	Nondepolarizers	Depolarizers
Untreated	Sensitive	Resistant
Treated	Resistant	Sensitive (anticholinesterases inhibit pseudo-cholinesterase, too)

Preoperative Preparation

1. Continue anticholinesterase therapy
2. PFTs (vital capacity, inspiratory force, maximal breathing capacity)
3. EKG: can have myocardial changes with MG
4. Check electrolytes/fluid status if on maintenance steroids

Predictors for need for postoperative mechanical ventilation

1. Disease present > 6 years
2. Coexistent COPD
3. Pyridostigmine dose > 750 mg/day
4. Vital capacity < 2.9 L

Anesthetic management

1. Avoid relaxants if possible, otherwise use minuscule doses
2. Twitch monitor mandatory
3. Avoid respiratory depressants
4. Expect prolonged action of succinylcholine and early phase II block
5. Delay extubation until return to baseline muscle strength

Sample questions

A = 1, 2, 3   B = 1, 3   C = 2, 4   D = 4 only   E = all are correct

1. A 50-year-old, 65-kg female myasthenia gravis patient presents to the emergency department with complaints of weakness, dyspnea, and inability to manage her saliva. Her medications include Pyridostigmine 500 mg/day and Prednisone 60 mg every other day. Physical exam reveals diffuse wheezing bilaterally, respirations 50/min, inspiratory force −20 cmH$_2$O, vital capacity 1500 cc, pulse 50/min, and small pupils. Correct statements regarding her management include
    1. Immediate endotracheal intubation and mechanical ventilation are indicated.
    2. Plasmapheresis is indicated.
    3. Intravenous atropine is indicated.
    4. Administration of 5 mg Edrophonium will improve her weakness.

2. True statement regarding myasthenia gravis and neuromuscular relaxants include
    1. Treatment with anticholinesterases can prolong the action of succinylcholine.

2. Untreated patients have increased sensitivity to nondepolarizing agents.
3. Untreated patients are resistant to succinylcholine.
4. Treated patients are resistant to nondepolarizing agents.

3. Which of the following drugs can exacerbate myasthenia gravis symptoms?
    1. Tetracycline
    2. Dilantin
    3. Chloroquin
    4. Levothyroxin

Answers: 1. B (this patient is in *cholinergic* crisis)   2. E   3. E

CHAPTER 21

Eaton–Lambert Syndrome

(Myasthenic Syndrome)

Lesion: Failure to release acetylcholine due to IgG antibodies against presynaptic calcium channels.

Patient population

Males > females

Coexisting diseases

Oat cell carcinoma of lung

Symptoms

1. Limb-girdle weakness, improves with activity
2. No cranial nerve involvement
3. Dry mouth
4. Paresthesia
5. Impotence

Treatment

1. 4-aminopyridine stimulates release of presynaptic acetylcholine.
2. Surgical removal of carcinoma.

- Table 21–1

	Myasthenic Syndrome	Myasthenia Gravis
Manifestations	Proximal limb weakness (legs > arms)	Extraocular, bulbar, facial weakness
	Exercise improves strength	Fatigue with exercise
	Myalgias common	Myalgias uncommon
	Reflexes absent/diminished	Reflexes normal
Gender	Male > female	Female > male
Coexisting disease	Oat cell lung carcinoma	Thymoma
Response to muscle relaxants	Sensitive to depolarizers and nondepolarizers	Sensitive to nondepolarizers
	Poor response to anticholinesterases	Resistant to succinylcholine
		Respond to anticholinesterases

From Stoelting RK, Dierdorf SF. Anesthesia and Co-Existing Disease, ed 3. New York: Churchill Livingstone, with permission.

Sample question

Single best answer

1. A 55-year-old male scheduled for bronchoscopy is evaluated in the preop clinic. He gives a history of leg pain and weakness that improves with walking. Deep tendon reflexes are diminished bilaterally in the lower extremities. True statements regarding his management include
   1. He will be resistant to succinylcholine.
   2. He should be placed on pyridostigmine preoperatively.
   3. He will demonstrate fade during electromyography with high frequency stimulation (50 Hz).
   4. He will require a smaller dose of vecuronium than usual.

Answer: 4

CHAPTER 22

Malignant Hyperthermia and Masseter Spasm

Malignant Hyperthermia

Pathophysiology

1. Causes a generalized hypermetabolic state.
2. Is due to an acute increase in intracellular Ca^{++}, activating metabolic pathways.
3. Leads to ATP depletion, acidosis, and cell death.
4. Support has been found for a genetic basis for MH.

Disorders thought to be associated with MH

1. Duchenne's muscular dystrophy
2. Myotonia congenita
3. Central core disease
4. King-Denborough syndrome
5. Heat stroke
6. SIDS
7. Osteogenesis imperfecta

Who should be tested for MH?

1. Patients with a history of MH-like event or masseter spasm
2. First-degree relatives of anyone with documented MH episode
3. Patients with a history of muscle cramps and a family history suggestive of MH
4. Patients with unexplained elevated creatine kinase

Triggering agents

1. All inhalational agents except nitrous oxide
2. Succinylcholine
3. Decamethonium

Presentation

May occur within minutes or several hours after administering triggering agent.

1. Hypermetabolic state
    A. Hypercarbia: increased $ETCO_2$ earliest and most sensitive sign
    B. Increased O_2 consumption: hypoxia, cyanosis, decreased venous PO_2 (first sign)
    C. Acidosis: mixed metabolic and respiratory
2. Tachypnea: won't see if neuromuscular blockade in use
3. Tachycardia, dysrythymias, cardiac arrest
4. Fever/sweating: a late sign, if present at all
5. Muscle rigidity: only seen if neuromuscular blockade not in use
6. Hypercalcemia, hyperkalemia, hyperphosphatemia
7. Rhabdomyolysis, myoglobinuria, and elevated serum creatine kinase
8. DIC: late

Differential diagnosis

1. *Thyroid storm*
2. *Pheochromocytoma*
3. *Neuroleptic malignant syndrome*
4. Familial fever
5. Sepsis
6. Hypercarbia/hypoxia
7. Drug reactions
8. Factitious

Management

If episode mild or trigger exposure brief, discontinuing trigger may be sufficient treatment. *If fulminant:*

1. Stop all inhaled agents, hyperventilate with 100% oxygen
2. Instruct surgeon to finish quickly or abort procedure
3. Call for help
4. Dantrolene 2–2.5 mg/kg IV, repeat as necessary to decrease $ETCO_2$ and pulse
5. Cooling measures: ice packs, cool fluids, and irrigation, cooling blanket, gastric lavage
6. Establish arterial line, monitor acid–base status, give HCO_3^- as needed (mixed venous gases are a more accurate assessment of CO_2 because blood has just exited hypermetabolic tissues)
7. Treat hyperkalemia with insulin, glucose, HCO_3^-
8. Calcium to correct hypotension, cardiac failure

Pharmacology of Dantrolene

1. Reconstituted with sterile water and mannitol (to make it isoosmotic).
2. *Inhibits the release of calcium by sarcoplasmic reticulum,* but doesn't inhibit reuptake.
3. *Reverses storage of calcium by mitochondria.*
4. *May block transmission of electrical impulse from dihydropyridine (DHP) receptor to the ryanodine receptor so that it depresses resting intracellular calcium levels as well as those triggered by MH.*
5. *Half-life ~ 10 hr* (normally, impulse goes from endplate → transverse tubule → sarcoplasmic reticulum. In MH, it goes from endplate → DHP receptor on the transverse tubule → ryanodine receptor → sarcoplasmic reticulum).
6. *Produces mild muscle weakness, but not paralysis.*

After the acute episode is over, monitor for

1. Return of symptoms of MH
2. Disseminated intravascular coagulation
3. Myoglobinuric renal failure or acute tubular necrosis

Management of myoglobinuria

1. Osmotic diuretics with or without furosemide to maintain high RBF and GFR (UOP > 100 cc/hr)
2. Alkalinize urine to pH > 5.6 with HCO_3^- or acetazolamide

Masseter Spasm

Presentation

1. Jaw rigidity with flaccid limbs after the administration of succinylcholine
2. Isolated masseter spasm is usually a normal variant, but can be a harbinger of MH if other muscle rigidity exists
3. All patients with moderate to severe trismus should be tested for MH

Characteristics

1. Extreme rise in serum C.
2. May occur even with peripheral train-of-four 0/4.
3. Tends to be transient.
4. Additional doses of succinylcholine may exacerbate it.
5. Dysrythymias may accompany it.

Management

If isolated finding and

1. Mouth is mildly resistant to opening: observation only for 12–24 hr.
2. Mouth is impossible to open: terminate procedure.
3. Mouth is distinctly tight, but able to force open: either terminate procedure or continue with nontriggering agents.

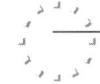

Sample questions

Single best answer

1. All of the following statements apply to both masseter spasm and malignant hyperthermia except
    1. It is triggered by succinylcholine
    2. It produces an increase in serum creatine kinase levels
    3. It is accompanied by generalized body rigidity
    4. Cardiac arrhythmias may accompany it
    5. May not occur every time the patient is exposed to a triggering agent

2. A 4-year-old child is undergoing inguinal hernia repair under general anesthesia. Forty-five seconds after the administration of succinylcholine to facilitate endotracheal intubation, attempted laryngoscopy reveals masseter spasm. The most appropriate measure at this time is to
    1. Give a second dose of succinylcholine

2. Perform blind nasal intubation and proceed
3. Proceed with surgery with general anesthesia via mask using nitrous, oxygen, and halothane
4. Cancel surgery, but advise parents a muscle biopsy is probably unnecessary
5. Cancel surgery, recommend muscle biopsy

A = 1, 2, 3   B = 1, 3   C = 2, 4   D = 4 only   E = all are correct

3. True statements regarding malignant hyperthermia include
   1. The earliest sign is an increased end-tidal CO_2
   2. The venous PO_2 falls before the arterial PO_2
   3. Disseminated intravascular coagulation is a common sequela
   4. Dantrolene is not indicated if the patient responds to external cooling (ice packs, cold IV fluids)

4. True statements regarding Dantrolene include
   1. It inhibits the release of calcium from the sarcoplasmic reticulum
   2. It blocks the reuptake of calcium by the sarcoplasmic reticulum
   3. It reverses mitochondrial storage of calcium
   4. It can produce skeletal muscle paralysis

Answers: 1. 3   2. 1   3. A   4. B

CHAPTER 23

Neuroleptic Malignant Syndrome

"Slow-onset malignant hyperthermia"

Defect: Derangement of dopaminergic receptors in the hypothalamus

Triggered by

1. Chronic administration of psychotropic drugs
    A. Phenothiazines (Thorazine)
    B. Butyrophenones (Haldol)
    C. Monoamine oxidase inhibitors
    D. Lithium
2. Acute withdrawal of Parkinson's medications (L-Dopa)

Signs/symptoms

1. Movement disorder: muscle rigidity/akinesis/extrapyramidal disturbance. (Muscle rigidity is a central effect, not peripheral like in malignant hyperthermia.)
2. Mental status changes: stupor/delirium/coma.
3. Loss of homeostatic function: hyperpyrexia/tachycardia/hyper- or hypotension.

Management

1. Discontinue neuroleptic medications
2. Dantrolene 3–10 mg/kg IV
3. Give dopamine receptor agonists: Bromocriptine, Amantadine
4. Supportive measures:
    A. Control temperature
    B. Correct acidosis
    C. IV hydration

● Table 23-1

	Neuroleptic Malignant Syndrome	Malignant Hyperthermia
Clinical signs	*Slow onset*	**Fast onset**
	Muscle rigidity *(central effect)*	Muscle rigidity *(peripheral effect)*
	Hyperpyrexia	Hyperpyrexia
	Acidosis	Acidosis
	Tachycardia	Tachycardia
	Hyper- or hypotension	Hyper- or hypotension
	Rhabomyolysis	Rhabdomyolysis
Diagnostic tests	Positive halothane/caffeine contracture test (can be normal, too)	Positive halothane/caffeine contracture test (can be normal, too)
Triggered by	Neuroleptic medications	Succinylcholine
	Abrupt discontinuation of L-Dopa	Decamethonium
		All inhaled agents except N_2O
Pharmacologic treatment	Dantrolene	Dantrolene
	Bromocriptine	
	Amantadine	

Muscular Dystrophy

Types

1. Pseudohypertrophic (Duchenne's)—**most common**
2. Myotonic dystrophy: has three subtypes, but for the purpose of boards, they're all the same

Duchenne's

Lesion

X-linked, recessive defect causes increased permeability of muscle membrane and fatty infiltration of muscle

Population

Males, clinically presents > 2 years of age

Manifestations

1. Kyphoscoliosis
2. Cardiopulmonary dysfunction
3. ↑ creatine kinase

Cardiac effects

1. Patients rarely have cardiac symptoms
2. Degeneration of myocardium (may be very sensitive to inhalational agents)
3. Mitral regurgitation (due to papillary muscle involvement)
4. Characteristic ECG changes (deep Q's in limb leads, short P-R interval, sinus tach, tall R in V1)

Pulmonary effects

1. Restrictive lung disease 2° to kyphoscoliosis
2. Recurrent pneumonia and decreased lung reserve 2° to weak respiratory muscles
3. Increased risk of sleep apnea

> **BEWARE:** Degree of pulmonary involvement not always obvious due to limited physical activity.

Anesthetic management

1. Regional is technique of choice.
2. Monitor for malignant hyperthermia (at very high risk for).
3. Monitor for rhabdomyolysis (at risk even without MH).
4. Avoid succinylcholine (profound hyperkalemia due to ↑ muscle membrane permeability).
5. Normal response to nondepolarizers, but should ↓ dose due to weakness.
6. Anticipate postoperative pulmonary dysfunction.

Myotonic Dystrophy

Lesion

Sustained muscle contracture after stimulation due to failure of calcium to return to sarcoplasmic reticulum.

Manifestations

1. Facial weakness
2. Dysarthria (increased risk of gastric aspiration)
3. Respiratory muscle weakness
4. Cardiomyopathy, dysrythymias, and conduction defects (common cause of death)
5. Central sleep apnea
6. Endocrine involvement (hypothyroidism, diabetes, adrenal insufficiency)

Anesthetic management

1. Suspect cardiomyopathy
2. Anticipate cardiac dysrythymias
3. Avoid succinylcholine: causes prolonged muscle contracture, making ventilation nearly impossible
4. Normal response to nondepolarizers
5. Presume at risk for malignant hyperthermia
6. Expect increased sensitivity to respiratory depressants (2° to sleep apnea)

Sample Questions

A = 1, 2, 3   B = 1, 3   C = 2, 4   D = 4 only   E = all are correct

1. An 8-year-old, 20-kg boy with Duchenne's muscular dystrophy is scheduled for a heel cord lengthening of his left lower extremity. He has no previous surgical history and has been NPO for 8 hours. Acceptable options for his anesthetic management include
   1. Mask induction with nitrous oxide, oxygen, and halothane
   2. IV induction with sodium thiopental and maintenance with nitrous oxide, oxygen, and isoflurane
   3. IV induction with propofol and succinylcholine

4. IV induction with propofol and maintenance with propofol, nitrous oxide, and oxygen

2. A 6-year-old, 15-kg male with Duchenne's muscular dystrophy is scheduled for bilateral contracture release of the upper extremity. Findings you would expect on preoperative evaluation include
   1. Sinus tachycardia and Q waves in leads I, II, and III on EKG
   2. Tachypnea and shortness of breath with patient at rest
   3. A systolic murmur, loudest at the apex
   4. A flattened expiratory portion of the flow-volume curve with a normal inspiratory portion

3. Statements that are true regarding both Duchenne's muscular dystrophy and myotonic dystrophy include
   1. Cardiac complications are a frequent cause of death
   2. There is a suspected link with malignant hyperthermia
   3. Succinylcholine causes profound hyperkalemia
   4. There is an increased risk of gastric aspiration

4. All of the following statements regarding myotonic dystrophy are true, *except:*
   1. The muscle contractures can be relieved with regional anesthesia
   2. The muscle contractures are relieved by local anesthetics
   3. The muscle contractures are relieved by general anesthesia
   4. Cardiac complications are the most frequent cause of death

Answers: 1. D   2. B   3. C   4. A

CHAPTER 25

Parkinson's Disease

Lesion: Loss of dopaminergic fibers in the extrapyramidal system resulting in unopposed acetylcholine activity.

Signs/symptoms

1. Cogwheel rigidity
2. Shuffling gait
3. Esophageal dysfunction (↑ risk of aspiration)
4. Mask facies
5. Resting tremor

Treatment

1. **Levodopa** (↑ dopamine levels)
2. **Anticholinergics** (↓ acetylcholine levels)
3. Antihistamines (↓ extrapyramidal effects)
4. MAO inhibitors

Fun facts to know about L-Dopa

1. Is immediate precursor of dopamine and can cross blood–brain barrier (dopamine can't)
2. Converted to dopamine by dopa-decarboxylase in periphery *and* centrally
3. Peripheral conversion →↑ systemic dopamine levels →↓ systemic norepinephrine stores → orthostatic hypotension
4. Carbidopa is added to inhibit *peripheral* enzyme activity

Side effects of L-Dopa

1. Cardiac stimulation: tachycardia, increased contractility and irritability
2. Depleted norepinephrine stores
3. Increased renal blood flow, GFR, renin → intravascular depletion and orthostatic hypotension
4. Nausea/vomiting
5. Central effects: agitation, psychosis, dyskinesia

Anesthetic Management

1. Continue medications (withdrawal of L-Dopa can ↑ rigidity and make ventilation difficult).

2. Avoid dopamine antagonists (butyrophenones and phenothiazines).
3. Anticipate orthostatic hypotension (ephedrine may not be effective due to depleted norepinephrine).
4. Anticipate dysrythymias (avoid Halothane?).
5. Anticipate intravascular volume depletion.

Drugs you shouldn't give to Parkinson's patients

All antagonize dopamine are common antiemetics

1. Droperidol (Inapsine)—a butyrophenone
2. Promethazine (Phenergan) ⎫
3. Prochlorperazine (Compazine) ⎬ phenothiazines
4. Chlorpromazine (Thorazine) ⎭
5. Metoclopramide (Reglan)—a benzamide

Sample question

A = 1, 2, 3   B = 1, 3   C = 2, 4   D = 4 only   E = all are correct

1. When treating nausea in patients with Parkinson's disease, drugs you should avoid include
   1. Metoclopramide
   2. Droperidol
   3. Prochlorperazine
   4. Hydroxyzine

Answer: A

Glaucoma

Defect: Obstructed efflux of aqueous humor from anterior chamber, causing increased intraocular pressure

There are two types

1. Open angle **(most common):** idiopathic obstruction of flow through trabecular meshwork, treated medically
2. Closed angle: iris blocks flow through trabecular meshwork, treated surgically with iridectomy

Goal of medical therapy is to lower intraocular pressure by

1. ↓ resistance to efflux of aqueous humor
2. ↓ production of aqueous humor
3. ↓ volume of aqueous humor via osmotically active agents

Drugs that promote efflux

By producing miosis that increases the size of the outflow tract

1. Acetylcholinesterase inhibitors (ecothiophate). Systemic effects: salivation, bronchospasm, hypotension, bradycardia, respiratory arrest, seizures, inhibit pseudocholinesterase.
2. Parasympathomimetics (pilocarpine, carbachol).
3. Epinephrine. Systemic effects: tachyarrythymias, angina, anxiety.

Drugs that reduce production of aqueous humor

1. Carbonic anhydrase inhibitors (acetazolamide). Systemic effects: metabolic acidosis, hypokalemia, increased respiratory rate, decreased production of cerebrospinal fluid, and lowered intracranial pressure.
2. β-blockers (**timolol,** propanolol). Systemic effects: bradycardia (refractory to atropine), hypotension, bronchospasm, lethargy.

Osmotic Agents

Mannitol, urea, glycerin, isosorbide. Systemic effects: dehydration, hyperglycemia.

Sample questions

A = 1, 2, 3   B = 1, 3   C = 2, 4   D = 4 only   E = all are correct

1. A 65-year-old man is undergoing a trabeculectomy with a retrobulbar block. His medications include timoptic drops and ecothiophate. During the surgical procedure, his pulse acutely drops from 70/min to 40/min. Likely causes for this include
   1. Excessive β-blockade
   2. Acute cholinergic crisis
   3. Local anesthetic toxicity
   4. Excessive stimulation of the trigeminal nerve

Single best answer

2. Same patient, different scenario: His resting pulse is 50/min at the beginning of the case. During surgical manipulation, it falls to 45/min, and the blood pressure is unchanged at 105/75 mmHg. The pulse does not increase with discontinuation of manipulation and does not respond to atropine. The most likely cause of this is
   1. Excessive β-blockade
   2. Acute cholinergic crisis
   3. Local anesthetic toxicity
   4. Excessive stimulation of the trigeminal nerve

Answers: 1. D   2. 1

Chapter 27

Transurethral Resection of the Prostate

Procedure: Utilizes a resectoscope, visualization aided by distention of the bladder and continuous irrigation to remove blood and tissue from visual field.

Irrigation fluid

Usually Cytal (mannitol and sorbitol) or Glycine

1. Must be a nonelectrolyte solution: prevents dispersion of electric current
2. Must be isoosmotic: prevents hemolysis following absorption of hypotonic fluid

Complications

1. **Intravascular absorption of irrigating fluid: most common.** Effects:
   A. Volume overload (leads to HTN, bradycardia, congestive heart failure, pulmonary edema)
   B. Serum hypo-osmolality (leads to hemolysis, pulmonary edema, and cerebral edema)
   C. Dilutional hyponatremia:
      –At ~120 meq/L, restlessness and confusion occur
      –At ~115 meq/L, widening of QRS and ST segment elevation are seen
      –At ~110 meq/L, dysrythymias, hypotension, seizures, coma, or death
   D. Elevated glycine and ammonia levels (both are thought to produce CNS symptoms, glycine in particular is an inhibitory neurotransmitter and causes visual disturbances)
   E. Hemolysis: due to hypo-osmotic irrigating solution

   NOTE: All of the above are lumped together as "TURP syndrome."

   F. Hypothermia: due to large volume of cold irrigation used
2. **Bacteremia:** can cause sudden cardiovascular collapse
3. **Bladder perforation:**
   A. Extraperitoneal (most common): c/o suprapubic/periumbilical/inguinal pain
   B. Intraperitoneal: c/o upper abdominal or shoulder pain
   C. Can have significant hemodynamic compromise

4. **Excessive bleeding:** Degree of blood loss difficult to evaluate due to irrigating fluid
   A. Coagulopathy is possible and has been attributed to:
   B. Prostatic release of plasminogen activator and activation of fibrinolytic system
   C. Disseminated intravascular coagulation

Factors affecting amount of fluid absorption

1. Hydrostatic pressure (how high is the irrigation bag?)
2. Length of procedure
3. Degree of exposed venous sinuses
4. Degree of bladder distention

Treatment of TURP syndrome

1. Loop diuretics
2. Hypertonic saline *rarely* indicated (can cause central pontine myelinolysis)

Sample questions

A = 1, 2, 3   B = 1, 3   C = 2, 4   D = 4 only   E = all are correct

1. One hour after transurethral resection of the prostate under spinal anesthesia with 100 mg lidocaine, a 60-year-old male is in the PACU on a 2-L nasal cannula. You are called to the bedside because the patient is disoriented and somewhat combative. Vital signs include blood pressure of 148/85, pulse oximeter of 94%. Possible etiologies of this scenario include:
   1. Cerebral edema
   2. Hypernatremia
   3. Pulmonary edema
   4. High spinal level

2. Effects of glycine absorption during transurethral resection of the prostate include
   1. Cardiac dysrythymias
   2. Transient blindness
   3. Hypertension
   4. Confusion

Single best answer

3. A 65-year-old male is undergoing transurethral resection of the prostate under spinal anesthesia with 12 mg hyperbaric tetracaine. After 30 minutes of resecting, he complains of periumbilical pain. The most likely reason for this is
   1. The spinal is wearing off
   2. Bladder perforation
   3. Bladder distention
   4. Nausea related to hyponatremia
   5. Mesenteric hypoperfusion

Answers: 1. B   2. C   3. 2

Chapter 28

Extracorporeal Shock Wave Lithotripsy

Technique: Immersion in water bath and ultrasonic destruction of nephrolithiasis.

Advantages

1. Low morbidity
2. Outpatient or short-stay procedure

Disadvantages

1. Painful
2. Stone must remain immobile (moves with diaphragmatic excursion)

Contraindications

1. Coagulopathy
2. Pregnancy

Anesthetic techniques

1. Spinal/epidural (hypotension usually offset by hydrostatic forces which help increase venous return)
2. General (must decide between spontaneous and controlled ventilation)
3. Intercostal block with sedation

Respiratory maneuvers to minimize movement of the stone

1. Jet ventilation (very little diaphragmatic movement, but risks outweigh benefits)
2. Controlled ventilation (use low respiratory rate, diaphragm is still during expiration)

Complications

1. Congestive heart failure (hydrostatic forces on abdomen/chest increase venous return to heart)
2. Arrhythmias (shock waves are triggered by R-wave, delivered during absolute refractory period to decrease risk of arrhythmia)
3. Hypoxia (impaired ventilatory mechanics from hydrostatic forces or due to pulmonary contusion)
4. Hypothermia (keep water warm)

28 ■ Extracorporeal Shock Wave Lithotripsy

5. Hypotension (risk of profound vasodilation upon emergence from water bath)
6. Electrocution (if grounded equipment fails)

Sample questions

Single best answer

1. During extracorporeal shock wave lithotripsy for nephrolithiasis under epidural anesthesia with 0.5% bupivicaine, a 33-year-old male develops frequent, sustained premature ventricular beats on EKG. Blood pressure is 135/72 mmHg, and SaO_2 is 98% on a 2-L/min nasal cannula. The most appropriate immediate therapy is
   1. Synchronized defibrillation starting at 200 joules
   2. Lidocaine bolus 1 mg/kg IV
   3. Discontinue epidural anesthesia, convert to general anesthesia, and send blood specimen to determine serum bupivicaine level
   4. Discontinue lithotripsy
   5. Administer a precordial thump

   A = 1, 2, 3   B = 1, 3   C = 2, 4   D = 4 only   E = all are correct

2. Alterations in respiratory parameters seen during extracorporeal shock wave lithotripsy include
   1. Decreased vital capacity
   2. Decreased functional residual capacity
   3. Decreased tidal volume
   4. Increased pulmonary blood flow

Answers: 1. 4   2. E

Chapter 29

Anesthetic Implications of Liver Disease

• **Table 29–1**

Liver Function	Product/Result	Effect If Function Is Impaired
Glucose homeostasis	Glycogen storage	Hypoglycemia
	Glycogenolysis	OR: hyperglycemia
Fat metabolism		Fatty liver infiltration
Protein synthesis	Albumin	Decreased drug binding, with increased sensitivity to drugs
	Coagulation factors	Decreased levels of factors II, VII, IX, X (vitamin K dependent)
		Decreased levels of factors V, XI, XII, XIII (not vitamin K dependent)
		Decreased prothrombin production
		Decreased fibrinogen production
	Plasma cholinesterase	Impaired hydrolysis of drugs containing ester-linkages (succinylcholine, atracurium, mivacurium, ester local anesthetics)
Drug metabolism		Decreased metabolism due to reduced hepatic blood flow or reduced enzyme activity OR:
		Increased metabolism due to enzyme induction

Interpretation of liver function tests

1. Bilirubin (conjugated in liver)

    ↑ unconjugated fraction = prehepatic problem (hemolysis, hematoma resorption, blood transfusion)
    ↑ conjugated fraction = hepatic or posthepatic problem

2. Transaminases (AST, ALT)
    A. Prehepatic problem = normal
    B. Hepatic problem = marked ↑
    C. Posthepatic problem = normal to slight ↑
3. Alkaline phosphatase present in bile duct cells
    A. Hepatic problem = normal to slight ↑
    B. Posthepatic problem = marked ↑
4. Albumin: level < 2.5 g·dL −1 indicates severe parenchymal liver disease. Plasma $t_{1/2}$ = 14–21 days, so levels are normal in early acute liver failure.

Additional tests

In addition to perturbations in any of the functions listed above, preoperative evaluation of the patient with liver disease should include a search for:

1. Portal hypertension and coexisting esophageal varices, ascites, or splenomegaly
2. Cardiac/circulatory changes and coexisting cardiomyopathy, increased cardiac output, increased intravascular volume, and anemia
3. Arterial hypoxemia due to massive ascites, intrapulmonary shunting, pneumonia, or concurrent COPD
4. Renal insufficiency (hepatorenal syndrome)
5. Encephalopathy with dysarthria, asterixis, and hyperreflexia

Preoperative tests

1. Electrolytes, BUN, creatinine, glucose
2. Bilirubin, AST, ALT, alkaline phosphatase, albumin
3. Coagulation: H/H, PT/PTT, fibrinogen, platelets (they can sequester if splenomegaly present)
4. Arterial blood gases
5. Chest x-ray
6. ECG and optional echocardiogram (if cardiomyopathy suspected)

Liver blood supply

% of total flow	Vessel	% total oxygen supplied
25%	Hepatic artery	45–50%
75%	Portal vein	50–55%

Factors regulating liver blood flow

1. Hepatic artery flow will increase to maintain oxygen delivery to the liver if:
   A. There is a decrease in portal venous blood flow, oxygen tension, or pH.
   B. There is systemic arterial hypoxemia, hypercarbia, or alkalosis.
2. Sympathetic stimulation decreases liver blood flow (diverting flow to muscles and heart for fight/flight).
3. Autoregulation: flow is maintained despite blood pressure fluctuation (plays a negligible role).

Intraoperative determinants of hepatic blood flow

1. Type of inhalational agent: halothane causes the largest drop (isoflurane actually increases hepatic artery flow)
2. Surgical stimulation
   A. Upper abdominal procedures mechanically impair blood flow > lower abdomen.
   B. Abdominal procedures cause local release of vasoconstricting substances.
3. Anything that decreases cardiac output will decrease hepatic blood flow.
4. Positive pressure ventilation/PEEP.
5. Regional anesthesia with sympathectomy (decreased perfusion pressure).

Pharmacologic implications of hepatic disease

1. Induction agents: dose is usually unchanged, because the increased volume of distribution offsets the decreased metabolism. In fact, sober cirrhotics tend to require larger than normal doses.
2. Muscle relaxants: increased volume of distribution necessitates higher initial doses; repeat doses are dictated by elimination pathways:

A. d-Tubocurare and pancuronium have prolonged elimination.
B. Vecuronium and atracurium elimination is unaltered.
C. Succinylcholine effect is prolonged in theory, not clinically significant.
3. Opioids: meperidine clearance greatly reduced. Morphine and fentanyl clearance unchanged.
4. Benzodiazepines: all have greatly reduced clearances.

Anesthetic implications of the acutely intoxicated alcoholic

1. MAC is decreased (alcohol is a CNS depressant).
2. Brain is less tolerant of hypoxia.
3. Increased risk of regurgitation/aspiration (ETOH delays gastric emptying and decreases lower esophageal sphincter tone).
4. Increased risk of coagulopathy (ETOH impairs platelet aggregation).
5. Serum catecholamines are increased (? Increased risk of dysrythymias).

Differential diagnosis of postoperative jaundice

Try to categorize source as prehepatic, intrahepatic, or posthepatic.

1. Prehepatic:
   A. ↑ bilirubin load (hemolysis of transfused or native blood, hematoma resorption)
   B. Impaired bilirubin metabolism (Gilbert's syndrome, Crigler-Najar disease)
2. Hepatic:
   A. Preexisting liver disease
   B. Intraoperative hypoxemia, hypotension
   C. Intrahepatic cholestasis
   D. Drug-induced dysfunction (halothane, methoxyflurane . . . **a diagnosis of exclusion!!**)
3. Posthepatic:
   A. Common duct injury or stone
   B. Pancreatitis with common duct obstruction

Sample questions

A = 1, 2, 3   B = 1, 3   C = 2, 4   D = 4 only   E = all are correct

1. True statements regarding muscle relaxants in patients with cirrhosis include
   1. Pancuronium will have a prolonged effect
   2. Vecuronium clearance is unaffected if the dose is kept below 0.1 mg/kg
   3. Atracurium clearance is unaffected if the dose is kept below 0.6 mg/kg
   4. Succinylcholine metabolism is markedly impaired

2. Intraoperative factors that may affect hepatic blood flow include
   1. The surgical site
   2. Congestive heart failure
   3. Controlled mechanical ventilation
   4. Systemic hypotension

3. True statements regarding hepatic perfusion are
   1. The liver receives most of its oxygen supply from the hepatic artery

2. Autoregulation is the principal mechanism for maintaining hepatic perfusion
3. The liver receives most of its blood supply from the hepatic artery
4. A decrease in portal venous blood flow will be met by a compensatory increase in hepatic artery flow

4. Hepatic artery flow will increase in response to
   1. Systemic alkalosis
   2. Isoflurane
   3. Portal venous acidosis
   4. Systemic hypoxemia

Single best answer

5. The inhalational agent that best preserves hepatic blood flow is
   1. Enflurane
   2. Desflurane
   3. Isoflurane
   4. Halothane
   5. Nitrous oxide

Answers: 1. A   2. E   3. D   4. E   5. 3

CHAPTER 30

Hepatitis B Infection

Incubation: 6 weeks to 6 months

Mode of transmission

Parenteral, oral-oral, or sexual

Tests

1. HBsAg: presence indicates contagious state. Detectable within 2 weeks after parenteral infection. If present > 6 months, patient is chronic carrier and is infectious.
2. Anti HBs: antibody to surface antigen. Appears 2–4 months after infection, after HBsAg no longer detectable. Confirms immune status.
3. HBcAg: indicates presence of HBV in blood. Patient highly contagious.
4. AntiHBc: antibody to core antigen. Is a marker of prior infection. Confirms immune status.

Prophylaxis

1. Vaccine is useless in HBV carriers.
2. Unnecessary if blood has anti-HBc or anti-HBs.
3. Provides lifelong immunity, except to immunocompromised patients (they need boosters).

Treatment after exposure to patient known to be HbsAg positive

1. Pooled gamma-globulin injection immediately (contains low titers of anti-HBs)
2. Vaccinate immediately

Sample questions: None . . . it's pretty straightforward.

CHAPTER 31

Liver Transplant

Procedure has four stages

Stage 0: Preincision:
      A. Establish vascular access
      B. Insert cannulae for venovenous bypass
      C. Begin correcting coagulopathy (DDAVP, epsilon-aminocaproic acid, FFP)

Stage 1: After incision, before removal of diseased liver

Stage 2: Anhepatic phase, venovenous bypass utilized to maintain renal perfusion, cardiac preload

Stage 3: Neohepatic (reperfusion phase), accompanied by following derangements:
      A. Metabolic acidosis
      B. Hyperkalemia
      C. Hypocalcemia
      D. Hypovolemia/anemia
      E. Hypothermia
      F. Hypotension/bradycardia

Special considerations beyond the normal patient with liver disease

1. May have increased intracranial pressure 2° to encephalopathy (worsens with inferior vena cava cross-clamping and reperfusion).
2. Renal dose dopamine may afford some renal protection.
3. Aggressive warming is essential.
4. Arms must be positioned in particular way . . . beware of peripheral nerve injury.

Venovenous bypass

Portal vein to femoral vein (flow in the two limbs doesn't have to be equal)

1. Purposes:
      A. Maintains preload to right ventricle
      B. Maintains renal perfusion during anhepatic phase
      C. Prevents splanchnic and abdominal venous congestion
2. Pitfalls:
      A. May not maintain cardiac output
      B. Air or thrombi can gather in the tubing

Sample questions: None . . . this has a pretty limited focus on the exam.

CHAPTER 32

Cocaine Intoxication

Class: Ester local anesthetic

Mechanism of action

1. Release of norepinephrine, epinephrine, and dopamine
2. *Inhibits reuptake of **norepinephrine**, epinephrine, and dopamine*
3. Chronic use depletes catecholamines

Systemic effects of overdose

CNS	Cerebral edema, stroke, seizures
CVS	Systemic hypertension 2° to intense coronary and systemic vasoconstriction; tachycardia; high risk of myocardial ischemia, dysrythmias
Pulmonary	Pulmonary edema
Hematologic	Platelet dysfunction
Pregnancy	Risk of abruption, spontaneous abortion

Anesthetic management

1. Esmolol: titrate to pulse < 100/min
2. Expect increased amounts of volatile agents to attenuate sympathetic responses due to high levels of circulating catecholamines
3. Use direct-acting sympathomimetics or sympatholytics since stores of catechols are unreliable

Sample questions

A = 1, 2, 3   B = 1, 3   C = 2, 4   D = 4 only   E = all are correct

1. A 24-year-old, 65-kg male with a gunshot wound to the abdomen is undergoing emergent exploratory laparotomy. A serum drug screen is positive for cocaine, and his vital signs include blood pressure 108/86 mmHg, pulse 122/min. Appropriate choices for induction agents include
   1. Thiopental 200 mg IV
   2. Etomidate 10 mg IV
   3. Propofol 130 mg IV
   4. Ketamine 130 mg IV

2. Same patient. A lumbar epidural is placed after induction for a combined regional/general anesthetic. General anesthesia is maintained with halo-

thane 1.1% end-tidal and oxygen. The epidural is injected with 15 mL of 0.5% bupivicaine with 1:200,000 epinephrine. ST segment depression and premature ventricular contractions are then noted on the EKG. In combination with the cocaine, possible causes of these EKG changes include
1. Halothane
2. Bupivicaine
3. Epinephrine
4. Hypotension

Answers: 1. A 2. E

CHAPTER 33

Renal Disease

• Table 33-1

	Tests of Renal Function				
Tests of Glomerular Filtration Rate			Tests of Renal Tubular Function		
Test	Normal value	Factors altering results	Test	Normal value	Factors altering results
BUN	10–20 mg·dL^{-1}	Increased with: high protein diet, GI bleeding, ↑ catabolism, dehydration	Urine concentrating ability (specific gravity)	1.003–1.030	Concentration low with: hypokalemia, hypercalcemia, high serum fluoride, diuretics
Creatinine	0.7–1.5 mg·dL^{-1}	Decreased with decreased muscle mass	Urine sodium	<40 mEq·L	
Creatinine clearance	110–150 mL·min	**Most reliable test of GFR**	Urine osmolarity	40–1400 mOsm·L	
Proteinuria	Minimal	Increased with: exercise fever CHF			

Anesthetic effects on renal function

1. All volatile anesthetics reduce GFR in parallel to reductions in blood pressure. Beware that fluoride from volatile agent metabolism is nephrotoxic, but toxicity is rare, because the fluoride is rapidly taken up by bone (methoxyflurane >> enflurane = sevoflurane > isoflurane = halothane = desflurane).
2. No intravenous anesthetic causes significant changes in GFR.

Differential diagnosis of perioperative oliguria

Most easily divided into prerenal and renal causes

● Table 33–2

Parameter	Prerenal	Renal
Urine Na+ (mEq·L)	<20	>40
Urine osmolarity (mOsm·L)	>400	<400
BUN/creatinine ratio	>10	≤10
Etiology	Hypovolemia	Ischemia
	Hypotension	Toxins
	Low cardiac output	Hemoglobin/myoglobin

Manifestations of chronic renal disease

1. Anemia: due to decreased erythropoietin production, reduces solubility of volatile agents and speeds rate of rise F_A/F_i
2. Coagulopathy: uremia-induced platelet dysfunction despite normal platelet count, PT/PTT
3. pH/electrolyte disturbances:
   A. Metabolic acidosis: often accompanied by hyperkalemia, treat with dialysis
   B. Hyperkalemia: treat with:
      –Insulin (drives K+ back into cells)
      –Glucose (prevents hypoglycemia from insulin)
      –Calcium (restores normal cardiac conduction)
      –NaHCO$_3$ (drives K+ back into cells)
      –Hyperventilation
4. Intravascular volume derangements: depletion/overload common, depending when last dialyzed

Pharmacologic considerations in renal disease

1. Barbiturates: ↑ available drug due to decreased protein binding in renal patients, so ↓ induction dose.
2. Narcotics: *all* narcotics have unchanged clearance in renal disease, but the *metabolites* of morphine and meperidine have decreased clearance and thus, prolonged effects.
3. Muscle relaxants:
   A. Succinylcholine: risk of hyperkalemia (but *amount* of K+ released is same as in nonrenal patients)
   B. Duration unchanged: mivacurium, pipecuronium, atracurium
   C. Duration prolonged: doxacurium, pancuronium, laudanosine (active metabolite of atracurium)
   D. Caveat: initial dose of vecuronium has normal duration but accumulates with additional doses
4. Reversal agents: duration doubled for neostigmine, pyridostigmine, edrophonium, so *recurarization* due to decreased clearance of neuromuscular blockers is unlikely
5. Nitroprusside: decreased thiosulfate excretion lowers risk of cyanide toxicity (must have thiosulfate to convert cyanide to thiocyanate)

Sample questions

A = 1, 2, 3   B = 1, 3   C = 2, 4   D = 4 only   E = all are correct

1. True statements regarding fluoride nephrotoxicity include
   1. Uptake by bone will prevent nephrotoxic serum levels of fluoride, even in patients with renal impairment
   2. Urine osmolality will be > 400 mOsm

3. It is resistant to vasopressin
4. It presents with oliguria

Single best answer

2. A 65-kg patient with impaired renal function undergoes placement of a ureteral stent under general anesthesia with thiopental 325 mg, atracurium 30 mg, and isoflurane. He has one out four twitches by nerve stimulator, and is reversed with neostigmine 5 mg and glycopyrolate 0.6 mg and is extubated. One hour later, his spontaneous tidal volume is 200 mL, pulse oximetry is 90% on F_iO_2 0.21, and he cannot sustain a 5-sec head lift. The most likely cause of this is
   1. Reoccurrence of neuromuscular blockade by atracurium
   2. Sedation due to residual thiopental
   3. Inadequate dose of neostigmine
   4. Acute cholinergic crisis due to neostigmine
   5. Neuromuscular blockade by residual atracurium metabolites

3. A 55-kg patient with renal impairment undergoes laparoscopic cholecystectomy under general anesthesia. Ten cmH$_2$O are applied to maintain oxygenation after insufflation of the abdomen. Two hours later, the urine output drops to 25 cc/hr, pulse 90/min, blood pressure 105/65 mmHg, CVP 9 mmHg, SaO$_2$ 96% on F_iO_2 0.55. The best treatment at this time would be
   1. Decrease the PEEP to 5 cmH$_2$0
   2. Discontinue PEEP and increase F_iO_2 to 0.8
   3. Dopamine infusion to increase renal blood flow
   4. Fluid bolus with 0.9% saline
   5. Furosemide 5 mg IV

Answers: 1. A   2. 5   3. 4

CHAPTER 34

Human Immunodeficiency Virus

Body fluids known to contain virus

Blood (principal mode of transmission)
Saliva
Tears
Semen
Cervical secretions
Urine
Cerebrospinal fluid
Breast milk

Methods of inactivation

1. 1:10 solution of sodium hypochlorite (household bleach)
2. Heat at 56° C for 10 minutes
3. Soak in ethylene oxide
4. Steam
5. Boil in water
6. Death by life outside host (can live 3–7 days outside host following big viral spill)

What you ought to know ANYWAY about risk of infection

1. After needle stick exposure to HIV-infected blood, risk is 1%.
2. Antibody testing of exposed person should be done immediately and repeated at 6, 12, and 24 weeks.
3. Prophylactic AZT has not been proven efficacious in preventing AIDS.
4. After needle stick exposure to Hepatitis-B infected blood, risk is 10%.

Sample questions: None . . . you don't need me to quiz you on this . . . it's for your own protection that you should know it.

CHAPTER 35

Laparoscopy

Technique: Endoscopic surgery aided by creation of pneumoperitoneum via insufflation of CO_2

Complications

Can be categorized into three main groups:

1. Ventilatory disturbances
2. Cardiovascular disturbances
3. Visceral injury

Ventilatory disturbances

1. ↑ **$PaCO_2$.** Degree of rise depends on:
   A. Anesthetic technique: general, spontaneously breathing > general, controlled ventilation > local
   B. Duration of pneumoperitoneum—CO_2 plateau reached in 20 minutes
   C. Intraabdominal pressure: high pressures limit peritoneal perfusion, thereby limiting CO_2 uptake
   D. Presence of cardiopulmonary disease

Mechanism of the rise in CO_2

Absorption of CO_2 from peritoneal cavity, which is dependent on:
   a. Diffusibility
   b. Peritoneal wall perfusion: limited by high intraabdominal pressure
Impaired ventilation (increased deadspace) due to:
   a. Patient position
   b. Abdominal distention

2. **Pneumomediastinum/pneumopericardium/pneumothorax**
   A. Happens with or without lung injury
   B. Because of rapid diffusibility of CO_2, can quickly become tension pneumo

Management of pneumothorax

Turn off N_2O
Adjust ventilation to correct hypoxia, PEEP if needed

Decrease intraabdominal pressure as able
Thoracentesis NOT INDICATED . . . will resolve within ~30 minutes 2° to high diffusibility of CO_2

3. Gas embolus
   A. Occurs during creation of pneumoperitoneum
   B. May be detected early if slow insufflation rate utilized
   C. CO_2 embolus produces more sudden and severe hypotension than air or O_2 embolus (due to vasodilation?)
   D. Symptoms tend to resolve quickly, 2° to high diffusibility of CO_2
   E. Will see paradoxical ↑ $ETCO_2$ before the acute ↓ due to CO_2 absorption from the blood

Management of CO_2 embolus

Stop insufflation and release pneumoperitoneum
Put patient head down with left lateral tilt (forces gas away from pulmonary artery outflow tract)
Hyperventilate with F_iO_2 1.0
Central venous catheter and CPR only as needed

Cardiovascular disturbances

Mainly, hemodynamic alterations due to:

1. Pneumoperitoneum
   A. ↓ venous return, therefore, ↓ cardiac output
   B. ↑ systemic and pulmonary vascular resistances
   C. Maintain or increase blood pressure usually
2. Patient position: head down: ↑CVP, cardiac output, cerebral blood volume, and ICP

Other complications you may see include

1. Cardiac arrest
2. Pneumopericardium
3. Vascular injury
4. Retroperitoneal hematoma
5. Parietal hematoma

Sample questions

A = 1, 2, 3   B = 1, 3   C = 2, 4   D = 4 only   E = all are correct

1. Which of the following changes in respiratory function are seen during laparoscopy?
   1. Increased arterial-to-alveolar carbon dioxide gradient
   2. Decreased total lung compliance
   3. Increased deadspace ventilation
   4. Increased intrapulmonary shunting

2. Absolute contraindications to laparoscopy include
   1. Increased intracranial pressure
   2. Ventriculoperitoneal shunt
   3. Peritoneojugular shunt
   4. Hypovolemia

Single best answer

3. During a laparoscopic procedure for treatment of endometriosis, your patient acutely develops cyanosis, her arterial oxygen saturation falls to 85%, and her peak inspiratory pressures increase from 25 to 50 cmH$_2$O. Current ventilator settings are tidal volume 700, rate = 12, F$_i$O$_2$ 0.3. Hemodynamically, she remains stable. The most appropriate action at this time is to
   1. Perform a tube thoracostomy
   2. Perform needle aspiration of the thorax
   3. Have the surgeon change from CO$_2$ to air for the insufflating gas
   4. Increase the F$_i$O$_2$ to 100%
   5. Add 5 cmH$_2$O of positive end-expiratory pressure

Answers: 1. A   2. A (hypovolemia is a relative contraindication)   3. 4

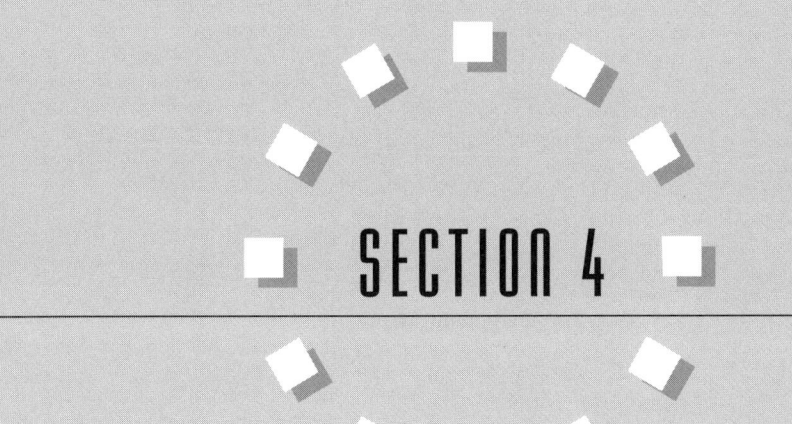

SECTION 4

Pediatric Anesthesia

CHAPTER 36

Respiratory Function: Infants versus Adults

Compliance and work of breathing

1. Must generate negative pressure 40–60 cmH$_2$O for first few breaths of life.
2. Work of breathing > adults due to increased chest wall compliance (minimal chest wall expansive forces) and decreased lung compliance.
3. Ribs are horizontally situated, allowing less chest expansion than the angled ribs of the adult. Therefore, the chest muscles are ineffective in assuming any work of breathing.
4. Diaphragm is main muscle of respiration and is comprised of easily fatigued fibers.

So what does this mean? It means neonates are at risk for respiratory failure whenever there is increased respiratory work.

Why? Because since the chest wall is so compliant, there is paradoxical movement whenever there is increased respiratory effort. The diaphragm must work harder to maintain tidal volume and it is easily fatigued because it lacks slow-twitch muscle fibers.

Pulmonary parameters

1. TLC in infants (60 cc/kg) < adults (80 cc/kg)
2. FRC is equal to adult on cc/kg basis (but absolute value is obviously smaller)
3. Closing capacity constitutes ~50% of infant TLC, whereas adult is only ~35%
4. Tidal volume is equal to adult (6–7 cc/kg)

   And:

5. O$_2$ consumption is 2 to 3 times adult values,

   So:

6. Alveolar ventilation must be at least twice as much as adult value, and this is achieved by an increased respiratory rate.

NOTE: When kids increase their respiratory rate, they increase not only alveolar ventilation, but also deadspace ventilation. **So,** they have more alveolar ventilation and deadspace ventilation than adults, but their VD/VT is the same as for adults.

Factors that contribute to rapid desaturation in infants

1. High O_2 consumption and smaller total volume at FRC.
2. FRC < closing capacity and closing volume is within the range of normal tidal breathing. **Therefore,** during tidal exhalation, they have airway closure occurring before they reach FRC (i.e., they have shunting during tidal breathing).
3. In infants, the elastic recoil of the lung exceeds the expansive forces of the chest wall, and if FRC were determined solely on these two factors, the infant's FRC would make up far less than the 40% of TLC that we see. (In other words, the lung wants to squish down and the chest wall alone can't prevent it.) Infants set their FRC by "auto-PEEPing" or laryngeal braking, *actively* ceasing their exhalation above the lung relaxation volume. When they are apneic, they are unable to "brake," and the lung deflates to a volume smaller than the awake FRC. **Therefore: in the apneic infant, there is a disproportionately smaller store to obtain oxygen from than in the apneic adult.**
4. Increased CO_2 production.

Physiologic causes of hypoxemia in neonates

1. Intrapulmonary shunting 2° to unexpanded areas of lung
2. Extrapulmonary shunting through patent foramen ovale or ductus arteriosus
3. Undiagnosed congenital heart disease
4. High resting O_2 consumption
5. Hypothermia—increases O_2 consumption even further

Mechanisms of *perioperative* desaturation in neonates

In addition to the above:

1. Airway obstruction
2. Apnea (see next list for causes of apnea)
3. Hypoventilation due to incomplete reversal of neuromuscular blockade, anesthetics
4. Decreased FRC due to general anesthesia (just like adults)

Factors predisposing neonates to postoperative apnea

1. Prematurity: risk remains increased until 44 to 60 weeks postconceptual age (depending on which study you read)
2. Immaturity of central respiratory drive centers
3. Hypothermia
4. Hypoglycemia
5. Hypocalcemia
6. Acidosis
7. Hypoxia (yes, they respond to hypoxia by going apneic . . . what are they thinking?)

Sample questions

A = 1, 2, 3   B = 1, 3   C = 2, 4   D = 4 only   E = all are correct

1. True statements regarding infant respiratory mechanics as compared to adults include
    1. Functional residual capacity, when based on weight, is larger in the adult

2. Work of breathing is less in infants
3. When apneic, the functional residual capacity is the same as during spontaneous ventilation in both infants and adults
4. The diaphragm is the main muscle of respiration

2. Which of the following comparisons of infant and adult respiratory volumes are correct?
   1. Total lung capacity is equal when based on cc/kg
   2. Functional residual capacity is equal when based on cc/kg
   3. Closing volume is less than functional residual capcity in both infants and adults
   4. Tidal volume is equal when based on cc/kg

3. Which of the following increase the risk of postoperative apnea in a neonate?
   1. Prematurity
   2. Hypoxia
   3. Hypocalcemia
   4. Anemia

Answers: 1. D   2. C   3. A

Pediatric Fluid Management

Formulae: Maintenance fluid requirements for children are based on body weight, average caloric expenditure, and the fact that each calorie burned results in the loss of 1 mL of water.[1]

≤10 kg   100 mL/kg
11–20 kg   1000 mL (for first 10 kg) + 50 mL/kg for each kg over 10 kg
≥20 kg   1500 mL (for the first 20 kg) + 20 mL/kg for each kg over 20 kg

Example: maintenance fluid for a 25-kg child:

1000 mL (first 10 kg) + 500 mL (second 10 kg) + 100 mL (last 5 kg)
= 1600 mL/day, **OR:** 66 mL/hr

Since pediatric cases are short, we just calculate hourly maintenance rates. The ratio of 24-hr fluids 100 mL:50 mL:20 mL is *about* 4:2:1. So, maintenance for kids is the same as adults:

4 mL/kg/hr for the first 10 kg
2 mL/kg/hr for the second 10 kg
1 mL/kg/hr for all remaining kg

Example for a 25-kg child:

40 mL (first 10 kg) + 20 mL (second 10 kg) + 5 mL (last 5 kg) = 65 mL/hr

Daily electrolyte requirements

~3 mEq/L each of Na^+, K^+, Cl^-

Replacement of electrolyte deficit

(Target value − present value) × kg × 0.3 = mEq needed

What fluid do you use?

1. Lactated Ringer's: all kids (has adequate amounts of electrolytes for healthy kids, and most have adequate glycogen stores so they don't need glucose)
2. Additives:
   A. Glucose 5% (healthy kids with prolonged preop fasting) or 10% for premies or neonates (limited glycogen stores)
   B. Electrolytes as needed (especially K^+)

Replacing fluid deficits

Normal healthy kids:

$$\text{\# hours of NPO status} \times \text{hourly maintenance} = \text{fluid deficit}$$

If patient is dehydrated: need ~10 mL/kg for each 1% of dehydration.
Clinical estimate of degree of dehydration:
- 5%: decreased skin turgor, "tacky" mucous membranes
- 10%: oliguria, tachycardia
- 15% hypotension, no lacrimation

Intraoperative fluid management

1. Replace deficit as in adults (½ in first hour, ½ over following 2 hr)
2. Provide maintenance in addition to deficit replacement
3. Replace insensible losses from evaporation based on degree of surgical exposure:
   A. Minimal exposure (like clubfoot repair): 2 mL/kg/hr
   B. Moderate exposure (like appendectomy): 3–5 mL/kg/hr
   C. Major exposure (like small bowel resection): 8–10 mL/kg/hr

No sample questions . . . I trust you to do math.

Reference

1. Holliday MA, Segar WE. The maintenance need for water in parenteral fluid therapy. Pediatrics 19: 823–832, 1957.

CHAPTER 38

Pyloric Stenosis

Lesion: Hypertrophy/hyperplasia of muscular layer of pylorus with resultant gastric outlet obstruction

Patient population

1. 2–6 weeks of life
2. Term or preterm
3. Males > females

Presentation

Nonbilious, projectile vomiting

Metabolic effects of vomiting

Lose H^+ and Cl^- ions → hypochloremic metabolic alkalosis → kidneys excrete K^+ in exchange for H^+ and excrete $NaHCO_3$ in an effort to retain Cl^- → hypokalemia and alkaline urine

Progressive volume and Na^+ depletion occurs → kidneys resorb Na^+ in exchange for H^+ and K^+, must also resorb HCO_3^- to maintain electroneutrality since there's no available Cl^- → paradoxical acidic urine and worsening of metabolic alkalosis, hyponatremia, and hypokalemia

Respiratory effects of pyloric stenosis

Metabolic alkalosis promotes hypoventilation (CO_2 retention)

Laboratory findings

Early	Late	Very Late
1. Hypokalemia	1. Hypokalemia	1. Severe dehydration
2. Hypochloremia	2. Hypochloremia	2. Hypovolemic shock
3. Metabolic alkalosis (mild)	3. Metabolic alkalosis (severe)	3. Metabolic *acidosis*
4. Alkaline urine	4. *Acidic* urine	
5. Normal Na^+	5. *Hyponatremia*	
	6. Hypocalcemia	

Anesthetic management

1. **Properatively**
    A. Not a surgical emergency!!
    B. Must rehydrate and correct metabolic derangements first
    C. Nasogastric or orogastric suction
2. **Induction:** Awake intubation or rapid sequence are equally acceptable
3. **Emergence:** Extubate only when fully awake with airway reflexes intact

Laboratory values defining surgical readiness

Cl^- > 88 mEq/L
HCO_3^- < 30 mmol/L
K^+ > 3.0 mEq/L
Urine output > 1–2 cc/kg/hr
Urine specific gravity < 1.020

Sample Questions

A = 1, 2, 3   B = 1, 3   C = 2, 4   D = 4   E = all are correct

1. Conditions that are associated with pyloric stenosis in an infant include
    1. Metabolic alkalosis
    2. Carbon dioxide retention
    3. Hyponatremia
    4. Hypokalemia

2. True statements regarding pyloric stenosis include
    1. The greater the degree of dehydration, the more urgent the need to proceed with surgery
    2. Respiratory acidosis may be seen
    3. Correction of electrolyte disorders should not delay surgical repair
    4. Metabolic acidosis is an indicator of severe dehydration

Answers: **1. E   2. C**

Tetralogy of Fallot

Tetralogy consists of

1. Pulmonary stenosis
2. VSD
3. Overriding aorta
4. Right ventricular hypertrophy

Physiology of TET spell (Hypercyanotic spells)

↑ right ventricular outflow tract obstruction and pulmonary vascular resistance → increased R to L shunting through VSD → cyanosis

Management of TET spells

1. Hyperventilate with 100% F_iO_2: ↓ pulmonary vascular resistance
2. Phenylephrine IV: ↑ systemic vascular resistance > pulmonary vascular resistance
    A. Results in L-to-R shunt
    B. Best used for *acute* treatment
3. Fluid bolus: 10–20 cc/kg
4. Propanolol: best used for *prevention*
5. Morphine: suggested in literature, but not particularly useful

Anesthetic Management

Must consider what will cause R-to-L shunting

1. ↓ SVR
2. ↑ PVR
3. ↑ myocardial contractility (worsens pulmonary outflow tract obstruction)

Anesthetic factors that ↓ SVR

1. Volatile agents
2. Histamine-releasing drugs

3. Ganglionic blockers
4. α-blockade

Anesthetic factors that ↑ PVR

1. Acidosis
2. Hypercarbia
3. Hypoxia
4. Positive pressure ventilation/PEEP
5. Loss of negative intrapleural pressure when chest is opened
6. Nitrous oxide

Preoperative management

1. Hydrate, especially if polycythemic
2. Continue β-blockers
3. Avoid noxious stimuli (crying)

Induction

1. Consider ketamine: increases SVR
2. Inhalational technique
   A. Direct myocardial depression prevents dynamic obstruction of pulmonary infundibulum
   B. Risk of increased PVR due to hypoxia and hypercarbia

Sample question

A = 1, 2, 3   B = 1, 3   C = 2, 4   D = 4   E = all are correct

1. During mask induction with N_2O, O_2, and halothane of a 5-day-old, 4-kg term infant with tetralogy of Fallot, the SaO_2 begins to fall and the mean arterial pressure is 35 mmHg. Appropriate responses at this time include:
   1. Hyperventilation with 100% O_2
   2. Atropine sulfate 0.5 mg IV
   3. Phenylephrine 4 µg IV
   4. Propanolol 50 µg IV

Answer: B

CHAPTER 40

Croup versus Epiglottitis

- **Table 40–1**

	Croup	Epiglottitis
Age	6 mo–6 yr	1–7 yr
Organism	Viral	Hemophilus influenza type B
Onset	Gradual	Rapid
Symptoms	**Low**-grade fver	**High**-grade fever
	Stridor	Stridor
	Retractions	Retractions
	Tachypnea	Tachypnea
	"Barking" cough	No cough
		Drooling
Physical exam	Cyanosis	Sitting up
	Retractions	Retractions
		Drooling
Neck X-ray	**Anterior** view:	**Lateral** view:
	"steeple sign"—narrowing of subglottic inlet due to edema	big, swollen epiglottis loss of vallecula

Airway management

Croup

1. Cool mist oxygen therapy
2. Racemic epinephrine nebulizer treatments: beware of rebound effect
3. Corticosteroids: longstanding controversy, but appear to help
4. If intubation necessary, should be done in operating room under general anesthesia, with smaller tube than usual to prevent subglottic stenosis.

Epiglottitis

1. Is an airway emergency
2. Laryngoscopy ONLY IN OPERATING ROOM . . . NEVER IN EMERGENCY ROOM!
3. ENT standby for emergent surgical airway
4. Premedicate with IV or IM atropine
5. Mask induction with patient in sitting position
6. Intubate under deep general anesthesia with patient breathing SPONTANEOUSLY
7. Use tube a full size smaller than appropriate for age

Sample questions

Single best answer

1. A 2-year-old child presents to the Emergency Department with respiratory distress. Physical exam reveals: T = 37.4C, resp = 40, mild suprasternal retractions with stridor and a loud, "honking" cough. The MOST appropriate first step would be
    1. Administer oxygen via cool mist mask, obtain a lateral chest X-ray
    2. Administer oxygen via nasal cannula, obtain a lateral neck X-ray
    3. Administer subcutaneous epinephrine
    4. Administer cool mist oxygen and obtain an anterior neck X-ray
    5. Administer oxygen and observe

2. A 5-year-old child presents with an 8-hr history of sudden onset of fever and respiratory distress. He is agitated and refuses to lie down to be examined. Physical exam reveals stridor, retractions, drooling, resp = 20, T = 39°C. After administering oxygen, the most appropriate action to take is
    1. Perform laryngoscopy in the emergency room to confirm the diagnosis
    2. Perform lateral X-rays of the neck to confirm the diagnosis
    3. Endotracheal intubation in the operating room following mask induction of general anesthesia
    4. Endotracheal intubation in the operating room following rapid-sequence induction
    5. Start an IV and institute antibiotic therapy

Answers: 1. 4   2. 3

Chapter 41

Diaphragmatic Hernia

Lesion: Herniation of bowel into thorax, resulting in pulmonary hypoplasia

Presentation

1. Respiratory distress
2. Scaphoid abdomen
3. Bowel sounds over chest (usually on left side)
4. Decreased breath sounds (usually on left side)

Initial management

1. Decompress bowel with oro/nasogastric tube (allows better ventilation)
2. Intubate
3. May require extracorporeal membrane oxygenation (ECMO) until medically stable enough to repair defect

Pearls of wisdom

1. Avoid mask ventilation . . . distends bowel, ↑ respiratory compromise
2. Do *NOT* try to reexpand the lung . . . may cause tension pneumothorax on the contralateral side (I hate it when that happens)

Anesthetic management

1. O_2, relaxant, potent agent . . . no N_2O
2. Standard monitors and arterial line
3. Avoid things that increase pulmonary vascular resistance (hypoxia, hypercarbia, acidosis)

Complications

1. Tension pneumothorax
2. Persistent pulmonary hypertension. Treatment includes vasodilators, hyperventilation, and/or ECMO

Sample questions

Single best answer

1. During repair of a left-sided diaphragmatic hernia in a 4200-g neonate, control ventilation is set at 60 cc and 25 breaths/min and F_iO_2 50%. A

blood gas reveals pH 7.2, PaCO$_2$ = 65 mmHg, PaO$_2$ = 60 mmHg. Which of the following is needed?
1. Needle thoracostomy of the right thorax
2. Increase tidal volume to 85 cc
3. Increase F$_i$O$_2$ to 75%
4. Increase respiratory rate to 45/min
5. Manually ventilate and try to reexpand the left lung

2. Immediately following normal spontaneous vaginal delivery, a 3800-g neonate is noted to be dyspneic with a scaphoid abdomen, diminished breath sounds on the left chest, and the oxygen saturation is 88% on blow-by O$_2$. What is the most appropriate therapeutic measure to undertake first?
1. Tube thoracostomy to left thorax
2. Mask ventilate with 100% O$_2$
3. Intubate
4. Insert a nasogastric tube
5. Institute extracorporeal membrane oxygenation

Answers: 1. 4   2. 4

Chapter 42

Omphalocele/Gastroschisis

- Table 42-1

	Omphalocele	Gastroschisis
Lesion	Failure of the gut to return to the abdominal cavity in utero	Abdominal wall dissolves due to interruption of omphalomesenteric artery
Abdominal contents	Abdominal contents are covered by membrane (↓ infection risk and fluid loss)	Abdominal contents *not* covered by membrane (↑ infection rate and fluid loss)
Associated anomalies	High incidence **Beckwith-Weidmann syndrome:** macroglossia, hypoglycemia, cardiac defects, omphalocele, retardation	Low incidence

Perioperative concerns

1. Fluid loss: both have huge fluid losses, omphalocele a little less because viscera is covered by membrane
2. Infection
3. Management of associated anomalies
4. Postoperative hypotension (hypovolemia) **OR** hypertension (due to decreased renal perfusion and resultant release of renin)

Anesthetic management

1. Vigorous volume resuscitation (0.9% NaCl: expect maintenance requirements ~100–200 cc/kg for entire case)
2. Avoid N_2O (aids return of gut to abdomen)
3. Monitor arterial line, CVP optional
4. Muscle relaxants (aid return of gut to abdomen)

There are two surgical options

1. Primary closure
2. Staged closure using a silo: necessary for large defects because of the respiratory and hemodynamic compromise caused by primary closure

Problems with primary closure and return of entire gut to abdomen

All are due to increased intraabdominal pressure

1. Postoperative respiratory failure: no room for diaphragmatic excursion.
2. Decreased venous return, and thus, decreased cardiac output and blood pressure. Leads to bowel ischemia and renal failure.

Sample questions

Single best answer

1. A 3500-g, full-term neonate is under general anesthesia using air, oxygen, neuromuscular blockade, and controlled ventilation for primary closure of a large gastroschisis defect. During return of the viscera to the abdominal cavity, the peak inspiratory pressures increase to 50 cmH$_2$O and the oxygen saturation falls to 75%. The twitch monitor reveals posttetanic facilitation. The most appropriate action at this time would be
   1. Administer more muscle relaxant
   2. Increase the minute ventilation
   3. Abandon primary closure
   4. Increase the F$_i$O$_2$
   5. Institute positive end-expiratory pressure

2. A 3850-g full-term neonate is undergoing primary surgical closure of a large omphalocele with general anesthesia using oxygen, air, pancuronium, and fentanyl. Two hours after the start of the procedure, his vital signs are: blood pressure 40/27, pulse = 195, Hct = 32%. He has received 115 cc of 0.9% NaCl. The most appropriate action at this time would be
   1. Fluid bolus with crystalloid
   2. Fluid bolus with colloid
   3. Transfuse with packed red blood cells
   4. Increase maintenance fluid rate
   5. Do not adjust fluid administration

Answers: 1. 3   2. 3

CHAPTER 43

Tracheoesophageal Fistula

Most common type: Blind esophageal pouch with distal fistula, fistula is usually posterior and immediately proximal to carina

Associated defects

1. Seen in 50% of patients
2. VATER syndrome:
   *V*ertebral and cardio*v*ascular defects
   *A*nal defects (imperforate)
   TE Fistula
   *R*adial and *r*enal anomalies

Presentation

1. Polyhydramnios in utero
2. Inability to pass feeding tube
3. Coughing/choking/drooling/cyanosis with first feeding

Preoperative management

1. Look for associated defects (especially cardiac)
2. Prevent the major preop complications, which are:
   A. Aspiration pneumonitis
      –Elevate head of bed to prevent aspiration
      –Continuous suction to pouch to prevent aspiration
   B. Dehydration: IV hydration mandatory

Anesthetic management

There are generally three surgical scenarios

1. Stable enough to undergo single-stage primary repair, gastrostomy not needed
2. Lung disease too severe to tolerate immediate thoracotomy, need gastrostomy to prevent aspiration until primary repair can be done
3. Will need staged repair to reanastomose esophagus, so fistula ligation and gastrostomy are done as first stage

Anesthetic technique

1. Gastrostomy alone can be done under local (preferred) or general anesthesia

2. Primary or staged repair is via left-sided thoracotomy under general anesthesia
3. If general anesthesia is required:
   A. Do an awake intubation.
   B. Advance tube into R. mainstem, then withdraw slightly so that tip is above carina and below fistula (allows ventilation of lungs, but not fistula).
   C. Maintain spontaneous ventilation until gastrostomy completed (prevents gastric distention seen during positive pressure ventilation due to gas following path of least resistance through fistula).
   D. Muscle relaxation for thoracotomy **only after proper ETT placement is verified.**

A setup for disaster

Patient with poor lung compliance and high PIPs has gastric distention and surgeons do a "decompressing" gastrostomy before ligation of fistula. Now all your positive pressure ventilation vents to atmosphere via gastrostomy! (Ooops!)

What do you do? Put Fogarty balloon tipped catheter into fistula to occlude it, either retrograde through gastrostomy or alongside ETT in trachea.

Sample questions

Single best answer

1. A 1-day-old full-term infant is undergoing gastrostomy and primary repair of a tracheoesophageal fistula. During inhalational induction, the abdomen becomes distended. The most appropriate course of action at this time would be
   1. Intubate and control ventilation
   2. Intubate and gently assist ventilation
   3. Do not intubate, continue spontaneous ventilation until gastrostomy performed
   4. Pass an orogastric tube

2. A 48-hour-old infant is undergoing primary surgical repair of a tracheoesophageal fistula via a left-sided thoracotomy. During controlled, positive pressure ventilation, the peak inspiratory pressures acutely change from 20 cmH$_2$O to 50 cmH$_2$0, the oxygen saturation falls to 60%, and there is no chest rise with ventilation efforts. The most likely reason for these changes is
   1. Tension pneumothorax
   2. The endotracheal tube is in the fistula
   3. Inadvertent extubation has occurred
   4. Bronchospasm

Answers: **1. 3   2. 2**

Chapter 44

Necrotizing Enterocolitis

Defect: Mucosal or transmural intestinal necrosis

Population

Low-birthweight infants (<1500 g) and premature infants (<32 weeks gestation)

Presentation

A wide spectrum of findings, ranging from guaiac-positive stools to sepsis, including:

1. Feeding intolerance
2. Abdominal distention
3. Frankly bloody stools
4. Metabolic acidosis
5. Sepsis

Radiologic diagnosis

1. Pneumatosis intestinalis (pathognomonic)
2. Pneumoperitoneum (2° to perforated bowel)
3. Portal venous gas (death likely)

Laboratory studies

1. Metabolic acidosis
2. Thrombocytopenia
3. Elevated PT/PTT
4. Hypofibrinogenemia
5. Leukopenia
6. Hypocalcemia
7. Hypoglycemia

Management

1. Attempt medical management (stop feeding, decompress bowel with orogastric tube, volume resuscitate, antibiotics, serial X-rays)
2. Surgical resection of necrotic bowel

Anesthetic management

1. Ensure adequate intravascular volume (high degree of third spacing, use balanced salt solution)

2. Correct coagulopathy (preop if possible)
    A. RBCs: transfuse to Hct ~40 to maintain oxygen delivery
    B. FFP: 10 mL/kg
    C. Platelets: 0.1 unit/kg
    D. Cryoprecipitate: 0.1 unit/kg
3. Rapid-sequence induction vs. awake intubation (equally acceptable, but preemies often have significant lung disease and poor reserve, so awake intubation may be better. Often not an issue, because they're usually already intubated).
4. Narcotic/relaxant/oxygen technique (avoid N_2O, lowest F_iO_2 tolerated to decrease risk of retinopathy)
5. Expect high peak airway pressures (respiratory distress syndrome, pulmonary hemorrhage, abdominal distention all contribute)
6. Correct:
    A. Hypocalcemia (10–30 mg/kg CaCl or 100 mg/kg Ca^{++} gluconate)
    B. Hypoglycemia (4–7 mcg/kg/min)
    C. Metabolic acidosis (normal is ~18–22 meq/L, dilute $NaHCO_3$ 1:1 or 1:2 to ↓ risk of CSF acidosis)
7. Aggressive warming measures

Complications

1. Intracranial hemorrhage (due to excessive fluid administration)
2. Reopening ductus arteriosus (excessive fluid administration)
3. Pulmonary edema (excessive fluid administration)
4. Acute renal failure (inadequate fluid administration and hypoperfusion)
5. Hepatic dysfunction (inadequate fluid administration)
6. Worsening of all preop problems (acidosis, coagulopathy, pulmonary status)

Sample questions

A = 1, 2, 3   B = 1, 3   C = 2, 4   D = 4 only   E = all are correct

1. Laboratory abnormalities commonly seen in infants with necrotizing enterocolitis include
    1. Hypocalcemia
    2. Hyponatremia
    3. Hypoglycemia
    4. Hypercarbia

Single best answer

2. A 1200-kg, 30-week-gestational-age infant is undergoing exploratory laparotomy for necrotizing enterocolitis. Maintenance fluids are normal saline at 8 mL/hr. Pressure cycled ventilation is maintained with a respiratory rate 20/min and peak inspiratory pressures of 28 cmH_2O. Initial intraoperative arterial blood gases reveal a $PaCO_2$ of 34 mmHg and an end-tidal CO_2 of 31 mmHg. After 1 hour of surgery, the end-tidal CO_2 reads 22 mmHg. The most appropriate therapy at this time is
    1. Reduce the compliance of the ventilator circuit
    2. Decrease the respiratory rate to 15/min
    3. Decrease the peak inspiratory pressure to 22 cmH_2O
    4. Administer normal saline bolus of 8 mL
    5. Recalibrate the capnograph

Answers: 1. E   2. 4

CHAPTER 45

Pierre–Robin Syndrome

Lesion: Microretrognathia and glossoptosis, with entire larynx being more *posterior* than normal. Thus, angle between base of tongue and laryngeal inlet is very acute.

Associated Defects

1. Cleft palate (50%)
2. Cardiac and skeletal defects (25%)
3. Choanal atresia
4. Stickler syndrome (myopia, retinal detachment, blindness)

Presentation

1. Airway obstruction, **especially when supine**
2. Cor pulmonale and congestive heart failure 2° to unrelieved airway obstruction, hypercarbia, and hypoxia
3. Aspiration pneumonitis
4. Failure to thrive

Preop management

1. Maintain prone position (tongue falls forward and relieves obstruction)
2. Tube feeds (unable to eat normally)

Surgical treatment

Glossopexy via a lip-tongue adhesion (mandibular hypoplasia will correct over time). Tracheotomy rarely done.

Anesthetic management

1. Maintain prone position.
2. Avoid sedation (aggravates airway obstruction).
3. Atropine premedication (blocks vagal reflex, dries secretions, which are copious).
4. Surgical standby for emergent tracheotomy.
5. Establish IV access with infant awake.
6. Preoxygenate while prone.
7. Turn supine, place roll under shoulders, insert oral airway (expect obstruction).
8. Awake intubation via direct laryngoscopy, blind or fiberoptic.

Emergence and postoperative management

1. Insert bilateral nasopharyngeal airways before emergence.
2. Extubate in OR awake.
3. In PACU, maintain prone or lateral position (prevents obstruction).
4. Admit to ICU after PACU.

Similar syndromes

1. Treacher–Collins syndrome ⎫ Both have similar features and
2. Goldenhar syndrome ⎬ airway management is similar.

Sample question

Single best answer

1. All of the following are true statements regarding Pierre–Robin syndrome except
    1. Airway obstruction is relieved by assuming the prone position
    2. Intubation is more difficult because the larynx is more anterior than usual
    3. There is a high incidence of concomitant congenital defects
    4. The mandible will assume a near-normal architecture over time
    5. Closely resembles Treacher–Collins in its clinical presentation

Answer: 1. 2

CHAPTER 46

Infants Born to Myasthenic Women

There are two types of infantile myasthenia gravis

1. **Congenital myasthenia**
   A. Extremely rare
   B. First appears during infancy (beyond neonatal period), persists for life
   C. Usually mild, not requiring pharmacologic therapy
2. **Neonatal myasthenia**
   A. Due to placental transfer of maternal antibodies
   B. Symptoms appear within 24 to 72 hours after birth
   C. Resolves by 3 months of age

Symptoms of neonatal myasthenia

1. Generalized weakness
2. Difficulty feeding
3. Respiratory fatigue/distress

Management

1. Intubate and ventilate if necessary
2. Atropine (.02 mg/kg) and pyridostigmine (5.0 mg/kg), usually for ~ 3 to 4 weeks

Sample question

Single best answer

1. A full term 3500-g infant is delivered by C-section to a myasthenia gravis female under general anesthesia due to failed epidural block and cephalopelvic disproportion. Anesthesia was induced with thiopental and succinylcholine, followed by 50% nitrous, 50% oxygen, and 0.8% isoflurane. Immediately after delivery, the infant has regular, but shallow, respirations, a weak cough, and somewhat limp appearance. The most likely cause of this is
   1. Placental transfer of neuromuscular blockers
   2. Residual effect of inhalational agents
   3. Placental transfer of maternal antibodies
   4. Placental transfer of thiopental
   5. Hypoglycemia

Answer: **1. 3**

CHAPTER 47

Fetal and Neonatal Circulation

The umbilical vessels communicate with the placenta. There are two arteries, one vein. The PO_2 of the umbilical vein is 30–35 mmHg.

Pathway of fetal circulation:

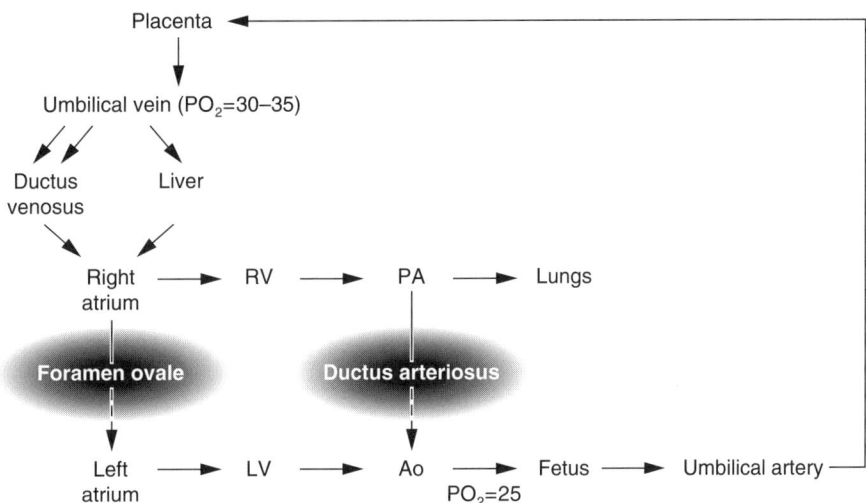

Figure 47–1.

Circulatory changes at birth (transitional circulation)

1. Placenta gone
2. R → L shunt exists at foramen ovale as long as PVR remains high
3. Bidirectional flow exists through patent ductus arteriosus
   A. *Functional* closure at 3 days old
   B. *Anatomic* closure at 3 weeks old
4. Pulmonary vascular resistance (PVR) falls to normal by 24 hours old. PVR falls in response to lung expansion and rise in PaO_2.

Once changes have occurred, the infant

1. Has "fixed" stroke volume, therefore cardiac output is heart rate dependent
2. Is more vagal than adults . . . prone to bradycardia

Factors that cause persistent fetal circulation (persistent transitional circulation)

1. Prematurity
2. Pulmonary disease: hypoxia, hypercarbia
3. Acidosis
4. Hypothermia
5. Congenital heart disease
6. Sepsis
7. High altitude
8. Diaphragmatic hernia, meconium aspiration (because are associated with respiratory failure)

Sample questions

A = 1, 2, 3   B = 1, 3   C = 2, 4   D = 4 only   E = all are correct

1. Factors that contribute to the persistence of fetal circulation include
   1. Living at high altitude
   2. Infant respiratory distress syndrome
   3. Gestational age < 36 weeks
   4. Hypothermia

2. True statements regarding the patent ductus arteriosus include
   1. Functional closure occurs by 3 days old
   2. In utero, high maternal PaO_2 leads to premature closure
   3. Anatomic closure of the ductus arteriosus occurs by 3 weeks old
   4. Closure of the ductus arteriosus is directly dependent on the increased PaO_2

Answers: 1. E   2. B

CHAPTER 48

Neonatal Temperature Regulation

There are four mechanisms of heat loss

1. Radiation: **most common** in babies *and* adults
2. Convection: second most common, all patients
3. Conduction: greater effect on infants 2° to large body surface area
4. Evaporation: more important in preemies with thin skin than in older infants

Anatomic factors that increase heat loss in infants

1. Relatively larger body surface area
2. Less keratin in skin (preemies)

There are three mechanisms by which to produce heat

1. Increased physical activity: can't do while anesthetized
2. Shivering: ability to shiver not present until ~3 months old, can't do while anesthetized
3. Nonshivering thermogenesis
    A. The only means of heat production in anesthetized neonate
    B. A result of brown fat metabolism

How does it work?

Cold body temperature ⇒ ↑ Norepinephrine production ⇒ Brown fat metabolism ⇒ Energy and heat

      ↙   ↘

   Peripheral   Pulmonary ⇒ Right-to-left shunting ⇒ Hypoxia
  vasoconstriction vasoconstriction
    ⇓
  Heat conservation

Figure 48–1.

Sample questions

A = 1, 2, 3 B = 1, 3 C = 2, 4 D = 4 only E = all are correct

1. Mechanisms by which anesthetized neonates produce heat include
    1. Erector pili activity
    2. Vasoconstriction
    3. Increased muscle activity
    4. Nonshivering thermogenesis

2. Possible consequences of intraoperative hypothermia in neonates include
   1. Acidosis
   2. Myocardial irritability
   3. Increased intrapulmonary shunting
   4. Greater absorption of inhalational agents

Answers: 1. D (gotcha)   2. E (also, prolonged neuromuscular blockade and respiratory depression)

CHAPTER 49

Prematurity

Perioperative concerns

1. Increased risk of hypothermia (see section on Neonatal Temperature Regulation)
2. Glucose homeostasis (may require 2–3 g/kg/day IV if NPO)
3. Risk of postoperative apnea—**a favorite topic on the boards**
4. Retinopathy of prematurity—**another favorite**
5. Coexisting pulmonary dysfunction

Types of apnea

1. Central: least common type in infants
2. Obstructive
3. Mixed (central and obstructive)

Factors that increase risk of postoperative apnea in infants

1. Prematurity (incidence inversely related to age, greatest risk is at < 50 weeks postconceptual age)
2. History of apnea
3. Hypothermia
4. Metabolic/electrolyte disorder (hypoglycemia, hypocalcemia, acidosis)
5. Hypoxemia
6. Airway obstruction (respiratory muscles fatigue easily, leads to apnea)
7. Anesthetic effects (less risk of apnea with regional vs. general)
8. Anemia (controversial, conflicting studies prove and disprove)

Preoperative pharmacologic management of apnea

Continue in perioperative period

1. Theophylline
2. Caffeine

Characteristics of retinopathy of prematurity

1. Etiology: multifactorial; no direct correlation with O_2 content or PaO_2 (has been reported in stillborns and children never on O_2 therapy)
2. Patient population: low-birthweight and premature infants (risk decreases after 44 weeks postconceptual age because the retina has matured)

Sample questions

A = 1, 2, 3   B = 1, 3   C = 2, 4   D = 4 only   E = all are correct

1. Factors predisposing to retinopathy of prematurity include
   1. High neonatal PaO_2
   2. Maternal oxygen therapy
   3. Persistent fetal circulation
   4. Gestational age less than 35 weeks

Single best answer

2. Premature infants undergoing general anesthesia are at particular risk to develop postoperative
   1. Apnea
   2. Airway obstruction
   3. Gastroesophageal reflux
   4. Postextubation croup
   5. Bradycardia

Answers: 1. D   2. 1

CHAPTER 50

Meconium Aspiration

Lesion: Aspiration of fetal feces

Population

Any infant with fetal distress (hypoxemia, acidosis, etc.)

Management

1. If vaginal delivery, suction pharynx before delivery of thorax
2. *Vigorous infant* with only lightly stained amniotic fluid: *Don't intubate*
3. *Depressed infant OR thick, particulate meconium:*
   A. Immediate laryngoscopy, intubate, and suction endotracheal tube (single pass)
   B. Spontaneous (preferred) or gentle manual ventilation for ~15 sec in between repeat passes of suction catheter
   C. Repeat suctioning until aspirate is clear

Pearl of Wisdom

If pulse < 60/min at delivery, bag-mask or bag-tube ventilation and resuscitation should take precedence over treatment for meconium aspiration

Sample questions

Single best answer

1. A 36-week-gestation, 2500-g infant is delivered by emergent C-section for fetal distress. The amniotic fluid contains thick meconium. Immediately after delivery, the infant's pulse is 60, his extremities are blue, and he is limp. The most appropriate first step would be
   1. Intubate and suction trachea for meconium
   2. Blindly suction pharynx for meconium prior to instituting bag-mask ventilation
   3. Obtain a heelstick to check glucose levels
   4. Administer atropine 0.02 mg/kg IM and perform external cardiac compressions
   5. Intubate and ventilate with 100% oxygen

2. A full-term, 3850-g double footling breech infant is delivered vaginally and the amniotic fluid is stained with meconium. The infant has a strong

50 ■ Meconium Aspiration

cry and is actively moving all extremities. The most appropriate management is
1. Intubate and suction trachea for meconium
2. Bulb suction naso/oropharynx and observe
3. Administer prophylactic antibiotics
4. Administer prophylactic synthetic surfactant
5. Apply warm humidified oxygen by hood with F_iO_2 0.3

Answers: 1. 5   2. 2

CHAPTER 51

Neonatal Resuscitation

Fetal assessment at delivery is via the Apgar score. This is a gimmee . . . memorize it! If you can't remember what things you're supposed to evaluate, remember this stupid mnemonic:

Appearance (color)
Pulse
Grimace (reflexes)
Activity (muscle tone)
Respirations

● Table 51–1

	Apgar Score		
Parameter	0	1	2
Color	Pale, blue	Body pink, limbs blue	Pink
Pulse (120–160/min)	Absent	<100	>100
Reflex	Absent	Grimace	Cough, sneeze
Muscle tone	Limp	Flexion	Moving
Respiration (30–60/min)	Absent	Irregular	Crying

Management of the abnormal Apgar

7–10: Warm the baby, nasal/oral suction only
4–6: Stimulate baby, suction airway, bag-mask ventilation with F_iO_2 1.0 if respiration remains irregular or HR < 100
0–3: Bag-mask ventilate with F_iO_2 1.0; if HR stays < 60, intubate. If HR remains < 80, begin compressions; additional resuscitation as needed (described below)

Differential diagnosis for neonatal depression

Not the complete list, just the common stuff

1. Drug addiction (avoid naloxone . . . precipitates withdrawal)
2. Perinatal drug therapy (did the mom get narcotics or other sedatives?)
3. Hypovolemia (treat with blood or albumin) ⎫
4. Hypocalcemia ⎪
5. Hypoglycemia (treat with a 2-mL/kg bolus of <30 mg/dL) ⎬ 3–6 cause hypotension
6. Hypermagnesemia (treat with calcium gluconate 100–200 mg/kg) ⎭

Neonatal effects of hypermagnesemia

1. Hypotonia
2. Ventilatory depression
3. Hypotension
4. Increased sensitivity to depolarizing and nondepolarizing muscle relaxants

Neonatal resuscitation drugs

1. Volume expansion: 5% albumin or O-negative blood, 10 mL/kg (hypovolemia common)
2. Epinephrine: 10–30 μg/kg of 1:10, 000
3. Naloxone: 10 μg/kg
4. NaHCO$_3$: rarely indicated; most neonatal acidosis is metabolic 2° to hypovolemia. Dose: 1–2 mEq/kg *OR* 0.3 × weight in kg × base deficit. Indications: pH < 7.0 or base deficit > 15 mEq. Effects of administration (besides raising pH):
    A. Hypercarbia (remember: $HCO_3^- + H^+ \leftrightarrows H_2CO_3 \leftrightarrows H_2O + CO_2$)
    B. Hypotension (acidosis-induced vasoconstriction maintains blood pressure until you correct the acidosis)
    C. Intravascular volume overload and intracranial hemorrhage (bicarb solution is very hypertonic, draws fluid intravascularly)
    D. Decreased hematocrit (normal Hct ~50%, decrease due to hypertonic hemodilution as described above)
    E. Increased PaO$_2$

Do you get the feeling they like to ask about bicarb?

> **NOTE:** Atropine, calcium, and HCO$_3^-$ not routinely useful in acute resuscitation.

Since we're talking about bicarb, what is a normal arterial blood gas for an infant?

- Table 51–2

	pH	PCO$_2$	PaO$_2$
Fetus (umbilical vein)	7.30–7.35	~40	~36
Infant (2 min old)	7.20	~45	~60
Infant (1st hr)	7.30–7.36	~40	~60
Infant (24 hr old)	7.33–7.40	~33	~75

Sample questions

Single best answer

1. You are asked to evaluate a 2500-g infant 3 hr after vaginal delivery. The mother received butorphanol 1 mg IV 1 hr prior to delivery. His respiratory rate is 40/min, pulse is 118. Arterial blood gases on room air reveal pH 7.30, PCO$_2$ 45 mmHg, PO$_2$ 55 mmHg. Appropriate management is:
    1. Oxyhood at F$_i$O$_2$ 0.3
    2. Observation only
    3. Naloxone 0.25 mg intravenously
    4. Intubate and positive pressure ventilate with F$_i$O$_2$ 0.4
    5. Caffeine infusion to stimulate respiratory rate

A = 1, 2, 3   B = 1, 3   C = 2, 4   D = 4 only   E = all are correct

2. One minute after birth, a 2000-g term infant has a pink trunk and cyanotic fingers and toes, irregular respiratory pattern, grimaces with nasal suctioning, is immobile, but has flexion of the elbows and knees and the heart rate is 80/min. True statements about this infant include
   1. The Apgar score is consistent with mild intrauterine asphyxia
   2. Atropine 40 µg via the umbilical vein is indicated
   3. Bag-mask ventilation with pure oxygen should be initiated
   4. Chest compressions should be initiated

Answers: 1. 2   2. B

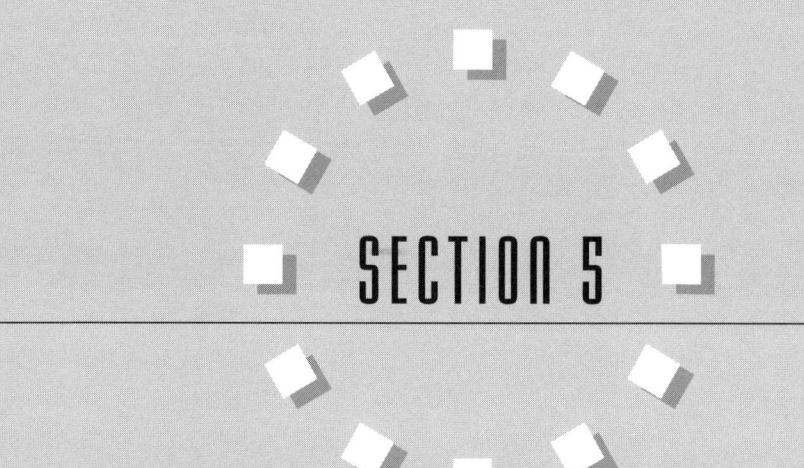

SECTION 5

Obstetric Anesthesia

Chapter 52

Fetal Monitoring

Usual parameters monitored

1. Baseline heart rate (normal 120–160 beats/min, accelerates with stimulation)
2. Beat-to-beat variability
3. Periodic patterns (accelerations, decelerations)
4. Uterine activity

Abnormalities of fetal heart rates and their significance

1. **Fetal tachycardia**
   A. Maternal fever, sepsis, thyrotoxicosis
   B. Maternal drug therapy with tocolytics, atropine, ephedrine
   C. *Chronic* fetal asphyxia (utero-placental insufficiency)
2. **Fetal bradycardia**
   A. *Acute* fetal asphyxia
   B. Fetal acidosis
   C. Periodic bradycardia with head compression, cord compression, and utero-placental insufficiency (see section on decelerations)
   D. Local anesthetic toxicity from paracervical block
   E. Maternal β-blockers
   F. Hypothermia
   G. Congenital AV block or CMV infection

Factors decreasing beat-to-beat variability

Ephedrine increases beat-to-beat variability

1. Fetal CNS hypoxia and acidosis
2. Narcotics
3. Barbiturates
4. Anticholinergics
5. Local anesthetics
6. Benzodiazepines
7. Inhalational agents

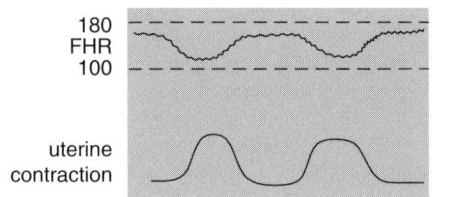 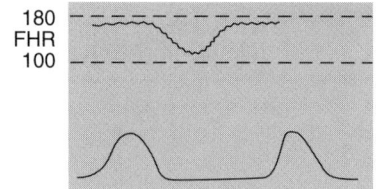 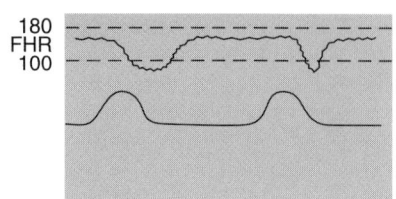

Figure 52–1. Periodic patterns and their significance.

● Table 52–1

	Early Decelerations	Late Decelerations	Variable Decelerations
Cause	Head compression	Utero-placental insufficiency	Cord compression
Features	"U"-shaped onset with contraction Peaks with contraction HR stays > 100 O_2 not therapeutic Atropine preventative	"U"-shaped onset after contraction starts Peaks after contraction HR stays > 100 O_2 therapeutic	Shape varies Onset time varies Peak varies HR goes < 100 O_2 not therapeutic Atropine preventative

Just in case they ask you, fetal scalp pH correlates with umbilical vein pH.

Normal values   7.25–7.45
Mild distress   7.20–7.24
Severe distress <7.20 (requires immediate delivery)

Sample question

Single best answer

1. A 19-year-old primigravida has cervical dilation to 5 cm. A lumbar epidural is injected with 10 mL 0.25% bupivicaine, and then an infusion is started with 0.125% bupivicaine at 6 cc/hr. Initial blood pressure is 112/82 mmHg, and 15 min later it is 80/45 mmHg with the patient in the supine position. The fetal monitor reveals late decelerations. All of the following are indicated EXCEPT
   1. Oxygen face mask
   2. Left uterine displacement
   3. Bolus 1000 mL normal saline
   4. Discontinue the bupivicaine infusion
   5. Phenylephrine 50 µg IV

Answer: 1. 5

CHAPTER 53

Physiologic Changes of Pregnancy

There's nothing tricky here . . . just memorize!

Respiratory system

1. ↑ V_E: due to increased VT and rate, but *primarily VT* (i.e., alveolar ventilation)
2. ↑ VO_2: duh.
3. ↑ O_2 delivery: due to right shift of oxyhemoglobin curve from increased 2,3 DPG
4. ↓ FRC: due to decreased ERV and RV; however, IRV is increased so TLC is unchanged
5. ↓ O_2 content: due to anemia
6. Also: ↓ airway resistance, ↑ AP and transverse diameter of thorax

Typical parturient ABGs at term

1. Normal pH, mildly low CO_2 (~32 mmHg due to increased V_E)
2. Mild base deficit (~22 mEq, due to HCO_3^- loss in compensation for respiratory alkalosis)
3. Mild hyperoxia (due to hyperventilation)

So what does this mean to you?

1. Combination of ↓ FRC and ↑ alveolar ventilation → speeds rate of rise F_A/F_I (speeds inhalational induction)
2. Combination of ↓ FRC and ↑ VO_2 → rapid desaturation when apneic

Fetal effects of maternal hyperventilation and hypocarbia during labor

Vasoconstriction of uterine and umbilical vessels coupled with some left shifting of oxyhemoglobin curve → ↓ blood flow and O_2 delivery to fetus → fetal hypoxemia and acidosis

Cardiovascular system

1. ↑ blood volume: due to increased plasma volume and red cell mass, but mainly *plasma volume* (thus, the dilutional anemia of pregnancy)
2. ↑ cardiac output
   A. Due to increased stroke volume and pulse, mainly *stroke volume*
   B. Increased all three trimesters

C. Additional increase with uterine contractions (autotransfusion)
D. Greatest increase immediately postpartum (↓ "reservoir" size)
3. ↓ blood pressure: (MAP, SBP, DBP) a decrease in SVR outweighs the effect of increased cardiac output

Hepatic system

1. ↑ SGOT, LDH, alkaline phosphatase
2. ↓ pseudocholinesterase level (but normal *function of enzyme*)
3. ↓ albumin (decreased available protein for drug binding)

Gastrointestinal system

↑ gastric acid volume (due to increased gastrin production) delayed gastric emptying (early effect of progesterone, later due to gravid uterus)

Sample question

A = 1, 2, 3   B = 1, 3   C = 2, 4   D = 4 only   E = all are correct

1. Pulmonary function changes that occur in pregnancy include
    1. Decreased inspiratory reserve volume
    2. Decreased diffusion capacity
    3. Decreased total lung capacity
    4. Increased alveolar ventilation

Answer: D

CHAPTER 54

Utero-Placental Blood Flow

Perfusion: The uterus is not capable of autoregulation; thus, perfusion is dependent on:

1. An adequate driving pressure (mom's MAP)
2. Low uterine venous pressure (promotes forward flow through placenta)
3. Low uterine vascular resistance

So, there is a decrease in utero placental flow if

1. Uterine artery pressure (maternal MAP) is decreased
2. Uterine venous pressure is increased (impedes forward flow)
3. Uterine vascular resistance is increased (impedes forward flow)

What might cause such nastiness?

- Table 54–1

Low Uterine Artery Pressure	High Uterine Venous Pressure	High Uterine Vascular Resistance
Hypovolemia Inadequate hydration prior to epidural Aortic compression by gravid uterus	Vena cava compression	Uterine contractions Preeclampsia Sympathomimetics (think Neo) High local anesthetic concentrations Diabetes mellitus

What is this thing called aortocaval compression?

Becomes important in second trimester

IVC compression by gravid uterus ⇒ Impaired venous return to maternal heart
  ↙   ↓   ↘
↑ Uterine venous pressure   maternal cardiac output, MAP
          ↘   ↙
      utero-placental flow and mother exhibits:
      nausea, vomiting, hypotension, sweating (shock)
                ↓
            Fetal distress

Figure 54–1.

1. See Figure 54–1.
2. Aortic compression by gravid uterus → uterine artery hypotension → fetal asphyxia and distress (mother may not be symptomatic).

Management of maternal hypotension

1. Oxygen (to maintain delivery to fetus)
2. Establish left uterine displacement (gets gravid uterus off aorta and vena cava)
3. Fluid bolus
4. Ephedrine (has both α- and β-effects, less increase in uterine vascular resistance)
5. Consider phenylephrine (pure α-effect may worsen hypoperfusion by raising uterine vascular resistance)

Sample questions

Single best answer

1. A 28-year-old multiparous patient is having a repeat C-section under epidural with 20 mL 2% lidocaine with 1:200,000 epinephrine and a T4 level. 25 mg ephedrine was given IM for a blood pressure of 100/65 mmHg immediately following initiation of the epidural. Upper extremity blood pressure was 128/77 mmHg at incision and increased to 145/88 mmHg during the procedure. A 3000-g infant with Apgars of 2 at 1 min and 5 at 5 min was delivered. The most likely explanation for the Apgar score is
   1. Fetal cardiac toxicity from excessively high levels of lidocaine
   2. Excessive uterine artery vasoconstriction due to synergy of epinephrine and ephedrine
   3. Utero-placental insufficiency due to compression of aorta
   4. Utero-placental hypoperfusion due to epidural-induced vasodilation
   5. Epinephrine-induced fetal hypoglycemia

   A = 1, 2, 3   B = 1, 3   C = 2, 4   D = 4 only   E = all are correct

2. A 30-year-old parturient receives a saddle block while in the seated position with 50 mg hyperbaric lidocaine in dextrose. She remains seated for 5 min. Immediately after assuming the lithotomy position, she becomes short of breath and complains of light-headedness. True statements about this situation include
   1. Her legs should be removed from the stirrups
   2. Intravenous ephedrine 5 mg should be administered immediately
   3. Her dyspnea is due to loss of chest wall proprioception
   4. The uterus should be displaced to the left

Answers: 1. 3   2. D

CHAPTER 55

Placental Transfer of Drugs and Oxygen

Factors affecting placental transfer of drugs

1. **High maternal concentration of drug due to**
   A. High total dose
   B. Highly vascular site of administration
   C. Slow maternal metabolism
   D. Maternal pH (acidotic pH ionizes local anesthetics, prevents placental transfer)
2. **Drug diffusion constant, which is increased by**
   A. Low molecular weight
   B. Low protein binding (only free drug crosses the placenta)
   C. High lipid solubility
   D. Low degree of ionization (only unionized drugs can cross the placenta)
3. **Anything altering placental perfusion** (aortocaval compression, hypovolemia, vasoconstrictors)

Factors affecting fetal drug concentration

1. Characteristics of fetal circulation: ~60% of umbilical vein blood passes through the liver as soon as it enters the fetus and is diluted with blood returning from the extremities. The remaining 40% of blood goes through the ductus venosus to the heart, where it's diluted by blood from the SVC and the coronary sinus. Once diluted, though, blood entering the heart via the ductus venosus is preferentially "streamed" across the foramen ovale, to the left heart and ultimately, the brain. Blood exiting the liver is further diluted in the heart in the same manner as blood arriving via the ductus venosus. Thus, very little of the blood entering the fetus ever gets to the brain or systemic circulation.
2. Metabolism: immature metabolic pathways can contribute to elevated drug levels.
3. Fetal protein binding: low protein binding capacity can lead to high free drug levels.
4. Fetal pH: local anesthetics can ionize in acidotic fetus, get "trapped," and cause high levels. 2-Chlorprocaine is the drug of choice for epidural with fetal distress due to short $t_{1/2}$.

Drugs that don't cross the placenta to a significant degree

1. Neuromuscular blockers (ionized and not lipid soluble)
2. Heparin

3. Insulin
4. Trimethephan

One drug they like to ask about is maternal-fetal distribution of bupivicaine

Compared to lidocaine, bupivicaine transfer to fetus is limited due to high protein binding and high pKa. However, over time the fetal concentration of FREE drug will equilibrate with mother. (So there's less *total* drug than mom, but equal amount of *active* drug).

Another favorite is the maternal-fetal distribution of thiopental

Maternal thiopental redistributes quickly, so very little gets delivered to the placenta. Because thiopental is very lipid soluble, virtually all of the drug delivered to the placenta rapidly crosses. Once across, though, it undergoes a first pass through the liver. The small amount that goes through the ductus venosus is quickly redistributed, so the baby never attains a high brain concentration.

Factors favoring placental oxygen transfer

Besides the things governing placental perfusion

1. Maternal oxyhemoglobin curve shifts right, favors unloading of O_2 to fetus
2. Increased maternal cardiac output and thus, increased O_2 delivery
3. Fetal oxyhemoglobin curve shifts left, favors picking up O_2
4. High fetal hematocrit increases O_2-carrying capacity

Sample questions

A = 1, 2, 3   B = 1, 3   C = 2, 4   D = 4 only   E = all are correct

1. Factors altering the fetal brain level of anesthetic agents administered to the mother include
    1. Blood flow patterns within the fetal heart
    2. The amount of umbilical venous blood flow to the fetal liver
    3. Fetal pH
    4. Placental metabolism

2. Fetal asphyxia can be worsened by
    1. The presence of maternal diabetes mellitus
    2. Maternal hypocarbia
    3. Maternal hypotension
    4. The use of α-adrenergic agonists

Single best answer

3. When a drug is administered IV to a parturient with normal uteroplacental blood flow, all the following are true except
    1. The drug perfuses the fetal liver prior to the fetal heart
    2. The primary mechanism for immediately lowering fetal drug levels is fetal hepatic metabolism
    3. Fetal protein binding is less than maternal protein binding
    4. Maternal arterial concentration is greater than umbilical artery concentration
    5. Umbilical venous concentration exceeds umbilical artery concentration

Answers: 1. A   2. E   3. 2

Chapter 56

Labor Analgesia

First stage of labor: Pain due to uterine contractions and cervical dilation. Pathways: visceral afferents run with sympathetic fibers at T10-L1.

Second stage of labor: Pain due to uterine contractions and perineal stretching. Pathways: S2–S4.

Systemic medications

1. Narcotics: best systemic pain relievers, but degree of relief limited by risk of respiratory depression
   A. Morphine: peak $1\frac{1}{2}$ hr after IM dose, lasts ~5 hr, causes the most neonatal respiratory depression
   B. Meperidine: peak 1 hr after IM dose, lasts ~4 hr, neonates born <1 hr or > 4 hr after dose aren't at risk of respiratory depression
   C. Fentanyl: peak 5 min after IV dose, lasts ~1 hr, little risk of accumulation in neonate
   D. Butorphanol, Nalbuphine: respiratory depression < morphine at large doses, but causes neonatal behavioral and cardiac changes
2. Phenothiazines: poor analgesics, good sedatives, also are antiemetics, commonly use promethazine (phenergan) and prochlorperazine (compazine)
3. Benzodiazepines: poor analgesics, good sedatives, all cause neonatal depression. Depression due to diazepam = lorazepam > midazolam

Regional analgesia

1. Paracervical block: effective for first stage of labor only. Disadvantages: high risk of fetal bradycardia, causes highest maternal serum levels of all the techniques.
2. Lumbar epidural: effective for first and second stage of labor, may be given by bolus or infusion, avoids risk of respiratory depression. Disadvantages: motor block, hypotension, risk of intravascular or intrathecal injection.
3. Epidural narcotics: effective for first and second stage of labor, combination with local anesthetics improves analgesia. Disadvantages: risk of maternal and fetal respiratory depression. Efficacy of fentanyl > meperidine > morphine. Complication rate morphine > mepereidine > fentanyl.
4. Intrathecal narcotics: effective for first stage and uncomplicated second stage no fetal respiratory depression. Disadvantages: inadequate for

episiotomy repair or forceps delivery. Same type and severity complications as systemic opioids.

Local anesthetics commonly used in obstetrics

1. Lidocaine: short acting, low risk of cardiotoxicity, more likely to have "ion trapping" in the short term due to low protein binding (high degree of placental transfer).
2. Bupivicaine: long acting, minimal motor block, high degree of protein binding limits placental transfer in the short term, but fetal/maternal equilibration of unbound drug concentration occurs with continuous infusions, and because of high pKa, bupivicaine is more prone to be "trapped."
3. Chlorprocaine: very brief action, minimal placental transfer due to rapid ester hydrolysis.

Sample questions

A = 1, 2, 3   B = 1, 3   C = 2, 4   D = 4 only   E = all are correct

1. The addition of epinephrine to subarachnoid narcotics for labor analgesia
   1. Prolongs the duration of analgesia
   2. Increases the incidence of nausea and vomiting
   3. Is a marker for intravascular injection
   4. Decreases the incidence of pruritis

Single best answer

2. To prevent pain during presentation of the fetal head, a nerve block must include at least
   1. T4-T12
   2. T12-S5
   3. T8-L2
   4. S2-S4
   5. T10-L1

3. Which of the following directly produces excessive fetal levels of lidocaine due to a labor epidural?
   1. Fetal acidosis
   2. Maternal acidosis
   3. Maternal sepsis
   4. Abruptio placenta
   5. Aortocaval compression

Answers: 1. C   2. 4   3. 1

Anesthesia for Cesarean Section

Available techniques: Regional anesthesia (spinal or epidural anesthesia), general anesthesia

Considerations with regional anesthesia

1. Risk for aspiration pneumonia . . . pretreat with nonparticulate antacid
2. Maintain left uterine displacement
3. Prehydrate with 1–2 L crystalloid to prevent hypotension from sympathectomy
4. Need ≥ T4 sensory level
5. Additives
   A. 1:200,000 epinephrine prolongs block and increases analgesia
   B. Sodium bicarbonate speeds onset (1 mEq/10 mL lidocaine or chlorprocaine, 0.1 mEq/10 mL bupivicaine)

Specific considerations for spinal

Onset	Fast, may cause more hypotension than epidural
Agents	~70 mg lidocaine, 7–10 mg tetracaine, 8–12 mg bupivicaine, all hyperbaric
Additives	Fentanyl 6.25 µg or morphine 0.1 mg
Complications	Same as any other spinal (high level, failed block, hypotension, headache)

Specific considerations for epidural

Onset	Slow, but may reduce risk of hypotension
Agents	15–25 mL 2% lidocaine (best for nonurgent cases), 3% 2-chlorprocaine (best for fetal distress because little risk of achieving high fetal levels), 0.5% bupivicaine
Additives	Fentanyl 50 µg or morphine 5 mg

Contraindications to regional

1. Tocolytic therapy
2. Severe maternal hypertension   } relative contraindications due to risk
3. Morbid obesity   } of hypotension
4. Hypovolemia
5. Coagulopathy
6. Sepsis

Considerations for general anesthesia

1. Risk of aspiration pneumonia
2. Risk of airway difficulties
3. Risk of hypotension (less than regional)
4. Risk of neonatal depression from anesthetic agents (more on this later)

Management of general anesthesia for cesarean section

1. Preoperative antacid
2. Adequate IV access
3. Left uterine displacement
4. Preoxygenate during surgical prep and drape
5. Rapid-sequence induction with cricoid pressure, succinylcholine 1.5 mg/kg, and either thiopental 4 mg/kg or ketamine 1 mg/kg
6. 50:50 $N_2O:O_2$ and ½ MAC agent until delivery, then change to 70:30 $N_2O:O_2$

Effects of anesthetic agents on mother and fetus

1. Thiopental: readily crosses placenta, quickly cleared or diluted by fetal liver, no advantage to delaying delivery after induction
2. Ketamine: risk of maternal hypertension, uterine rupture and hallucinations, crosses the placenta but no neonatal depression if dose ≤ 1 mg/kg
3. Propofol: risk of hypotension similar to thiopental
4. N_2O: crosses readily, fetal levels equilibrate with mom with prolonged exposure, so you should limit exposure by keeping at 50% and keep time from induction to delivery ≤ 15 min
5. Volatile agents: decrease uterine tone, but uterus retains responsiveness to pitocin
6. Locals: potential for fetal cardiac/CNS toxicity if prolonged exposure, high drug doses (epidurals), or acidotic fetus

Sample questions

Single best answer

1. A woman is undergoing cesarean section due to failure to progress. Rapid-sequence induction of general anesthesia is with thiopental 200 mg IV, succinylcholine 120 mg IV, nitrous oxide 70%, F_iO_2 0.3. Twenty-five minutes after induction, the infant is delivered with a 1-min Apgar of 6. The most likely cause of the abnormal Apgar is
   1. Neonatal pseudocholinesterase deficiency
   2. High serum thiopental levels
   3. High serum nitrous oxide levels
   4. Utero-placental insufficiency due to prolonged time to delivery
   5. Hypocalcemia

2. A 85-kg female is undergoing cesarean section for double footling breech. General anesthesia is induced with 250 mg thiopental and 130 mg succinylcholine and is maintained with nitrous oxide:oxygen (5 L/min:5 L/min) with a respiratory rate of 14, tidal volume 1400 mL. The infant is delivered 5 min after induction with an Apgar score of 5 at 1 min. The most likely cause of the low score is
   1. High serum thiopental levels
   2. High serum succinylcholine levels
   3. Placental hypoperfusion

4. High serum nitrous oxide levels
5. Cord compression by fetal presenting parts

3. A woman is undergoing cesarean section after failure of terbutaline to suppress preterm labor. Epidural anesthesia to a T4 level is established with 18 mL 2% lidocaine with epinephrine 1:200,000 after preloading her with 2000 mL lactated Ringer's. Just after incision, her blood pressure is 88/44 mmHg, which is treated with 500 mL crystalloid. Blood pressure is 105/72 mmHg, pulse 110/min, pulse oximeter 96%. She becomes agitated and restless. The most likely cause of her behavior is
   1. Excessively high epidural level
   2. Acute pulmonary edema
   3. Local anesthetic toxicity
   4. Hypoperfusion of the central nervous system
   5. High serum levels of terbutaline

Answers: 1. 3   2. 3   3. 2

Anesthesia for Breech Delivery

(who is Frank, anyway?)

Patient population: More common with premature infants

Anesthetic techniques for vaginal delivery of breech

1. Epidural: excellent perineal muscle relaxation, level can be extended if emergent caesarean section required
2. Spinal
3. Caudal
4. Narcotics, sedatives during labor and pudendal block at the time of delivery

Anesthetic techniques for caesarean section of breech delivery

1. Epidural
2. Spinal
3. General

Complications unique to breech delivery

1. Difficulty extracting infant due to uterine hypertonus or "tangled" presenting parts can occur with vaginal or caesarean delivery.
   Treatment: emergent general anesthesia with inhaled agents or IV nitroglycerin to relax uterus.
2. Head entrapment: seen with vaginal delivery, especially preemies.
   Treatment: IV nitroglycerin or emergent general anesthesia with inhaled agents to relax uterus
3. Cord prolapse: lower uterine segment isn't filled with baby, so cord can become the presenting part.

Sample question

Single best answer

1. A gravid female is in active labor with a term, frank breech fetus. She declines an epidural, instead receiving meperidine 12.5 mg IV 90 min prior to delivery. Variable decelerations are noted during placement of pudendal block with 20 mL 1% lidocaine with 1:100,000 epinephrine. Two minutes later, late decelerations are noted with a fetal heart rate 60/min not

recovering between contractions. Rapid-sequence induction is performed with thiopental 200 mg IV and succinylcholine 100 mg IV. The infant is delivered within 5 min with Apgars of 2 and 4. The most likely cause of the low Apgar is

1. High infant meperidine levels
2. Local anesthetic toxicity
3. Utero-placental insufficiency due to cord compression
4. Utero-placental insufficiency due to epinephrine in local anesthetic solution
5. High infant thiopental level

Answer: 1. 3

CHAPTER 59

The Bleeding Parturient

There are three main causes of antepartum hemorrhage

1. Placenta previa: presents with painless bleeding, risk of massive hemorrhage
2. Abruptio placentae: presents with painful bleeding, risk of massive hemorrhage, DIC, uterine irritability
3. Uterine rupture: presents with severe abdominal pain, risk of massive hemorrhage

Anesthetic management of placenta previa

1. ALWAYS be prepared for emergent C-section and have large-bore IV access established
2. For vaginal delivery or nonemergent C-section: regional okay, but beware of sympathectomy if massive bleeding occurs
3. For emergent C-section: general anesthesia, induce with drugs that maintain hemodynamic stability

Anesthetic management of placental abruption

1. Check coagulation studies (abruption is most common cause of coagulopathy during pregnancy)
2. If abruption is small, hemodynamically stable and no coagulopathy: regional and vaginal delivery
3. If abruption is severe, with massive bleeding and/or fetal distress: general anesthesia, replace blood and coagulation factors, emergent C-section

Anesthetic management of uterine rupture

1. Always requires emergent C-section and general anesthesia (sympathectomy would be dumb)
2. Beware of risk of uterine rupture in laboring patient with prior uterine surgery . . . be suspicious if she has an epidural and develops fetal distress, uterine irritability, or explained hypotension

Causes of postpartum bleeding

1. Lacerations (wahoo)
2. Retained placenta
3. Uterine atony: treatment includes
   A. Uterine massage

B. Oxytocin IV (causes hypotension, tachycardia, dysrythmias, H$_2$O intoxication, and uterine rupture)
C. Methergen IV (causes hypertension)
D. Prostaglandin F2α (causes bronchospasm, HTN)
E. Drugs that can reduce uterine contractility
    –magnesium
    –β-blockers
    –Ca^{++} channel blockers
    –indomethacin
    –halothane, isoflurane, enflurane
    –epinephrine (low dose)
4. Uterine inversion: treatment includes
    A. Resuscitation
    B. Relax uterus (volatile agents, nitroglycerin)
    C. Reduce inversion

Anesthetic management for retained placenta

They'll always ask you about anesthetic management for retained placenta: requires uterine relaxation (so avoid ketamine) and manual extraction of placenta (ouch!)

1. If surgical spinal or epidural already in place, use that.
2. Inhalational analgesia
3. General anesthesia with endotracheal intubation (improves uterine relaxation)
4. IV nitroglycerin (~50 μg IV)

Sample questions

Single best answer

1. A parturient with a small placental abruption documented by ultrasound has normal prothrombin time, partial thromboplastin time, and bleeding times, pulse 82/min, blood pressure 136/77 mmHg. After an uneventful test dose and negative aspiration of CSF, her lumbar epidural is dosed with 12 mL of 0.25% bupivicaine with epinephrine 1:200,000, resulting in a T8 sensory level. Twenty minutes later, she assumes the lithotomy position with left uterine displacement for vaginal delivery and complains of lightheadedness, feeling her heart racing, and nausea. Blood pressure is 65/45 mmHg, pulse 115/min. The most likely cause of these symptoms is
    1. Aortocaval compression
    2. Excessive sympathetic blockade
    3. Local anesthetic toxicity
    4. Acute extension of the abruption
    5. High serum epinephrine levels

2. Same patient. Same scenario. Initial management should be
    1. Remove her legs from the stirrups
    2. Bolus 1000 mL lactated ringer's
    3. Ephedrine 10 mg IV
    4. Esmolol 10 mg IV
    5. Place patient on her hands and knees

Answers: **1. 4   2. 2**

CHAPTER 60

Pre-Eclampsia/Eclampsia

Findings required for diagnosis

See Table 60–1.

• **Table 60–1**

	Mild-Moderate	Severe
Hypertension	Systolic ≥ 140 mmHg OR 30 mmHg > normal Diastolic ≥ 90 mmHg OR 15 mmHg > normal	Systolic ≥ 160 mmHg Diastolic ≥ 110 mmHg
Proteinuria	< 5 g/24 hr	5 g/24 hr
Generalized edema		

The addition of seizures to the above symptoms characterizes eclampsia.

Pathophysiology of pre-eclampsia

Decreased placental perfusion (mechanism unknown)
↓
Imbalance of prostaglandin and thromboxane
↓
Total body vasoconstriction → Hypertension, CHF
↙   ↓   ↘
Intravascular depletion despite   Decreased RBF, GFR, UOP   ↑ uterine vascular
total body Na⁺, H₂O retention   and glomerular fibrin deposits   resistance
↓   ↓   ↓
Decreased utero-placental   Proteinuria, oliguria   Utero-placental
perfusion   insufficiency

Figure 60–1.

Treatment of pre-eclampsia

1. Delivery of fetus is curative
2. Magnesium sulfate (seizure prophylaxis)
3. Antihypertensives (hydralazine, nitroprusside, etc.)

Effects of magnesium in mother

4–6 mEq/L therapeutic range	→ 5–10 mEq/L Prolonged PR, widened QRS	→ 10 mEq/L Depressed tendon reflexes	→ 15 mEq/L SA, AV node block, respiratory paralysis	→ 25 mEq/L Cardiac arrest

Side effects of magnesium and drug interactions

1. ↓ acetylcholine release
2. ↓ sensitivity of motor endplate to acetylcholine

  } ↑ sensitivity to depolarizing and nondepolarizing drugs

3. Placental transfer, causing poor neonatal muscle tone and respiratory depression
4. ↓ uterine contractility

Effects of pre-eclampsia on the different organ systems

1. CNS: visual disturbances, cerebral hemorrhage, seizures (eclampsia)
2. Airway: edema (avoid intubation if possible)
3. Pulmonary: edema (biggest risk is postpartum)
4. CVS: CHF, elevated systolic, diastolic and mean blood pressure, elevated SVR, mild tachycardia, decreased wedge pressure and cardiac index
5. Renal: decreased RBF, GFR, UOP, fibrin deposits leading to proteinuria
6. Liver: subcapsular bleeding, hepatic rupture, elevated SGOT, LDH, alk phos, coagulopathy, DIC

Anesthetic management

1. Epidural is method of choice for labor—may decrease catecholamine release and help contol BP. Remember high risk of hypotension if sympathectomy occurs
2. Avoid general if possible, big risk of airway complications

Sample questions

A = 1, 2, 3   B = 1, 3   C = 2, 4   D = 4 only   E = all are correct

1. Treatment of pre-eclampsia with magnesium is associated with decreased
   1. Dose requirement of succinylcholine
   2. Excitability of the muscle membrane
   3. Dose requirement of vecuronium
   4. Uterine contractility

Single best answer

2. A 22-year-old, 80-kg patient in active labor has a lumbar epidural and is having a C-section for late decelerations. Her labs show urine protein 4 g/dL over 24 hr, blood pressure 166/128 mmHg, and she complains of blurred vision and epigastric pain. The epidural is dosed with 15 mL 0.5% bupivicaine, but she complains of pain at incision and has a T11 sensory block. General anesthesia is induced with etomidate 8 mg, succinylcholine 120 mg, curare 3 mg and maintained with nitrous oxide, F_iO_2 0.5, and enflurane 1%. At induction, she develops myoclonic activity. The most likely cause is

60 ■ Pre-Eclampsia/Eclampsia

      1. Progression from pre-eclampsia to eclampsia
      2. Etomidate
      3. Enflurane
      4. Local anesthetic toxicity
      5. Succinylcholine

3. Same patient, same drugs. At emergence, she exhibits myoclonus. The most likely cause is
      1. Progression of pre-eclampsia to eclampsia
      2. Etomidate
      3. Enflurane
      4. Local anesthetic toxicity
      5. Intracranial hemorrhage

Answers: 1. E   2. 2   3. 1

CHAPTER 61

Tocolytic Therapy

Indications: Preterm labor

Agents used

1. β_2-agonists (terbutaline, ritodrine) **most common agents**
2. Magnesium sulfate
3. Prostaglandin inhibitors
4. Calcium channel blockers

Effects of β_2-agonist therapy

1. Decreased uterine contractility
2. Vasodilation
3. Bronchodilation
4. Release of antidiuretic hormone (ADH)

Side effects of tocolysis

1. Pulmonary edema
   A. Etiology: unknown (cardiogenic vs. noncardiogenic)
   B. Risk factors for:
      – Preexisting cardiac disease
      – Multiple gestation
      – Fluid overload
      – Tachycardia
      – Chorioamnionitis
2. Hypotension
3. Hypokalemia
4. Hyperglycemia
5. Metabolic acidosis
6. Fetal tachycardia and hypoglycemia

} Maternal side effects

Sample questions

A = 1, 2, 3   B = 1, 3   C = 2, 4   D = 4 only   E = all are correct

1. After a failed trial of magnesium sulfate, ritodrine, and verapamil for suppression of preterm labor, delivery of 35-week-gestation twins by cesarean section is performed under epidural anesthesia with 20 mL 0.5%

bupivicaine. After delivery, the mother has persistent uterine atony. Possible causes include
1. Magnesium sulfate
2. Verapamil
3. Large uterine size
4. Ritodrine

2. Same mother, blood pressure is 95/65 mmHg throughout procedure, despite ephedrine given in 5-mg IV aliquots. At delivery, both infants have irregular respiration, poor tone, and heart rates less than 100/min. Possible contributing factors include
1. Magnesium sulfate
2. Local anesthetic toxicity
3. Prematurity
4. Metabolic acidosis due to maternal hypotension

Answers: 1. E 2. E

CHAPTER 62

Anesthesia for Nonobstetric Surgery during the First Trimester

Common surgical procedures (anything, really)

1. Ovarian cystectomy: most common
2. Appendectomy: second most common

Anesthetic goals

1. Avoid teratogens: no anesthetic agent ever proven to be teratogenic in humans, but nitrous is often implicated (remember organogenesis is 15 days–2 mo).
2. Avoid fetal hypoxia and acidosis by preventing maternal hypercarbia, hypoxia, and hypotension.
3. Prevent preterm labor.

Anesthetic technique

1. Observe full stomach precautions.
2. Maintain left uterine displacement.
3. Fetal heart monitoring after 16 weeks' gestation.
4. Any technique is fine as long as you maintain utero-placental perfusion and oxygenation. Regional may be best, since it avoids maternal risk of aspiration.

Sample question

A = 1, 2, 3   B = 1, 3   C = 2, 4   D = 4 only   E = all are correct

1. A 25-year-old primigravida is having placement of a cervical cerclage at 24 weeks' gestation. You should tell her
   1. There is a risk that her baby may be malformed due to the anesthesia
   2. A paracervical block will pose less risk of fetal cardiotoxicity than a spinal
   3. That prophylactic terbutaline is indicated
   4. That she may go into premature labor, no matter what anesthetic technique is used

Answer: 1. D

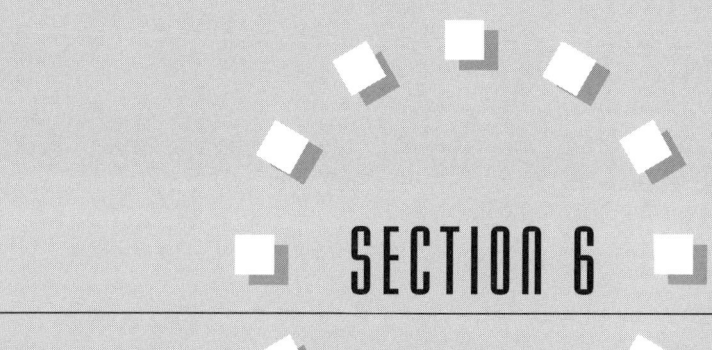

SECTION 6

Regional Anesthesia and Pain Management

Local Anesthetics

Structure: Weakly basic, hydrophilic tertiary amines linked via an ester or amide intermediate chain to a lipophilic aromatic ring

Figure 63–1. From Barash PG, Cullen BF, Stoelting RK. Clinical Anesthesia, ed 2. Philadelphia: Lippincott, 1992, p. 510. Reprinted with permission.

Activity

These weak bases are poorly water soluble; thus, they are manufactured as water-soluble salts. They ionize when placed in aqueous solution, forming a charged, quaternary amine that is at equilibrium with the uncharged tertiary amine (free-base form). The pH at which this equilibrium is attained is the pKa.

Translation: As environmental pH decreases, the amount of ionized drug increases. As environmental pH increases, the amount of ionized drug decreases.

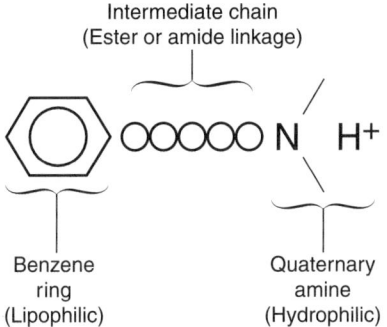

Figure 63–2. From Barash PG, Cullen BF, Stoelting RK. Clinical Anesthesia, ed 2. Philadelphia: Lippincott, 1992, p. 510. Reprinted with permission.

Mechanism of action

1. Axon is penetrated by nonionized free base, which dissociates to the cation form, the degree of dissociation being dictated by the drug pKa and tissue pH.

2. Cation form binds to receptor site within Na+ channel, blocking depolarization-induced influx of Na+ and propagation of nerve impulse.
3. Binding is dependent on the state of the Na+ channel:

   A. Open
   B. Inactive (partially open)
   } Phasic blockade, more intense and longer-lasting than tonic blockade, promoted by repetitive stimulation of the nerve

   C. Resting (closed): tonic blockade, not influenced by repeated stimulation of nerve

Translation: during phasic blockade, most channels are in the open state, exposing more receptor sites. Therefore, lots of binding occurs and lasts a long time because drug dissociation is slower from activated channels than from resting channels.

Comparison of local anesthetics

- **Table 63–1**

Characteristic	Esters		Amides	
1. pKa	≥8 (more basic)		≤8 (less basic)	
2. Stability in solution	Unstable		Stable	
3. Metabolism	Pseudocholinesterase		Hepatic degradation	
4. Significant metabolites	Para-amino benzoic acid (PABA)		None	
5. Allergenicity	Common		Rare	
6. Clinically employed agents and their pKa	Tetracaine	8.4	Mepivicaine	7.7
	Procaine	8.9	Lidocaine	7.8
	2-chlorprocaine	9.1	Etidocaine	7.9
			Prilocaine	8.0
			Bupivicaine	8.1

Factors determining the speed of onset

1. **pKa:** since nonionized form is more membrane-permeant, drugs with low pKa (closer to physiologic pH) have a faster onset. Altered by environment (pKa is lower *in vitro* than it is in solution)
2. **Lipid solubility:** the more lipid soluble the drug, the faster it penetrates the nerve
3. Alkalinization: add HCO_3^- to solution to raise pH, promoting the nonionized (permeable) form
4. Dose and concentration: high concentrations and total doses expose more drug to the nerve
5. How rapidly drug arrives at nerve: subarachnoid injection (immediate contact with nerve) has faster onset than brachial plexus (has to diffuse some distance to nerve)
6. Absence of neural sheath: speeds onset

Factors determining the duration of action

1. **Protein binding:** Na+ channel receptor site is a protein; thus, drugs with high protein binding have longer duration
2. Vascular effects: at clinically used doses, all locals except cocaine cause vasodilation, increasing perfusion and removal of drug from site. Adding a vasoconstrictor (epinephrine) decreases this effect and prolongs duration
3. Site of injection: highly vascular sites have shorter duration, as explained

4. Baricity: isobaric mixtures last longer than hyperbaric
5. Lipid solubility: increased lipid solubility increases duration

Factors determining plasma concentration

1. Total dose
2. Site of injection: the more vascular the site, the higher the systemic absorption. Plasma concentrations are: intercostal > paracervical > caudal > epidural > brachial plexus > subarachnoid > subcutaneous.
3. Vasoconstrictors: effective with lidocaine and mepivicaine, regardless of site. Ineffective for bupivicaine and etidocaine for epidural, but effective for brachial plexus.
4. Vasodilation: bupivicaine > lidocaine.
5. Lipid solubility: more soluble drug penetrates nerve ∴ not available for systemic absorption.
6. Renal disease: all local metabolites are renally excreted.
7. Hepatic disease: decreased enzymatic degradation of amides, decreased pseudocholinesterase.
8. Concomitant drug therapy: any drug depressing hepatic or renal function decreases clearance.
9. Congestive heart failure: poor perfusion, thus poor clearance.

Differential nerve blockade

Blockade of functions is progressive, with sympathetic blockade first, then sensory, then motor. Some agents produce more intense blockade of one function over another (e.g., motor > sensory). It was originally thought that this differential blockade was due to variable susceptibility of nerve fibers to blockade, with susceptibility inversely related to size. However, we now know that large, myelinated "A" fibers (motor, some sensory function) are actually intrinsically **more** sensitive than small, unmyelinated "C" fibers (sensory). No single explanation of differential blockade is available, but factors causing this phenomenon include:

1. "C" fibers are blocked faster than "A" fibers (no myelin sheath, ∴ not dependent on pKa or lipid solubility of agent). However, in high concentrations, even hydrophilic agents produce rapid blockade of "A" fibers, because of the concentration gradient across neural membrane.
2. Differences in the number of nodes of Ranvier: must block three consecutive nodes to stop impulse propagation. Small "C" fibers have nodes clustered more closely, so they are easier to block.
3. Frequency-dependence: sensory fibers fire more rapidly than motor, thus, more Na^+ channels are in the open (blockable) state.
4. Geographic location: sensory fibers are the outermost fibers of the nerve bundle, more readily accessible to the agent.

Toxicity of local anesthetics

Three categories
1. Systemic toxicity
2. Tissue toxicity
3. Miscellaneous

In general, the more potent the agent, the more toxic it is.

Systemic toxicity

Central nervous system toxicity is more common than cardiovascular toxicity.

1. **Central nervous system toxicity**
   A. Occurs at lower doses than cardiovascular toxicity
   B. Signs and symptoms: dizziness, visual disturbances, tinnitus, disorientation, and seizures
   C. Factors affecting CNS toxicity:
      1. More potent = more toxic
      2. Rate of IV administration (fast rate = more toxic)
      3. Hypercarbia: ↓ seizure threshold/↑ cerebral blood flow, thereby increasing tissue concentration/↓ intracellular pH, promoting ion trapping/↓ protein binding
      4. Acidosis: ↓ seizure threshold (respiratory > metabolic 2° to concomitant ↑ in $PaCO_2$)
2. **Cardiovascular toxicity**
   A. Signs and symptoms are progressive: hypertension, tachycardia → myocardial depression and mild hypotension → severe hypotension, conduction defects, dysrythmias
   B. Mechanical effects: direct depression of myocardium and vascular smooth muscle
   C. Electrical effects:
      1. Depressed rapid rate of depolarization (blockade of fast Na^+ channels) in Purkinje fibers and myocardial fibers
      2. Decreased duration of action potential
      3. Decreased effective refractory period
      4. Prolonged PR interval, widened QRS
      5. Depressed SA node activity
      6. Blockade of slow Ca^{++} channels (only proposed for bupivicaine)
   D. Factors affecting cardiovascular toxicity:
      1. Characteristics of the agent: margin between dose causing cardiovascular collapse (CC) and CNS toxicity (CC/CNS ratio) varies with the agent. CC/CNS margins: lidocaine > etidocaine > bupivicaine
      2. Pregnancy: increased sensitivity to neural blockade and narrowed CC/CNS ratio
      3. Hypoxia, hypercarbia, acidosis (all increase incidence of toxicity)

Tissue toxicity

1. Concentration to produce toxicity greatly exceeds clinically required dose
2. Additives can be the culprit: sodium bisulfite (a neurotoxic antioxidant preservative) used to be in chlorprocaine, was replaced with EDTA (non-neurotoxic antioxidant)
3. Back spasm: seen with chlorprocaine, thought 2° to chelation of paraspinous muscle Ca^{++} by EDTA
4. Skeletal muscle changes: reversible

Miscellaneous toxicity

1. **Allergic reactions**
   A. More common with esters (2° to PABA), but true allergy extremely rare
   B. Multidose vials of amides contain the antimicrobial preservative methylparaben, structurally similar to PABA, implicated in some allergic reactions

C. Skin testing is of questionable value (local anesthetic:carrier molecule complex is required to precipitate reaction, and these complexes are not commercially available)
2. **Methemoglobinemia**
   A. Causes cyanosis, particularly in neonates
   B. Only seen with prilocaine, requires dose > 500 mg (huge)
   C. Prilocaine is metabolized to O-toluidine, which then oxidizes hemoglobin to methemoglobin.
   D. Cyanosis is delayed 4–8 hr after prilocaine dose 2° to required metabolism to O-toluidine
   E. Treatment: methylene blue 1–5 mg/kg IV *or* ascorbic acid 2 mg/kg IV *or* spontaneous recovery

Sample questions

A = 1, 2, 3   B = 1, 3   C = 2, 4   D = 4 only   E = all are correct

1. Mechanisms by which hypercarbia increases local anesthetic toxicity in the central nervous system include
   1. Increased cerebral blood flow
   2. Promotion of ion trapping
   3. Decreased protein binding
   4. A rightward shift of the oxyhemoglobin curve

2. The onset of local anesthetic effect is enhanced by
   1. Selection of a drug with a low pKa
   2. Injection into alkalotic tissues
   3. Carbonation of the drug
   4. Addition of phenylephrine

3. Allergic reactions to local anesthetics
   1. Are more common with esters than amides
   2. Can be elicited by the preservative methylparaben
   3. Are usually due to para-aminobenzoic acid
   4. Can readily be diagnosed with skin testing

4. True statements regarding differential nerve blockade by local anesthetics include
   1. *In vivo*, large, myelinated "A" fibers are more sensitive to blockade than small, unmyelinated "C" fibers
   2. Sensory blockade precedes motor blockade
   3. The frequency at which a nerve fiber depolarizes influences its susceptibility to blockade
   4. "C" fibers tend to be blocked first *in vitro*

5. During continuous epidural infusion for labor analgesia, the advantages of equi-anesthetic doses of etidocaine over bupivicaine include
   1. More rapid onset
   2. Less toxicity with inadvertent intravenous administration
   3. More rapid hepatic metabolism
   4. Less motor block

6. Tissue acid–base balance affects local anesthetic activity by influencing the
   1. State of "openness" of the sodium channels

2. Quantity of nonionized drug
3. Degree of binding of drug to extracellular receptors
4. Rate of metabolism of amides
5. Degree of protein binding of the drug

Answers: 1. A   2. A   3. A   4. E   5. A   6. B

CHAPTER 64

Spinal Anesthesia

Anatomy

1. Caudal extent of spinal cord: L1 in adults, L3 in infants
2. Caudal extent of subarachnoid space: S2 (all patients)
3. A line connecting the superior edge of the iliac crests intersects the L4-5 interspace

Approaches to the subarachnoid space

1. Midline
2. Paramedian
3. Taylor

Anatomic structures encountered with the midline approach:

Supraspinous ligament → Interspinous ligament → Ligamentum flavum → Epidural space → Dura mater → Subdural space → Arachnoid mater → Subarachnoid space

Anatomic structures encountered with paramedian approach: omits supraspinous and interspinous ligaments, all other structures are the same

- **Table 64–1**

Paramedian Approach	Taylor Approach
Technique 1. Insert needle 1 cm lateral and 1 cm inferior to spinous process superior to desired interspace 2. Angle needle medially ~15 degrees, advance until subarachnoid space is encountered	Technique 1. Insert needle 1 cm caudal and 1 cm medial to posterior superior iliac spine 2. Direct needle cephalad and medially 3. Enter subarachnoid space via L5-S1 interspace (the largest interspace)
Advantages over midline approach 1. Avoids calcified ligaments of elderly patients 2. Pathway has larger diameter 3. Not dependent on patient's ability to flex lumbar spine	Advantages over midline approach same as paramedian approach

Physiologic effects of spinal anesthesia

1. **Cardiovascular:** *blockade of preganglionic sympathetic fibers is responsible for all changes in hemodynamic parameters.* The degree of sympathectomy depends on the height of block, sympathetic blockade exceeds sensory block by ≥ 2 dermatomes (not seen with epidural), and it produces venodilation more than arterial dilation (thus, total peripheral resistance only minimally decreased). Changes in hemodynamic parameters seen with ≥ T4 level:
   A. ↓ venous return (2° to venodilation) → ↓ cardiac output → ↓ MAP → ↓ coronary artery blood flow
   B. Decreased pulse 2° to blockade of cardiac accelerators at T1-T4 (block ≤ T5 *increases* pulse)
2. **Respiratory**
   A. Inspiratory function preserved (phrenic blockade rare ∴ diaphragmatic function intact)
   B. Expiratory function is impaired (intercostal muscles blocked)
   C. Dyspnea is common, 2° to loss of afferent input from chest wall and abdomen
   D. Changes in pulmonary function parameters: ↓ vital capacity (minimal), ↓ expiratory reserve volume, ↓ peak expiratory flow rates, impaired cough

> **PEARL:** Hypotension resulting in hypoperfusion of the brain is the mechanism of respiratory arrest during high spinal. Respiratory arrest resolves with volume resuscitation and normalization of blood pressure.

3. **Renal:** Renal blood flow (RBF) is maintained if MAP remains ≥ 80 mmHg. A decrease in RBF leads to decreased glomerular filtration and urine output.
4. **Gastrointestinal**
   A. Hyperperistalsis (unopposed parasympathetic activity) → nausea, vomiting. Treat nausea with atropine (anticholinergic). Contracted gut may actually improve surgical conditions.
   B. ↓ hepatic blood flow 2° to ↓ MAP, but is more affected by surgical site.

● Table 64–2

Drugs Commonly Used for Spinal Anesthesia

	Duration in Minutes			Effect on Spinal Cord Blood Flow	
Drug	Plain	With epinephrine	With Phenylephrine	Plain	With a Vasoconstrictor
Lidocaine	60	75–100	75–100	↑	No effect
Tetracaine	90	120–150	≥150	↑	No effect
Bupivicaine	90	120–150	120–150	↓	↓

Effects of adding vasoconstrictors on duration of anesthesia in summary

1. Lidocaine: epinephrine = phenylephrine > plain
2. Bupivicaine: epinephrine = phenylephrine > plain (only slightly)
3. Tetracaine: phenylephrine > epinephrine > plain (epi only prolongs lumbar and sacral block)

Baricity

Compares the density of local anesthetic to that of cerebrospinal fluid (CSF)
1. Isobaric
   A. Density = CSF
   B. Tends to remain at site of injection
   C. Ways to make solution isobaric: mix equal volumes of local and either CSF or NaCl
2. Hypobaric
   A. Density < CSF
   B. "Floats" to highest point (L3-L4 in the supine patient)
   C. Ways to make solution hypobaric: mix equal volumes of local and sterile water OR: warm the undiluted local
3. Hyperbaric
   A. Density > CSF
   B. Sinks to the lowest point (T5-T6 in the supine patient)
   C. Ways to make solution hyperbaric: mix equal volumes of local and dextrose OR: cool the undiluted local

Factors affecting height of subarachnoid block

- Table 64–3

Major Effect	Minor Effect	No Effect
1. Dose	1. Age	1. Height
2. Density (baricity)	2. Shape of spinal canal	2. Weight
3. Position of patient	3. Technique of injection	3. Gender
	4. Characteristics of CSF	4. Vasoconstrictors
	5. Temperature of local	5. Barbotage/rate of injection

Complications of subarachnoid block

1. **Hypotension**
   A. Cause: vasodilation (venous > arterial) and decreased venous return
   B. Management: prehydration as a preventative. Vasoconstrictors (ephedrine better than phenylephrine because it also boosts heart rate)
2. **Headache**
   A. Cause: continued loss of CSF through puncture site
   B. Increased incidence with:
      1. Females
      2. Parturients
      3. Age < 50 years
      4. Large needle
      5. Needle bevel perpendicular to dural fibers
      6. Cutting-type bevel
      7. Midline approach
      8. Dextrose-containing solutions
   C. Features: frontal or occipital location; worse with erect posture, improves with recumbency; associated with tinnitus/photophobia
   D. Treatment:
      1. Analgesics/bedrest/hydration
      2. Epidural blood patch
      3. Caffeine IV or PO
3. **High spinal**
   A. At risk: parturients in particular
   B. Symptoms: agitation/nausea/vomiting/hypotension

C. Treatment:
   1. Oxygen
   2. Fluids
   3. Trendelenburg (↑ venous return without significantly raising level of block further)
   4. Vasoconstrictors (ephedrine > phenylephrine)
   5. Intubate if necessary (but cervical blockade recedes quickly)
4. **Nausea/vomiting:** causes:
   A. Hypotension/cerebral hypoxia
   B. Hyperperistalsis (unopposed parasympathetic activity)
   C. Concurrent medications
   D. Surgical manipulation
5. **Backache:** proposed causes:
   A. Muscle spasm
   B. Ligamentous strain
   C. Hematoma
6. **Major neurologic injury** (extremely rare): Causes:
   A. Needle trauma (risk increases with repeated attempts)
   B. Contaminated injectate
   C. Chemical toxicity of injectate (remember sodium bisulfite?)
   D. Spinal cord ischemia

Sample questions

A = 1, 2, 3   B = 1, 3   C = 2, 4   D = 4 only   E = all are correct

1. In adults, structures that are caudad to a line drawn between the superior edge of the iliac crests are
   1. The termination of the spinal cord
   2. The spinous process of L2
   3. The L2-3 interspace
   4. The termination of the dural sac

2. An otherwise healthy 35-year-old patient receives a spinal anesthetic with a T4 sensory block. His mean arterial pressure decreases from 100 mmHg to 75 mmHg. You would expect this to cause a decrease in
   1. Cerebral blood flow
   2. Coronary artery blood flow
   3. Glomerular filtration rate
   4. Hepatic blood flow

Single best answer

3. Spinal anesthesia with a T2 sensory block causes
   1. Decreased closing volume
   2. Decreased expiratory reserve volume
   3. Decreased minute ventilation
   4. Decreased expiratory flow rates

4. A 67-year-old man receives a subarachnoid block with 80 mg of hyperbaric lidocaine in dextrose for a cystoscopy and placement of ureteral stents. He has a history of hypertension and angina controlled with nifedipine and sublingual nitroglycerin. Shortly after the spinal is initiated, his blood pressure drops from 145/82 mmHg to 65/45 mmHg and his pulse increases from 80/min to 115/min. He is diaphoretic, complains of chest pain and of having difficulty breathing. After administer-

ing oxygen by face mask, the most appropriate next step in correcting this situation is
1. Administer sublingual nitroglycerin
2. Administer 1000 mL lactated Ringer's solution IV
3. Place the patient in trendelenburg position
4. Give 100 μg phenylephrine IV
5. Give 5 mg ephedrine IV

5. A 22-year-old parturient receives a subarachnoid block with 75 mg hyperbaric lidocaine in dextrose for a caesarean section. She has received 1000 mL lactated Ringer's IV and left uterine displacement is initiated. Despite this, her blood pressure decreases from 118/77 mmHg to 78/55 mmHg. The most appropriate therapy at this time is
1. Lactated Ringer's 500 mL IV
2. Phenylephrine 50 μg IV
3. Ephedrine 7.5 mg IV
4. Head down tilt at ~20°
5. Place her on "all fours" (hands and knees)

Answers: 1. D   2. C   3. 3   4. 2   5. 1

CHAPTER 65

Epidural Anesthesia

Anatomy

1. Caudal extent of epidural space: S2
2. Cephalad extent of epidural space: foramen magnum
3. Epidural space bound by: dura mater and ligamentum flavum

Techniques for identifying epidural space

1. Loss of resistance with air- or saline-filled syringe
2. "Hanging drop" technique (fluid gets sucked into subatmospheric epidural space)

Onset of drugs

1. Sensory block occurs first, then sympathetic, then motor (compare this to spinals)
2. Chlorprocaine ~10 min, bupivicaine ~20 min, all other drugs onset is ~15 min

- Table 65–1

	Average Duration of Epidural Agents (min)				
	Bupivicaine 0.5%	Etidocaine 1%	Mepivicaine 2%	Lidocaine 2%	2-chlorprocaine 3%
Plain	200	150	110	100	50
Epinephrine	210	190	170	150	70

Mechanism of action of epidural local anesthetics

1. Blockade of dorsal and ventral spinal *roots* (surrounded by thin dura, easy to diffuse through)
2. Spinal *cord* blockade (minor effect). Caveats: sacral "sparing" common, due to thick size of sacral nerve roots regression of block is from cephalad to caudad (like spinal) differential block easier to achieve than with spinal

Physiologic effects of epidural anesthesia

1. **Cardiovascular:** *blockade of preganglionic sympathetic fibers is primarily responsible for the changes in hemodynamic parameters (like spinals). However,*

systemic absorption is higher than with spinals (2° to large volume of local), and some hemodynamic changes may be due to intrinsic vasodilation and cardiac depressant effects of the local. Sympathetic level doesn't exceed sensory level (unlike spinal) and venodilation > arterial dilation (same as spinal).

Changes seen in hemodynamic parameters with ≥ T4 level:
A. Venodilation → ↓ venous return → ↓ CVP and cardiac output (especially if flow is obstructed by gravid uterus)
B. Arterial dilation → ↓ total peripheral resistance → ↓ mean arterial pressure
C. Decreased pulse 2° to blockade of cardiac accelerators at T1–4 (block ≤ T5 *increases* pulse)

Greater degree of hypotension seen with:
A. Hypovolemic patients
B. Lipophilic drugs (better penetration and faster onset of sympathectomy)
C. Epinephrine-containing solutions (is a β_2 agonist, causes vasodilation that's not offset by β_1 activity)

PEARL: When epinephrine-containing solutions are used, *early* hypotension is due to epinephrine β_2 agonism and *late* hypotension is due to sympathectomy and intrinsic vasodilation and cardiac depressant effects of local.

2. **Respiratory effects:** extremely rare
3. **GI effects:** unopposed parasympathetic activity increases gut motility

Factors influencing quality of epidural block

1. Volume:
   A. In general, more volume = higher level (but relationship not linear)
   B. At equal volumes, there's greater spread with thoracic injection vs. lumbar
2. Mass:
   A. In general, same mass = same effect (i.e., 20 mL 1% lidocaine = 10 mL 2% lidocaine)
   B. Is most important determinant of *quality* of block
   C. If volume is held constant and concentration is increased, you get faster onset, denser block, longer duration
3. Vasoconstrictors:
   A. Increase duration of all drugs, and epinephrine is better than phenylephrine
   B. More pronounced effect with lower concentrations of bupivicaine than higher (because at low concentrations, bupivicaine has less intrinsic vasoconstriction)
4. Site of injection:
   A. At equal volumes, there is greater spread with thoracic vs. lumbar injection
   B. Compared to thoracic injection, lumbosacral injection causes greater cephalad spread (because epidural space is smaller here, so drug must spread cephalad)
5. Patient factors:
   A. Parturients are more sensitive to locals than nonparturients
   B. Age, height, patient position have no effect on quality of block

Test doses

1. Purpose: to rule out subarachnoid or intravascular injection
2. Volume and agents: ~4 mL 1.5% lidocaine with 1:200,000 epinephrine
3. If subarachnoid: is an adequate volume to give unequivocal block
4. If intravascular: will produce tachycardia (although lack of tachycardia doesn't rule it out)

Complications of epidural blockade

1. Intravascular injection:
    A. Usually due to injection into an epidural vein
    B. Can occur despite the absence of blood during aspiration test
    C. Systemic toxicity same as that outlined in section on local anesthetics
2. Subarachnoid injection:
    A. Can occur despite the absence of CSF during aspiration test
    B. Produces rapid onset of profound motor and sensory block, hypotension, bradycardia, respiratory depression, and possible pupillary dilation if level extremely high
    C. Support airway and volume resuscitate PRN, sedation not usually required
3. Subdural injection: takes ~15–30 min to "set up"; results in a higher than expected level
4. Neurologic injury: EXTREMELY RARE. Possible causes:
    A. Trauma
    B. Anterior spinal artery thrombosis: rapid onset, painless, flaccid paralysis
    C. Adhesive arachnoiditis: follows painful injection of chemical irritant
    D. Hematoma: rapid-onset backache, progressive loss of function, no change in WBC
    E. Abscess: slow onset (days) of backache, progressive loss of function, ↑ WBC
5. Systemic toxicity
    A. Is usually due to inadvertent intravascular injection (toxicity due to systemic absorption is extremely rare)
    B. CNS toxicity more likely than cardiovascular
    C. Fractionated, slow injection minimizes risk
6. Dural puncture
    A. Factors increasing risk of headache are same as those following intentional dural puncture
    B. Conservative management is indicated . . . prophylactic blood patch not indicated

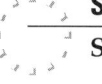

Sample questions

Single best answer

1. During removal, the tip of a lumbar epidural catheter breaks off, remaining in the patient. The most appropriate course of action is
    1. Leave the tip in and initiate broad spectrum antibiotics
    2. Urgent surgical removal of the catheter tip
    3. Leave the tip in place and inform the patient that no further treatment is needed
    4. Flouroscopically guided removal under local anesthesia
    5. Call your lawyer

2. Most of the local anesthetic injected into the epidural space will
   1. Be retained in the epidural fat
   2. Be absorbed into the blood
   3. Produce blockade of the spinal roots
   4. Produce blockade of the spinal cord
   5. Diffuse into the intrathecal space

A = 1, 2, 3   B = 1, 3   C = 2, 4   D = 4 only   E = all are correct

3. In elderly patients, the reduction in local anesthetic requirement for the same segmental spread and the faster onset time as compared to young patients is due to
   1. Decreased numbers of nerve fibers
   2. Deterioration of the myelin sheath
   3. Diminished egress through the intervertebral foramina
   4. Changes in the shape of the epidural space

Answers: 1. 3   2. 2   3. E

Chapter 66

Pediatric Regional Anesthesia

Metabolism of local anesthetics compared to adults

1. Amides: ↓ oxidation, reduction, conjugation, protein binding, BUT: ↑↑ volume of distribution. Net effect: for a given dose, serum concentration in kids < adults
2. Esters: ↓ plasma cholinesterase activity

Maximum recommended doses in children

1. Tetracaine 1.5 mg/kg
2. Bupivicaine 3 mg/kg
3. Lidocaine 7 mg/kg

Anatomic differences for spinal/caudal anesthesia compared to adults

1. Spinal cord ends at lower level (L3 vs. L1)
2. Paramedian landmarks not as easily palpated (midline approach is best)
3. Sacrum is narrower and flatter
4. Higher risk of accidental dural puncture because of:
   A. Shorter distance from skin to subarachnoid space (dural sac extends to ~S3)
   B. Angle of approach is more direct

Physiologic differences for spinal/caudal anesthesia compared to adults

1. Cardiovascular stability (rarely get hypotensive, even with T2 levels)
2. Relatively higher dose requirement (due to greater volume of CSF/body weight)
3. Fast injection more likely to produce high level (due to proximity of vertebral levels)

Spinal anesthesia in children

1. **Technique:**
   A. Short needle improves detection of CSF
   B. Midline approach at L4-5 or L5-S1
   C. DO NOT ELEVATE LEGS ABOVE HEAD . . . RISK OF TOTAL SPINAL!!
   D. Start IV after spinal in (low risk of hypotension)

2. **Doses** (for T4 level)

● Table 66–1

Drug	Dose	Duration
Lidocaine	2 mg/kg	45 min (plain)
Bupivicaine	0.6–0.8 mg/kg	70 min (plain)
Tetracaine	0.4–1.0 mg/kg	80 min (with epi)

3. **Complications:**
   A. Headache: rare if < 13 yrs old (2° to low CSF pressure?)
   B. Backache: incidence unknown
   C. Total spinal: patient exhibits apnea without hypotension

Caudal anesthesia in children

1. **Technique:** single shot or continuous infusion, access through sacral hiatus
2. **Doses:** 0.05 mL/kg/number of dermatomes to be blocked[1]
3. **Drug:** 0.25% and 0.125% bupivicaine produce similar analgesic effects and are equally acceptable, but motor block less likely with 0.125%.
4. **Complications:** higher risk of accidental dural puncture for reasons described

Sample questions

A = 1, 2, 3   B = 1, 3   C = 2, 4   D = 4 only   E = all are correct

1. A 4-yr-old, 18-kg child is having a bilateral inguinal hernia repair under general anesthesia. The surgeon requests that a caudal block be placed for postoperative analgesia. True statements about appropriate doses include
   1. The volume of 0.25% bupivicaine required for an adequate sensory block will exceed the toxic dose
   2. Equal volume doses of .0125% and 0.25% bupivicaine will produce similar degrees of motor block
   3. Total volume of drug will exceed that required for bilateral ilioinguinal/iliohypogastric nerve blocks
   4. Equal volume doses of 0.125% and 0.25% bupivicaine will produce similar degrees of analgesia
2. Compared to adults, infants undergoing spinal anesthesia
   1. Require larger doses when based on body weight
   2. Are at greater risk of postdural puncture headache
   3. Will have a shorter duration of action for any given local anesthetic
   4. Will exhibit the same degree of hypotension following accidental subarachnoid injection as adults

Single best answer

3. A 2-month-old, 2.5-kg premature infant is scheduled for inguinal hernia repair under spinal anesthesia. He has a history of apnea and bradycardia treated in the past with theophylline and caffeine, which he no longer receives. Spinal anesthesia is induced with 2.5 mg hyperbaric tetracaine and sedation is achieved with ketamine 0.5 mg IV. Shortly after placing the electrocautery pad on the infant's back, he is noted to

be apneic. Pulse oximeter reads 88% on 1L/min nasal cannula, pulse 110/min, blood pressure 68/45 mmHg. The most appropriate treatment at this time is

1. Loading dose of theophylline 12.5 mg IV, followed by maintenance infusion
2. Loading dose of caffeine 25 mg IV, followed by intermittent maintenance doses
3. Place patient in reverse trendelenburg and mask-ventilate with oxygen until apnea resolves
4. Atropine 0.05 mg IV
5. Remove the cold electrocautery pad, which has stimulated the baby to hold his breath

Answers: 1. D   2. B   3. 3

Reference

1. Takasaki M, Dohi S, Kawabata Y, Takahashi T. Dosage of lidocaine for caudal anesthesia in infants and children. Anesthesiology 47: 527, 1977.

Epidural and Intrathecal Opioids

Site of action: Mu, delta, and kappa receptors in laminae I and V of dorsal horns (in substantia gelatinosa)

Factors affecting onset

1. Epidural onset speed limited by: rate of dural penetration, fat absorption, and systemic uptake
2. Lipophilic, nonionized drugs (fentanyl) have fast onset, *but* as drug crosses dura, most gets trapped in epidural fat or absorbed into bloodstream, resulting in low CSF concentration
3. Hydrophilic, ionized drugs (morphine) have slow onset, but reach high CSF concentrations (once it gets into CSF, this water-loving drug tends to hang around)

Factors affecting dermatome spread

1. Hydrophilicity: the more water-soluble, the greater the spread (morphine is the most water-soluble)
2. Volume of injectate only affects spread of *lipophilic* drugs (degree of spread directly related to volume)

Factors affecting duration

1. Hydrophilicity: the more water-soluble, the longer the duration
2. Dose: increased dose = increased duration, but this is only true for hydrophilic drugs (morphine)

Complications

1. Pruritis: most common complication of both routes (>60%), treat with benedryl or naloxone
2. Urinary retention: males > females, may require catheterization, treat with naloxone or urocholine
3. Nausea/vomiting: incidence higher with morphine, treat with naloxone or scopolamine
4. Respiratory depression: least common complication, but most onerous. Has a biphasic incidence. Early respiratory depression is due to vascular absorption and redistribution and is more common with lipophilic drugs. Late respiratory depression (primarily seen with morphine) is due

to rostral spread of drug within the CSF to the respiratory centers of the brain. An increased incidence of respiratory depression is seen with:
A. Large doses of opioids
B. Elderly patients
C. Concomitant administration of systemic opioids
D. Coexisting pulmonary disease

Sample questions

A = 1, 2, 3   B = 1, 3   C = 2, 4   D = 4 only   E = all are correct

1. Respiratory depression following epidural injection of opiates is
   1. More likely to occur early following fentanyl administration
   2. Directly related to the potency of the opiate
   3. More likely to occur late following morphine administration
   4. Not influenced by concomitant parenteral administration of opiates

2. Respiratory depression following intrathecal administration of morphine
   1. Occurs early due to systemic absorption
   2. Occurs late due to bulk flow of cerebrospinal fluid
   3. Is similar in magnitude to the respiratory depression following equipotent parenteral doses
   4. Is dose dependent

3. Epidural morphine
   1. Has a duration that is dose dependent
   2. Results in a peak serum concentration equal to that seen following equipotent IV doses of morphine
   3. Has a longer duration at equipotent doses than intravenous morphine
   4. Results in a peak serum level less than that produced by epidural fentanyl

Answers: 1. B   2. E   3. A

Low Back Pain and Epidural Steroids

Most common source of low back pain: Mechanical compression of L5 or S1 by herniated disc, causing nerve root irritation/inflammation

Indications for epidural steroids

1. Acute radicular back pain due to herniated disc (should try a few days of bedrest and mild analgesics for 4–6 weeks first)
2. Chronic radicular pain failing conservative treatment (tend to respond poorly to steroids, though)
3. Metastatic cancer causing mechanical compression on nerve roots
4. Diagnostic blockade to elucidate the origin of pain when radiculopathy not clear-cut

Steroids employed

1. Methylprednisolone acetate (Depo-Medrol™), 80–120 mg
2. Triamcinolone diacetate (Aristocort™) 50–75 mg

Comparative efficacy of pain relief

Epidural steroids + local > local only > saline

Recommended intervention 2 weeks after initial injection of steroids

1. If complete pain relief was obtained, don't repeat injection (they're already pain-free)
2. If no pain relief was obtained: don't repeat injection (unlikely to provide relief)
3. If partial pain relief was obtained: repeat injection likely to give additional relief. Most experts recommend a maximum of three doses, 2 weeks apart

Contraindications to epidural steroids

1. Coagulopathy
2. Chronic therapy with NSAIDs or aspirin (risk of coagulopathy)
3. Infection at planned site of injection
4. Back pain due to bony abnormality (spinal stenosis, spondylosis, etc.)
5. Prior laminectomy with same pain as preoperatively

Complications of epidural steroids

1. Possible neural degeneration by high concentrations of polyethylene glycol (the vehicle for depot steroids)
2. Cushing's syndrome
3. Dural puncture
4. Epidural abscess

Sample question

A = 1, 2, 3   B = 1, 3   C = 2, 4   D = 4 only   E = all are correct

1. Epidural steroids
   1. Can induce congestive heart failure
   2. Produce better pain relief when coupled with local anesthetics
   3. Are indicated in the treatment of acute low back pain not responding to a trial of conservative therapy
   4. Are not particularly helpful in chronic radicular low back pain

Answer: 1. E

CHAPTER 69

Sympathetically Mediated Pain Syndromes

Two main syndromes

1. Reflex sympathetic dystrophy
2. Causalgia

Three features required

1. Pain
2. Autonomic dysfunction
3. Dystrophic changes

• Table 69–1

	Reflex Sympathetic Dystrophy	Causalgia
Antecedent event	1. Crush/laceration/fracture/sprain 2. Postoperative (usually median nerve distribution) 3. Stroke or MI	Incomplete injury to major nerve trunk (gunshot wound is most common mechanism)
Distribution	Nondermatomal Usually hand or foot	80% involve arm or thigh (injury usually to brachial plexus branch or sciatic nerve)
Onset and nature of pain	Gradual onset Is continuous/burning Tender to touch	Immediate onset is burning/crushing/sharp tender to touch
Manifestations of autonomic dysfunction	Early changes: skin is warm/red/dry	All changes seen earlier than in reflex sympathetic dystrophy
	Late changes: skin is cold/pale or cyanotic/sweaty/glossy	Skin is warm/red/dry (usually) *but can be* cold/cyanotic/sweaty
Dystrophic changes	Seen late Bone demineralization Joint stiffening	Seen early Bone demineralization Joint stiffening
Diagnostic tests	1. Stellate ganglion block 2. Lumbar sympathetic block	1. Stellate ganglion block 2. Lumbar sympathetic block

(Continued)

● **Table 69-1** *(Continued)*

	Reflex Sympathetic Dystrophy	Causalgia
Treatment (best results if instituted early)	1. Series of local anesthetic blocks of stellate ganglion or lumbar sympathetics 2. IV regional with guanethidine 3. Systemic alpha blockade with prazosin or phenoxybenzamine 4. Physical therapy	1. Surgical sympathectomy 2. Chemical neurolytic sympathectomy 3. Series of local anesthetic blocks of stellate ganglion or lumbar sympathetics (least successful)

Sample Questions

A = 1, 2, 3   B = 1, 3   C = 2, 4   D = 4 only   E = all are correct

1. A 26-year-old female who fractured her ulna and radius 6 months ago presents with a complaint of burning pain in her hand. Physical exam reveals decreased finger motion, cold, shiny skin, and osteoporosis by X-ray examination. Therapeutic options for her include
   1. Ipsilateral surgical stellate ganglion sympathectomy
   2. Serial ipsilateral sympathetic stellate ganglion blocks with local anesthetic
   3. Injection of phenol into the ipsilateral stellate ganglion
   4. IV regional blockade with guanethidine

2. Characteristics of acute reflex sympathetic dystrophy include
   1. Glossy skin overlying the affected area
   2. Osteoporosis
   3. Loss of sensation of light touch
   4. Pain not conforming to a dermatomal distribution

3. Statements that describe the pain of both reflex sympathetic dystrophy and causalgia include
   1. There is hyperalgia to light touch
   2. It tends to spread beyond the point of initial presentation
   3. It has a burning quality
   4. The onset is immediate

Answers: 1. C   2. D   3. A

CHAPTER 70

Stellate Ganglion Blockade

Indication: Treatment of reflex sympathetic dystrophy of the arm

Technique:

1. Patient is supine
2. Palpate the transverse process of C6 (Chassaignac's tubercle)
3. Displace carotid artery laterally
4. Insert 22-gauge short-bevel needle perpendicular to skin (anterior to posterior)
5. After contacting C6 transverse process, withdraw ~3 mm
6. Inject 8–12 cc local

Nearby anatomic structures

1. Recurrent laryngeal nerve
2. Phrenic nerve
3. Carotid artery
4. Epidural/subarachnoid space
5. Brachial plexus

Complications

Here's the world's geekiest mnemonic

"*Stella's horse is short of breath from seizing* and can't *raise his arm* to take his *blood pressure.*"
      (1)   (2)   (3)   (4)   (5)

1. Recurrent laryngeal nerve blockade—*hoarseness*
2. Phrenic nerve blockade—*dyspnea*
3. Intraarterial injection—*high plasma levels and seizures*
4. Brachial plexus blockade—*motor dysfunction of the arm*
5. Epidural/subarachnoid injection—causes profound *hypotension,* possible total spinal

Signs of successful blockade

1. Horner's syndrome (miosis, ptosis, anhydrosis)
2. Conjunctival injection
3. Nasal stuffiness
4. Vasodilation and warmth of affected limb

70 ■ Stellate Ganglion Blockade

Sample questions

A = 1, 2, 3   B = 1, 3   C = 2, 4   D = 4 only   E = all are correct

1. Possible complications of stellate ganglion block include
   1. Dyspnea
   2. Ptosis of the ipsilateral eye
   3. Hoarseness
   4. Vasodilation of the ipsilateral arm

2. Correct statements regarding stellate ganglion block include
   1. Chassaignac's tubercle is the principle landmark
   2. A paresthesia should be elicited before injection
   3. It is a useful technique in the treatment of reflex sympathetic dystrophy
   4. IV injection can cause seizures

Answers: 1. B   2. B

Celiac Plexus Blockade

Anatomy: Comprised of the greater and lesser splanchnic nerves, both of which are derived from thoracic sympathetic ganglion

Location

Lies in retroperitoneal space anterior to body of L1 and posterior to aorta (right) and inferior vena cava (left)

Function

Nociceptive innervation to pancreas, liver, stomach, viscera

Clinical uses of blockade

1. Neurolytic sympathetic blockade for relief of cancer pain
2. Supplemental anesthesia for abdominal procedures

Technique

1. Place patient prone with pillow under abdomen for thoracic flexion
2. Draw a triangle connecting the T12 spinous process (triangle's apex) with each 12th rib at a point on the rib ~8 cm from midline (triangle's corners)
3. After making skin wheals at each "corner," insert a 12.5-cm, 22-gauge needle, following line of the triangle, directing the needle anteriorly, cephalad, and medially until body of L1 is contacted
4. Partially withdraw and redirect needle anteriorly to "walk off" L1, advance ~2 cm beyond this point while aspirating (right-sided ganglion ~2 cm deeper than left)
5. Inject ~25 mL of either 0.25% bupivicaine or 0.75% lidocaine (each side)

Complications

1. Orthostatic hypotension
2. Somatic spread with impaired ambulation
3. Subarachnoid/epidural/intravascular injection
4. Diarrhea
5. Punctured organs (kidney most common)
6. Pneumothorax
7. Hematoma/bleeding

71 ■ Celiac Plexus Blockade

Sample questions

A = 1, 2, 3   B = 1, 3   C = 2, 4   D = 4 only   E = all are correct

1. Patients who would benefit from celiac plexus blockade include
   1. A 60-year-old male with end-stage pancreatic cancer
   2. A 55-year-old male undergoing total gastrectomy and jejunostomy tube placement
   3. A 48-year-old female with hepatocellular carcinoma
   4. A 35-year-old female with irritable bowel syndrome

2. A 45-year-old man with end-stage pancreatic cancer is being evaluated for possible neurolytic celiac plexus blockade. After careful placement of the needle with negative aspiration tests, each plexus is blocked with 15 mL of 0.25% bupivicaine with epinephrine 1:200,000. Ten minutes after injection, he is pain free and is unable to walk without assistance. His vital signs are blood pressure 85/50, pulse 108/min. Possible causes of these findings include
   1. Subarachnoid injection of local anesthetic
   2. Epidural injection of local anesthetic
   3. An excessively high concentration of bupivicaine
   4. Blockade of the celiac plexus and upper lumber somatic roots

Answers: 1. A   2. D

Chapter 72

Postherpetic Neuralgia

Presentation: Follows acute Herpes zoster, may last for several months. Often accompanied by profound depression, suicidal ideation

Pain characteristics

Stabbing, burning, itching pain that is unrelenting. Has elements of a central pain state

Treatment modalities for *acute* zoster which may reduce incidence of postherpetic neuralgia

1. Topical aspirin mixed with diethyl-ether applied to affected areas
2. Sympathetic blockade (via epidural or paravertebral approach)

Proposed treatment modalities for postherpetic neuralgia

1. Tricyclic antidepressants: may target the "central pain" aspect of the neuralgia, as well as alleviate depression (Elavil, prolixin)
2. Anticonvulsants (phenytoin, carbemazepine)
3. Steroids: subcutaneous at site of lesions or epidural
4. Sympathetic nerve block: thought to reduce neuralgia by improving circulation to neural structures, reducing inflammation and thereby preventing further nerve damage. Not particularly reliable

Additional treatments for neuralgia

Desperation measures, none particularly reliable

1. Acupuncture
2. TENS units
3. Cryotherapy
4. Lytic nerve blocks

Sample questions

A = 1, 2, 3   B = 1, 3   C = 2, 4   D = 4 only   E = all are correct

1. Appropriate therapy for postherpetic neuralgia includes
    1. Elavil
    2. Acyclovir
    3. Valproic acid
    4. Electroconvulsive therapy

2. True statements regarding postherpetic neuralgia include
   1. It is always preceeded by visible lesions
   2. It is a central pain state
   3. It only occurs in immunocompromised patients
   4. It is dermatomal in distribution

Answers: 1. B   2. C

CHAPTER 73

Neurolytic Nerve Blocks

Criteria
1. Malignant cancer pain (especially if life expectancy < expected duration of neurolysis)
2. Absence of a central pain state
3. Slowly progressive tumor (will stay within the boundaries of the block)
4. Degree of debilitation and life expectancy make patient a poor surgical candidate
5. Best suited for cancer involving cranial nerves, breast, chest, abdominal wall, and abdominal viscera

General guidelines for neurolysis
1. Must be preceded by prognostic blocks
2. Patient must understand that the permanency of block is relative and that pain can return even worse than before neurolysis
3. Preexisting neurologic deficits must be documented
4. Avoid peripheral neurolysis (poor success rate, high risk of postblock neuralgia)

Ideal clinical scenarios
1. Severe, localized perineal cancer pain
2. Bladder pain/spasm
3. Facial pain
4. Celiac plexus pain

Characteristics of neurolytic agents
- Table 73–1

Ethyl Alcohol	Phenol
1. Painful injection	1. Painless injection
2. Immediate neurolysis (within seconds)	2. Delayed neurolysis (~15 min)
3. Neurolysis more intense than phenol	3. Neurolysis less intense than ethyl alcohol
4. Long duration	4. Short duration
5. Intrathecal injection is undiluted and hypobaric	5. Intrathecal injection is diluted with glycerin and hyperbaric
6. High incidence of postblock neuralgia	6. Low incidence of postblock neuralgia
	7. Block is biphasic because phenol has a local anesthetic property, ∴ extent of neurolysis is not evident for ~24 hr
	8. Diluent effects potency (is more potent in saline than in glycerin)

Complications

1. Failure to relieve pain
2. Spillover to surrounding structures
   A. Especially common with lumbar and caudal injections
   B. Frequent sphincter dysfunction with resultant urinary retention and overflow incontinence and fecal incontinence
   C. Unintentional motor/sensory block
3. Axon regeneration and extreme pain worse than original pain
4. Development of a central pain state

Which agent is best for which block?

1. Peripheral nerve block: 5–20% phenol in NaCl or H_2O
2. Somatic nerve block: 100% ethyl alcohol
3. Sympathetic nerve block: 50% ethyl alcohol in NaCl
4. Subarachnoid blockade: undiluted ethyl alcohol or phenol in glycerin

Sample question

A = 1, 2, 3   B = 1, 3   C = 2, 4   D = 4 only   E = all are correct

1. Compared to alcohol for neurolysis, phenol
   1. Is hyperbaric when injected intrathecally
   2. Is painful on injection
   3. Has a shorter duration
   4. Has a high risk of postneurolysis neuralgia

Answer: 1. B

CHAPTER 74

Cervical Plexus Blockade

Anatomy: Plexus arises from C1-C4; has two components:

1. Deep cervical plexus innervates:
   A. Phrenic nerve
   B. Strap muscles
   C. Prevertebral muscles
   D. Cutaneous sensation from jaw line to T2 distribution
2. Superficial cervical plexus—innervates only cutaneous structures

Clinical uses

1. Carotid endarterectomy
2. Tracheotomy (must perform bilateral blocks)
3. Thyroidectomy (must perform bilateral blocks)

Technique for deep cervical plexus blockade

1. Single injection of ~10 cc local at C4 transverse process, **OR**
2. Three separate injections, one each at the level of the C2, C3, C4 transverse processes

Complications of deep cervical plexus blockade

1. Epidural/subarachnoid injection
2. Phrenic and superior laryngeal nerve blockade
3. Intravascular injection

Technique for superficial cervical plexus blockade

1. Insert needle at the midpoint of the posterior border of sternocleidomastoid muscle
2. Advance needle somewhat anteriorly, injecting along medial and posterior border of sternocleidomastoid

Complications of superficial cervical plexus blockade

Ipsilateral accessory nerve blockade with trapezius muscle paralysis

Sample questions

A = 1, 2, 3   B = 1, 3   C = 2, 4   D = 4 only   E = all are correct

74 ■ Cervical Plexus Blockade

1. Complications of superficial cervical plexus blockade include
   1. Epidural injection
   2. Phrenic nerve blockade
   3. Horner's syndrome
   4. Trapezius paralysis

Single best answer

2. A complication of deep cervical plexus blockade is
   1. Ipsilateral mydriasis
   2. Horner's syndrome
   3. Hoarseness
   4. Hyperventilation
   5. Bradycardia

Answers: 1. D   2. 3

Chapter 75

Brachial Plexus Anatomy and Blockade

Anatomy

"Robert   Taylor   drinks   cold   beer."
(roots)   (trunks)   (divisions)   (cords)   (branches)

Mneumonic

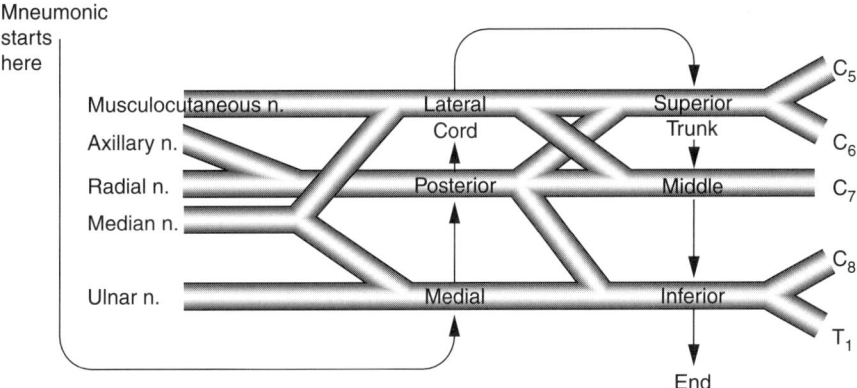

Figure 75–1.

Branches	"**M**uscular	(musculocutaneous)
	Arms	(axillary, radial, median)
	up	(ulnar)
Cords	**m**y	(medial)
	pant	(posterior)
	leg	(lateral)
Trunks	**s**atisfy	(superior)
	me	(middle)
	infinitely"	(inferior)

(Thanks to Kathy Schwock, MD, for her twisted imagination and help in contriving this mneumonic!)

75 ■ Brachial Plexus Anatomy and Blockade

Plexus consists of anterior rami of cervical roots C5-T1

1. **Roots** form trunks:
   - C5, 6   superior trunk
   - C7   middle trunk
   - C8, T1   inferior trunk
2. **Trunks** have anterior and posterior divisions
   Posterior divisions of all three trunks form the *posterior* cord
   Anterior division of inferior trunk forms *medial* cord
   Anterior division of middle and superior trunks form *lateral* cord
3. **Cords** form branches (terminal nerves)
   - Lateral cord   musculocutaneous n.
   -                    median n.
   - Medial cord   median n.
   -                    ulnar n.
   - Posterior cord   axillary n.
   -                     radial n.

Cutaneous innervation of the arm (4 nerves)

1. Axillary n.: shoulder and upper arm
2. Intercostobrachialis n.: medial aspect of arm
3. Radial n.: lateral aspect of lower arm
4. Medial brachial cutaneous n.: thin strip in middle of arm

Cutaneous innervation of the forearm (3 nerves)

1. Medial antebrachial cutaneous n.: medial 1/2 of forearm
2. Musculocutaneous n.: lateral 1/2 of forearm
3. Radial n.: thin strip in middle of posterior forearm

Innervation of the hand

● Table 75–1

Nerve	Roots	Sensory	Motor
Median	C5, 6	Palm (except ulnar distribution)	Opposition of thumb with little finger
Radial	C6, 7	Dorsum (except ulnar distribution	Extension of thumb
Ulnar	C8	5th finger and medial 1/2 of hand fingers and 4th finger	Ab/adduction of fingers

● Table 75–2

Interscalene Block		
Advantages	Disadvantages	Landmarks/Anatomy
1. Good for shoulder surgery	1. Misses **ulnar** nerve (inferior trunk)	1. Posterior border of sternoleidomastoid
2. Can do with arm in any position	2. Inadvertent blockade of: phrenic, vagus, recurrent laryngeal n., and cervical plexus	2. Roll fingers over anterior scalene into interscalene groove
3. Low risk of pneumothorax	3. Inadvertent epidural, spinal, intravascular injection	3. Draw a line laterally from cricoid to the intersection with transverse process of C6
4. Paresthesia not required		4. External jugular vein often overlies this point, but unreliable

• **Table 75–2** *(Continued)*

Supraclavicular Block		
Advantages	**Disadvantages**	**Landmarks/Anatomy**
1. Small volume 2. All three trunks in close proximity 3. Blockade reliable 4. Do with arm in any position	1. Requires paresthesia 2. High risk of pneumothorax 3. Frequent phrenic block, Horner's syndrome, neuropathy: avoid in patients with respiratory compromise	1. 3 trunks are clustered *vertically* over the 1st rib, *posterior* to subclavian artery 2. Trunks are *inferior* to clavicle at its midpoint 3. Palpate interscalene groove ~1.5 cm posterior to clavicular midpoint 4. Direct needle caudad and posteromedially, seek paresthesia 5. If artery hit, redirect posterolaterally
Axillary Block		
1. Paresthesia not required 2. No risk of pneumothorax	1. Misses **musculocutaneous** nerve 2. Not suitable for shoulder surgery 3. High-risk intravascular injection 4. Rare neuropathy 5. Must abduct arm	1. Neurovascular bundle is multicompartmental: multiple injections improve reliability 2. Relationship to axillary artery Median: superior ulnar: under (inferior) radial: posterior

Anatomic relationships of structures in axillary sheath

They LOVE this stuff!

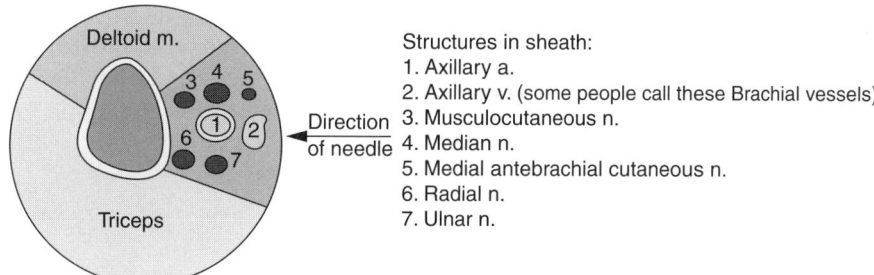

Structures in sheath:
1. Axillary a.
2. Axillary v. (some people call these Brachial vessels)
3. Musculocutaneous n.
4. Median n.
5. Medial antebrachial cutaneous n.
6. Radial n.
7. Ulnar n.

Figure 75–2.

I remember things in relation to the Axillary artery: m&m's on top (with median in middle), and **U**lnar **u**nder.

Rescue blocks for failed axillary block

1. **If you missed the ulnar nerve:** palmar and dorsal sensory to 3rd, 4th fingers and palm, motor spreads fingers
   A. Elbow approach: 5 mL local fanned 3 cm proximal to ulnar groove
   B. Wrist approach: 5 mL local injected immediately lateral OR medial to flexor carpi ulnaris tendon at the level of the pisiform bone
2. **If you missed the radial nerve:** sensory to dorsal surface of thumb and first 3½ fingers, motor abducts thumb
   A. Elbow approach: 5 mL local, insert needle perpendicular to skin 2 cm lateral to biceps tendon at intercondylar line until it contacts bone

B. Wrist approach: 3 mL local superficially injected along the extensor pollicis tendon and across anatomic "snuffbox"
3. **If you missed the median nerve:** sensory to palmar surface of thumb and first 3½ fingers, motor adducts thumb
   A. Elbow approach: 5 mL local medial to brachial artery at intercondylar line, elicit paresthesia
   B. Wrist approach: 3 mL local, insert needle perpendicular to skin 3 cm proximal to wrist crease between flexor carpi radialis and palmaris longus tendons

Sample questions

Single best answer

1. The axillary approach to the brachial plexus
   1. Uses the axillary vein as a landmark
   2. Uses the insertion of the teres major as a landmark
   3. Has a risk of a pneumothorax
   4. Produces paresthesias of the median and ulnar but not the radial nerve
   5. Anesthetizes the musculocutaneous nerve

A = 1, 2, 3   B = 1, 3   C = 2, 4   D = 4 only   E = all are correct

2. Distal spread of local anesthetic following axillary block is discouraged by
   1. Internally rotating the arm
   2. Digital pressure distal to the injection site
   3. Cephalad direction of the needle
   4. Adduction of the shoulder after injection

3. Forty minutes after axillary blockade with 40 cc of 1.5% mepivicaine, a 70-kg man reports sensation over the lateral surface of the forearm, the anterior and posterior surfaces of his 4th and 5th fingers, and the dorsum of the hand. On motor exam, he is able to adduct his thumb and abduct his fingers. Nerves that were incompletely blocked include
   1. Radial
   2. Musculocutaneous
   3. Ulnar
   4. Median

4. During brachial plexus nerve block
   1. Phrenic nerve block occurs with the interscalene and supraclavicular approaches
   2. Infiltration of the coracobrachialis muscle will block the nerve most often missed with the axillary approach
   3. The nerve most often missed with the interscalene approach arises from the inferior trunk of the plexus
   4. Triceps weakness is an early sign of radial nerve anesthesia with the axillary approach

Answers: 1. 4   2. C   3. E   4. E

CHAPTER 76

Lower Extremity Nerve Blocks

The lower extremity receives all its innervation from the lumbar plexus and the sacral plexus.

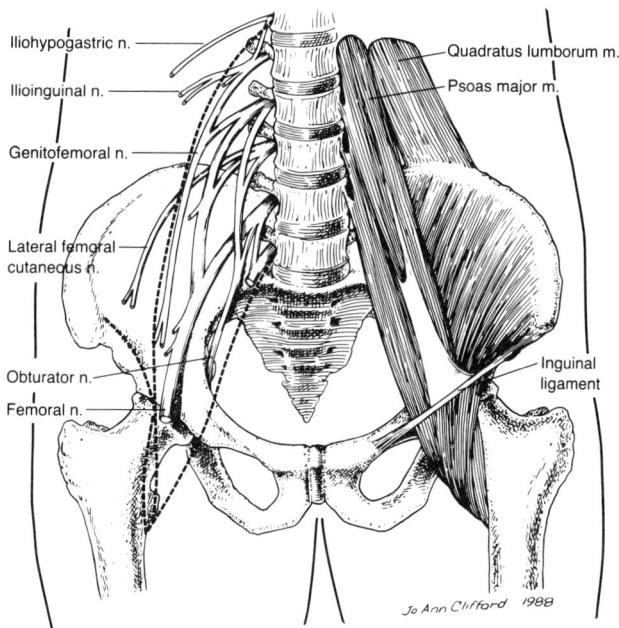

Figure 76–1. From Miller RD, Cucchiara RF, Miller ED, Jr, Reves JG, Roizen MF, Savarese JJ. Anesthesia, ed 4. New York: Churchill Livingstone, 1994. Reprinted with permission.

Lumbar plexus anatomy

1. Ventral rami of T12 (variable)
2. Ventral rami L1-L4
3. Ventral rami of L5 (variable)

Psoas compartment blockade

The lumbar plexus nerves can be anesthetized individually or "en bloc" by injecting the psoas compartment.

● Table 76–1

Posterior Approach	Winnie "3-in-1" Approach[1]
1. Patient is prone
2. Identify L4 spinous process
3. Insert 22-gauge spinal needle perpendicular to skin ~5 cm lateral to L4 spinous process
4. Verify needle position via loss of resistance or paresthesia
5. Inject 20–40 mL of 1.5% lidocaine or 0.5% bupivicaine	1. Patient is supine
2. Identify inguinal ligament and femoral artery
3. Insert 1½-inch 22-gauge needle perpendicular to skin just lateral to arterial pulse, seeking paresthesia
4. Apply distal pressure during injection of 20–40 mL local anesthetic

Complications of both approaches

1. Inadequate block (Winnie approach tends to miss obturator nerve)
2. Hematoma
3. Neuropathy

Techniques of blocking individual terminal nerves of lumbar plexus (all are in supine position)

● Table 76–2

Femoral n.	Lateral Femoral Cutaneous n.	Obturator n.
1. Identify inguinal ligament and femoral artery pulse
2. Insert 1½-inch, 22-gauge needle perpendicular to skin ~ one fingerbreath lateral to pulse
3. Do not seek paresthesia
4. Inject 5–10 mL of local	1. Make a mark ~1 cm both caudal and lateral to pubic tubercle
2. Insert needle perpendicular to skin, contact bone
3. Redirect laterally and caudally while injecting	1. Identify anterior superior iliac spine
2. Insert needle two fingerbreadths medially and inferiorly
3. Direct needle laterally to pierce fascia lata, then fan local laterally and medially

Sacral plexus blockade (sciatic nerve blockade)

● Table 76–3

Posterior Approach	Supine Approach
1. Patient lies on nonoperative side, with operative leg flexed at hip and knee and rolled anteriorly
2. Draw an acute angle, with the apex at the greater trochanter and the two sides extending to the sacral hiatus and the posterior superior iliac spine
3. At a right angle, bisect the line between the greater trochanter and the iliac spine and extend the bisecting line until it contacts the line connecting the trochanter and the sacral hiatus (point "A")
4. Insert a spinal needle at point "A," eliciting paresthesias of leg and foot
5. Inject ~25 mL 1.5% lidocaine or 0.5% bupivicaine	1. Patient supine, hip flexed 90° to torso
2. Draw a line between ischial tuberosity and greater trochanter and mark the midpoint
3. At midpoint, insert spinal needle perpendicularly, seeking paresthesias
4. Inject ~25 mL of local

Ankle block

1. Paresthesias not necessary
2. Each of the five nerves is blocked separately
3. All nerves arise from sciatic nerve except saphenous (from femoral nerve)

● **Table 76-3**

Nerve	Sensory Distribution	Approach
Posterior tibial n.	Sole of foot, nailbeds	Infiltrate behind medial malleolus
Sural n.	Lateral aspect of both foot and proximal sole	Infiltrate behind lateral malleolus
Deep peroneal n.	Skin between 1st and 2nd toes	Insert needle perpendicularly just lateral to the tendon of the extensor hallucis longus, inject deep to fascial planes
Superficial peroneal n.	Dorsum of foot excluding area between 1st and 2nd toes	Direct needle laterally from its point of insertion for the deep peroneal block, make a wheal
Saphenous n.	Medial aspect of foot	Direct needle medially from its point of insertion for the deep peroneal block, make a wheal

Sample questions

A = 1, 2, 3   B = 1, 3   C = 2, 4   D = 4 only   E = all are correct

1. Psoas compartment blockade
    1. Must be combined with sciatic blockade to provide complete anesthesia for lower extremity surgery
    2. Produces no sympathetomy when performed correctly
    3. Can be achieved via a single injection
    4. May be performed in both the supine or prone position

2. Transmetatarsal amputation of the great toe requires blockade of the
    1. Superficial peroneal nerve
    2. Posterior tibial nerve
    3. Deep peroneal nerve
    4. Saphenous nerve

Single best answer

3. All of the following nerves are derived from the lumbar plexus except
    1. Ilioinguinal
    2. Lateral femoral cutaneous
    3. Saphenous
    4. Posterior cutaneous nerve of the thigh
    5. Obturator

Answers: 1. E   2. E   3. 4

Reference

1. Winnie AP, Ramamurthy S, Durrani Z. The inguinal paravascular technique of lumbar plexus anesthesia: The "3-in-1 block." Anesth Anal 52: 989, 1973.

CHAPTER 77

Intravenous Regional Anesthesia

(Bier Block)

Advantages

1. Easy to do
2. Rapid onset
3. Rapid recovery (best for procedures <90 min)
4. Good muscle relaxation

Disadvantages

1. Tourniquet pain
2. Quick onset of postop pain
3. Can't provide a bloodless field
4. Requires exsanguination (painful to injured limb)

Complications

1. Local anesthetic toxicity (via accidental or early deflation of tourniquet)
2. Compartment syndrome (rare)
3. Loss of limb (rare)

Technique

1. Place IV as distal as possible in operative limb (doesn't have to be distal to surgical site, though)
2. Place double tourniquet proximally
3. Exsanguinate arm
4. Inflate proximal cuff ~150 mmHg > than systolic pressure (confirm loss of pulse)
5. Inject 4–6mg/kg of 0.5% *plain* lidocaine or prilocaine
6. When patient complains of tourniquet pain, inflate distal cuff and deflate proximal (distal cuff overlies anesthetized area)

Technique for tourniquet release

1. <20 min since injection: do not release.
2. At 20–40 min after injection: release and immediately reinflate. Wait for signs of toxicity. If none, wait 1 min and release.
3. 40 minutes or more: release in a single maneuver.

Sample question

Single best answer

1. Factors determining the duration of a Bier block of the upper extremity include
   1. Duration of tourniquet inflation
   2. Concentration of the local anesthetic solution
   3. Whether or not epinephrine is added
   4. Volume of local anesthetic injected
   5. Which local anesthetic agent is used

Answer: 1. 1

CHAPTER 78

Retrobulbar Block and Oculocardiac Reflex

Technique

1. Short-bevel needle (protects against ocular perforation)
2. Have patient look straight ahead (less risk of bleeding, nerve injury, or CNS injection)
3. Enter inferior fornix of conjunctiva
4. Advance ~1.5 cm, then angle superiorly, advancing until muscle cone is penetrated
5. 6–10 cc (1:1) mix of 2% lidocaine (fast onset) and 0.75% bupivicaine (long-lasting)
7. Additives: hyaluronidase (promotes tissue penetration); epinephrine (vasoconstricts, reduces bleeding, prolongs orbital akinesia)

Results

1. Akinesis and anesthesia of globe and orbit
2. Intorsion during downward gaze, because superior oblique is outside muscle cone and may be missed

Complications

1. Hemorrhage/hematoma—**most common**
2. Brainstem anesthesia: apnea, tachycardia, hypertension, cardiac arrest, shivering, loss of consciousness, dilated contralateral pupil, amaurosis, gaze palsy (occurs via spread of local along optic nerve sheath)
3. Direct trauma to eye
4. Local anesthetic toxicity: IV toxicity unlikely . . . dose is too small; intraarterial injection can cause high brain levels via retrograde carotid flow
5. Oculocardiac reflex, *a favorite of the boards,* so . . .

Oculocardiac Reflex

Afferent limb

Trigeminal nerve (CN 5)

Efferent limb

Vagus nerve (CN 10)

Pathway

Orbit → ciliary ganglion → trigeminal n. (opthalmic div.)
→ sensory nucleus (CN 5) → vagus

Triggered by

1. Traction on extraocular muscles, especially medial rectus
2. Pressure on globe or orbit
3. Retrobulbar block

Effect

Bradycardia, AV block, ventricular ectopy, asystole

Incidence

1. Usually an isolated event . . . tends to fatigue with repeated stimulation
2. Exacerbated by hypercapnia and hypoxia

Prophylaxis

1. Atropine oral premedication will not prevent—chronologically too far removed from stimulus
2. IV glycopyrolate *may* prevent in patients with history of conduction defects

Management

1. Ask surgeon to stop surgical manipulation. This usually terminates reflex.
2. Assess respiratory status.
3. Administer IV atropine 2–5 µg/kg if bradycardia is persistent or severe.

Sample Questions

A = 1, 2, 3   B = 1, 3   C = 2, 4   D = 4 only   E = all are correct

1. A healthy 2-year-old, 15-kg child undergoing strabismus repair is given atropine 0.3 mg and midazolam 7 mg po 20 min prior to induction of general endotracheal anesthesia with nitrous oxide, F_iO_2 0.3 and 1% halothane. Twenty minutes after the beginning of the procedure, his pulse changes acutely from a sinus rate of 115/min to a sinus rate of 60/min. True statements regarding this event include
    1. Discontinuation of the halothane is the treatment of choice
    2. A larger dose of the atropine premed would have prevented the event
    3. It is likely to recur frequently throughout the surgical procedure
    4. The pulse will likely return to normal with cessation of surgical stimulus

2. A 65-year-old male has undergone retrobulbar block with 8 cc of 2% lidocaine and 0.75% bupivicaine in a 1:1 ratio for debridement of a previously enucleated orbit. Ten minutes into the procedure, he develops frequent ventricular ectopy and first-degree AV block, but otherwise has no other symptoms. Possible causes of his dysrythymia include

78 ■ Retrobulbar Block and Oculocardiac Reflex

   1. Brainstem anesthesia due to intraarterial injection
   2. Excessive intraocular pressure from the retrobulbar block
   3. Local anesthetic toxicity due to IV injection
   4. Oculocardiac reflex due to stimulation of the empty orbit

3. The oculocardiac reflex is mediated by the
   1. Facial nerve
   2. Trigeminal nerve
   3. Glossopharyngeal nerve
   4. Vagus nerve

4. Possible complications of retrobulbar block include
   1. Oculocardiac reflex
   2. Hemorrhage
   3. Damage to the globe
   4. Akinesis of the eye

Answers 1. D   2. C   3. C   4. A

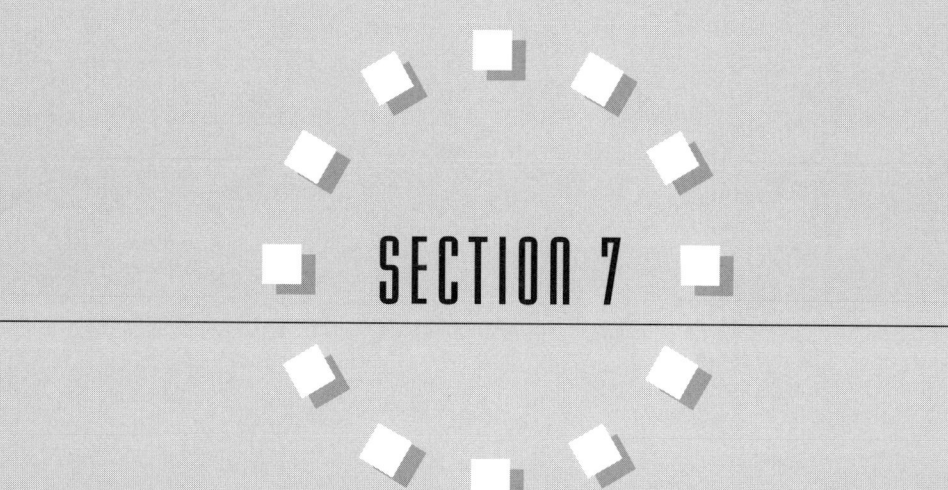

SECTION 7

Cardiothoracic Anesthesia

CHAPTER 79

Coronary Blood Flow and Myocardial Oxygenation

Determinants of coronary artery blood flow

1. Ventricular pressures:
   A. Left coronary artery is perfused only during diastole because high left ventricular systolic pressures compress the artery.
   B. Right coronary artery is perfused during both systole and diastole because lower ventricular pressures do not completely compress artery during either phase of contraction.
2. Coronary artery perfusion pressure (expressed as LVEDP—aortic diastolic pressure)
3. Location of coronary vessels: endocardial vessels are most affected by high intraventricular pressures, and thus, most at risk for ischemia.
4. Coronary artery stenosis: blood flow is reduced by stenosis. Stenotic vessels will vasodilate to increase flow, but this ability is limited.
5. Autoregulation: range is 50–120 mmHg. Mediated by many factors, most important is autonomic nervous system. (Parasympathetic stimulation causes direct vasodilation, sympathetic stimulation increases O_2 demand and thus, causes vasodilation)

Determinants of myocardial oxygenation

Extraction of oxygen from the coronary arteries is nearly maximal at rest (coronary vein saturation ~30%), so there's little ability to improve oxygenation through increased extraction. Hence, myocardial oxygenation is determined by the balance of supply and demand.

Factors that increase myocardial oxygen demand

1. Tachycardia: double jeopardy . . . it increases demand while reducing diastolic time for coronary perfusion
2. Increased contractility (work)
3. Increased preload: increases wall tension (work), which also reduces coronary perfusion
4. Increased afterload: increases LV wall tension (work) and reduces coronary artery perfusion pressure (reduces the pressure gradient between LVEDP and aortic diastolic pressure)

Factors that decrease myocardial oxygen supply

1. Anything that decreases coronary artery blood flow:
   A. Decreased artery lumen: atherosclerosis, arterial spasm, vasoconstriction due to ↑ PaO_2, ↓ $PaCO_2$, PGE_2
   B. Decreased perfusion pressure: ↑ LVEDP or ↓ aortic diastolic pressure
   C. Tachycardia: decreases diastolic time for perfusion
2. Anything that decreases oxygen availability
   A. Decreased delivery due to left shift of oxyhemoglobin curve (see Chapter 21)
   B. Decreased oxygen content: hypoxia, anemia

How do you detect intraoperative myocardial ischemia?

1. Transesophageal echo: regional wall motion abnormalities are *earliest* indicators of ischemia
2. EKG: ST segment depression (or elevation) in leads V5 or V6, but not as sensitive as TEE
3. Hemodynamic instability by PA catheter: ↑ wedge pressure, ↓ cardiac output, large A waves (poor ventricular compliance), or large V waves (papillary muscle dysfunction . . . poor indicators of ischemia)

Treatment of postoperative ischemia

1. Decrease the demand for O_2: correct tachycardia with β-blockers, correct hypertension with β-blockers or vasodilators
2. Increase oxygen supply:
   A. Increase aortic diastolic pressure with vasoconstrictor
   B. Increase coronary flow with nitroglycerin
   C. Prevent further reduction in supply (heparin to prevent thrombosis of coronary artery, Ca^{++} channel blockers to prevent spasm)
   D. Intraaortic balloon pump or bypass

And just for clarification, what is coronary steal?

Suppose that a single coronary artery supplies two distal branches, one of which is stenotic. The stenotic vessel is already maximally dilated, while the normal one is not. If a coronary artery vasodilator is given (like isoflurane), only the normal vessel is able to dilate, resulting in diversion of blood flow from the stenotic vessel to the normal vessel.

Sample questions

A = 1, 2, 3   B = 1, 3   C = 2, 4   D = 4 only   E = all are correct

1. A 60-year-old man with a history of angina is in the recovery room following a hernia repair. Blood pressure 140/90 mmHg, pulse = 100/min, Hgb 8.6 gm/dL, temperature 35.5°C, and the patient is shivering. The EKG has ST segment depression in lead V5. Maneuvers that may relieve the ST segment depression include
   1. Propanolol
   2. Warm the patient
   3. Transfuse two units packed erythrocytes
   4. Administer morphine

2. Coronary artery blood flow is
   1. Directly proportional to aortic diastolic pressure
   2. Equally distributed throughout the myocardium

3. Increased by halothane
4. Only present during diastole

3. Myocardial oxygenation is significantly increased by
   1. Increasing the hemoglobin from 8 gm/dL to 10 gm/dL
   2. Increasing the amount of oxygen extraction
   3. An increased P_{50}
   4. Increasing the left ventricular end-diastolic pressure

Answers: 1. E   2. B   3. B

Ventricular Function Curves

You are expected to understand normal ventricular function versus the function of a failing ventricle. The two basic principles to understand are:

1. In the normal heart, contractility increases as the muscle fiber starting length increases. From this, it is easy to see that, although afterload can affect cardiac output somewhat, the MOST important determinant of contractility and cardiac output is PRELOAD. Bear in mind, though, that there is an optimum length beyond which contractility will fall (point "A" on Figure 80–1).
2. For a given increase in preload, there will be a lesser increase in output by the failing heart than by the normal heart. (Compare point "B" to point "A.")

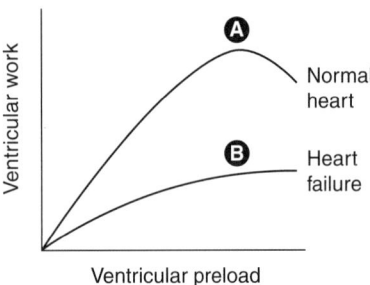

Figure 80–1.

Be familiar with all the possible labels that can be applied to this figure

Alternate labels for PRELOAD axis	Alternate labels for WORK axis
1. LVEDV	1. LV stroke work index
2. LVEDP	2. SV
3. LAP	3. Cardiac output or index
4. PCWP or PAOP	4. Blood pressure

Another way to evaluate contractility is by using ventricular pressure-volume curves. A normal cardiac cycle looks like this:

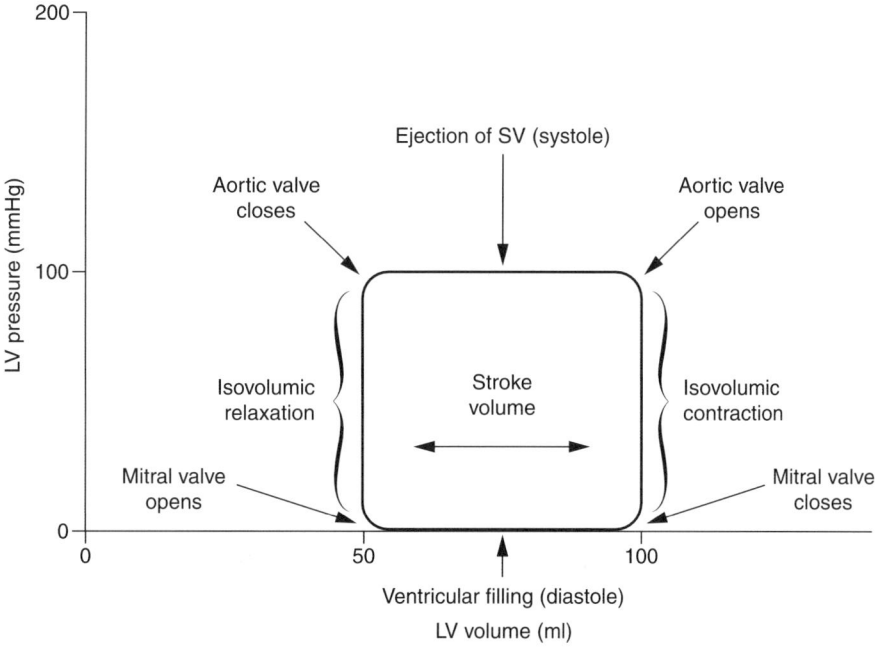

Figure 80-2.

You should know how pharmacologic interventions and abnormal states will affect this curve

Draw them yourself so you'll really understand:

1. ↓ preload (nitroglycerin effect): loop is shorter and shifted left
2. ↑ preload (volume effect): loop is wider . . . SV is increased
3. ↓ afterload (nitroprusside effect): loop is shorter . . . less pressure required to eject SV
4. ↑ afterload, normal ventricular compliance (phenylephrine effect): loop is taller, width unchanged . . . high ventricular pressure required but SV unchanged
5. ↑ afterload, poor ventricular compliance (aortic stenosis effect): loop is tall and narrow . . . high pressure required, and SV is low due to poor filling

If you understand all this, then you can take a logical approach to the management of hypotension

If blood pressure is low, then look at filling pressures and cardiac output:

● Table 80–1

	Cardiac Output	Cause	Remedy
Filling pressure high	High	"Off the curve" or too vasodilated	Inotrope or vasoconstrictors
	Low	Poor contractility	Inotropes, LVAD, IABP
Filling pressure low	High	Low SVR	Vasoconstrictors
	Low	Hypovolemia	Give volume

Sample questions

Single best answer

1. Following coronary artery bypass surgery, a 70-year-old man has the following hemodynamic parameters: sinus rythym 100/min, blood pressure 90/50 mmHg, pulmonary capillary occlusion pressure 17 mmHg, cardiac output 3.5 L/min, hemoglobin 10 g/dL. You should:
   1. Start dobutamine at 5 µg/kg/min
   2. Administer propanolol
   3. Transfuse with two units packed red blood cells
   4. Administer nitroprusside
   5. Administer nitroglycerin

   A = 1, 2, 3   B = 1, 3   C = 2, 4   D = 4 only   E = all are correct

2. True statements regarding congestive heart failure include
   1. Decreased myocardial contractility reduces oxygen consumption
   2. Diuresis may improve cardiac output
   3. Afterload is the most important determinant of cardiac output
   4. For a given increase in preload, there will be less improvement in cardiac output than in the normal heart

Answers: 1. 1   2. C

Blood Pressure Monitoring

Effect of site of measurement: Compared to the ascending aorta, peripheral arteries create significant impedance to flow, generating reflected waves and resulting in:

1. Higher systolic pressures
2. Lower diastolic pressures
3. Similar mean arterial pressures

How do pressure transducers work?

Arterial pulses containing a wide range of frequencies are transmitted via a fluid-filled tube to a transducer that converts the mechanical energy of the arterial pulsation into voltage.

Factors affecting accuracy

1. Damping: the tendency of a system to reduce oscillations via frictional and viscous forces
2. Natural frequency: if the arterial pressure signal approaches the natural frequency of the system, the peaks and troughs of the signal will be exaggerated (resonance or "ringing" occurs). Ideally, the natural frequency of the system exceeds the maximum frequency of the arterial signal, minimizing ringing.

Factors that cause ringing

Anything that reduces the natural frequency of the system

1. Long tubing
2. Narrow tubing
3. Viscous fluid
4. Large volume in the transducer
5. Air bubbles in the system
6. Compliant tubing

Factors that increase damping

1. Short tubing
2. Viscous fluid
3. Air in system
4. Kinked tubing

Zeroing transducers

You can zero anywhere you want and use any reference point you want. Typically, the right atrium is the reference point for arterial pressure and the system is zeroed by opening the stopcock at the level of the right atrium, disregarding the position of the transducer. Just remember that the pressure perceived at the transducer is the sum of the arterial pressure and the weight of the water column between the reference point and the transducer.

Sample questions

A = 1, 2, 3   B = 1, 3   C = 2, 4   D = 4 only   E = all are correct

1. "Ringing" is found in arterial pressure transducer systems having
   1. Short tubing
   2. Low natural frequency
   3. Noncompliant tubing
   4. Low damping coefficients

Single best answer

2. In an intraarterial pressure transducing system with low natural frequency, the most accurately measured parameter is
   1. Systolic blood pressure
   2. Mean arterial pressure
   3. Diastolic pressure
   4. Resonance
   5. The dicrotic notch

Answers: 1. C   2. 2

CHAPTER 82

Temperature Correction of Arterial Blood Gases

Regardless of patient temperature, the sampling electrode is always heated to 37°C. Solubility of gases, ion dissociation, and hemoglobin function are all affected by temperature. Therefore, PaO_2, $PaCO_2$, and pH are all temperature dependent.

Effect of temperature on arterial blood gas values

• Table 82–1

Patient Temperature	In vivo	In Sampling Bath at 37°C
<37°C	↓PaO_2, $PaCO_2$ ↑pH	Falsely high PaO_2, $PaCO_2$ Falsely low pH
>37°C	↑PaO_2, $PaCO_2$ ↓pH	Falsely low PaO_2, $PaCO_2$ Falsely high pH

Explanation

The solubility of gas increases as temperature decreases; therefore, there are fewer molecules in the gas phase, so there is less partial pressure exerted. Thus, *in vivo*, the PaO_2 and $PaCO_2$ are lower in a hypothermic patient than they would be in a normothermic patient. If you then take the hypothermic patient's blood and warm it up to 37° for analysis, more gas molecules will enter the gas phase, causing an increase in pressure and falsely elevating the PaO_2 and $PaCO_2$.

Sample questions

A = 1, 2, 3   B = 1, 3   C = 2, 4   D = 4 only   E = all are correct

1. During cardiac bypass at 33°C, an arterial blood gas is drawn. Analysis is performed at 37°C. Values which will be higher than the *in vivo* values include
   1. PaO_2
   2. HCO_3^-
   3. $PaCO_2$
   4. pH

2. Same patient. Which values would be lower than the actual *in vivo* situation?

1. PaO_2
2. HCO_3^-
3. $PaCO_2$
4. pH

Single best answer

3. A large air bubble in an arterial blood gas sample drawn from a patient breathing room air will cause which of the following perturbations?
   1. PaO_2 increased, $PaCO_2$ decreased
   2. PaO_2 decreased, $PaCO_2$ increased
   3. PaO_2 increased, $PaCO_2$ increased
   4. PaO_2 decreased, $PaCO_2$ decreased
   5. PaO_2 increased, $PaCO_2$ no change

Answers: 1. B   2. D   3. 1

Central Venous and Pulmonary Artery Catheters

How a PA catheter works: A balloon-tipped catheter follows the path of blood flow through the RA and RV into the pulmonary artery, where it "wedges," creating a static column of blood between the catheter tip and the left atrium. The resultant pressure measurement is the pulmonary artery occlusion pressure (PAOP).

What does the PAOP tell us?

Clinically, we view PAOP as being equal to LVEDP. This view makes the folowing assumptions:

1. There is no abnormal pressure gradient across the mitral valve
2. LV compliance is normal; and thus, LVEDP = LVEDV (LVEDV is the best indicator of LV preload)
3. The catheter tip is West's zone III (where Pa > Pv > PA; and thus, the catheter tip lies in the middle of an uninterrupted column of blood)

How else can we evaluate LV preload?

Clinically, we often use CVP as an indicator of LV preload. This view makes the following assumptions:

1. There are no abnormal pressure gradients across the tricuspid, pulmonary, or mitral valves
2. Pulmonary vascular resistance is normal
3. RV and LV function and compliance are normal

In other words, we assume:

$$CVP \approx PA_D \approx PAOP \approx LAP \approx LVEDP \approx LVEDV$$
$$\uparrow \quad \uparrow \quad \uparrow \quad \uparrow \quad \uparrow$$
RV function   PVR   airway pressure   mitral valve   LV compliance

Factors that alter the accuracy of PA catheter measurements

1. "Whip" of catheter during cardiac cycle causes artifact
2. Overwedging creates falsely high PAOP
3. Failure to measure at end exhalation
4. Physical misplacement of catheter tip in zone II or I
5. Anything that increases pulmonary vascular resistance, converting zone

III ($Pa > Pv > P_A$) to zone II ($Pa > P_A > Pv$) or zone I ($P_A > Pa > Pv$), such as:

- –hypoxia
- –hypercarbia
- –hypothermia
- –hypovolemia
- –PEEP (increases P_A)
- –pneumothorax
- –acidosis
- –COPD
- –tachycardia (limited diastolic runoff)

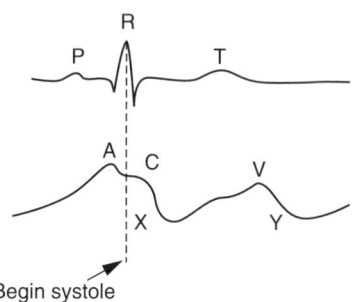

Figure 83–1.

Significance of various portions of central venous waveform

1. A wave: atrial contraction, follows EKG p wave
2. C wave: isovolumic ventricular contraction against closed tricuspid valve causes valve to encroach on RA, producing pressure wave
3. X descent: ventricular ejection, tricuspid valve recedes from atrium, causing atrial pressure to fall
4. V wave: atrial filling while tricuspid valve is still closed
5. Y descent: opening of tricuspid valve allows egress of atrial blood, and atrial pressure falls

Abnormal CVP waveforms and their significance

1. Loss of A waves: atrial fibrillation/atrial flutter
2. Cannon A waves: anything that increases resistance to right atrial emptying: nodal rythms, tricuspid stenosis, RV hypertrophy, pulmonary hypertension
3. Cannon V waves: tricuspid regurgitation, ventricular noncompliance as with ischemia or failure

Abnormal CVP/PAOP/LVEDP gradients and their significance

1. CVP > PAOP:
   A. ↑ PVR (due to any of the factors listed)
   B. Tachycardia
2. PAOP > LVEDP:
   A. Mitral stenosis
   B. PEEP
   C. Tip in zone II or I
   D. LA myxoma
3. PAOP < LVEDV:
   A. Noncompliant LV
   B. Aortic insufficiency causing early mitral closure

Complications of PA catheters

Besides all the bad things that come from shoving a needle into someone's neck
1. Cardiac dysrythmias
2. Pulmonary hemorrhage
3. Pulmonary infarction
4. PA rupture: presents with hemoptysis, treat with PEEP, attempt to isolate the lung, reduce pulmonary artery pressure
5. Looping, knotting
6. Embolization of vegetations, clots

Sample questions

A = 1, 2, 3   B = 1, 3   C = 2, 4   D = 4 only   E = all are correct

1. Inaccurate pulmonary artery occlusion pressures will be found during
   1. Spontaneous ventilation at end exhalation
   2. Hypothermia
   3. Intermittent mechanical ventilation at 8/min
   4. The use of positive end-expiratory pressures of 12 cm H_2O

Single best answer

2. Following coronary artery bypass grafting, a patient in the intensive care unit undergoes measurement of serial pulmonary artery occlusion pressures. The nurse inflates the balloon with 1 mL air and immediately notes bright red blood in the endotracheal tube. The most appropriate first step is to
   1. Suction the endotracheal tube
   2. Add another 1 mL to the balloon
   3. Perform endobronchial intubation
   4. Initiate positive end-expiratory pressure 10 cm H_2O
   5. Administer nitroprusside

Answers: 1. C   2. 5

CHAPTER 84

Thermodilution Cardiac Output

Technique: A known quantity of cool or room-temperature solution is injected into a central vein and a thermistor in the pulmonary artery measures the temperature change over time.

Calculation

Cardiac output is proportional to the difference between blood and injectate temperatures divided by the area (volume) under the curve. Thus, calculation of cardiac output assumes:

1. Constant flow
2. Complete mixing of injectate with blood
3. No recirculation
4. Injectate is delivered as a bolus

Sampling errors are due to

1. Injectate factors: incorrect volume, incorrect temperature, speed of injection, type of injectate
2. Dilutional factors: intracardiac shunt, coadministration of IV fluids, valvular regurgitation
3. Respiratory phase: best measurements are at apnea or full inspiration . . . respiratory action causes cooling of pulmonary tree
4. Patient position: cardiac output is higher in left and right lateral positions than supine
5. Catheter position: both too proximal and too distal alter cardiac output

Falsely high cardiac output

1. Small injectate volume
2. Injectate too warm
3. Thrombus
4. Catheter wedged
5. Tricuspid regurgitation
6. Left-to-right shunt

Falsely low cardiac output

1. Large volume injectate
2. Injectate too warm

3. Catheter too proximal (permits backflow)
4. Right-to-left shunt

Don't kill yourself trying to memorize all these . . . just understand that anything causing less "cold" to reach the thermistor will overestimate the cardiac output, and vice versa.

Sample question

A = 1, 2, 3   B = 1, 3   C = 2, 4   D = 4 only   E = all are correct

1. Thermodilution cardiac output
    1. Is falsely high if an inadequate injectate volume is used
    2. Is falsely high if the catheter tip is "wedged"
    3. Is falsely low if the rate of injection is too slow
    4. Measures left ventricular stroke volume

Answer: 1. A

CHAPTER 85

Mixed Venous Saturation

Clinical use: Provides an indication of tissue oxygenation and the balance between O_2 supply and demand

How do you get this information?

The Fick equation states:

$$\text{Cardiac output} = \frac{\text{Oxygen consumption}}{\text{Arterial } O_2 \text{ content} - \text{mixed venous } O_2 \text{ content}}$$

What can you glean from this?

If O_2 consumption and arterial O_2 content are unchanged, then changes in the mixed venous saturation are directly proportional to changes in cardiac output. In other words, as O_2 delivery decreases, O_2 extraction increases and mixed venous saturation falls.

Causes of low mixed venous saturation

1. Low O_2 delivery to tissues: low cardiac output, anemia, hypoxia, alkalosis, and methemoglobinemia (because methemoglobin can't bind O_2 and also causes a left shift of oxyhemoglobin curve, impairing release of O_2 to tissues)
2. Increased O_2 consumption: fever, shivering, hypermetabolic states like thyrotoxicosis

Causes of high mixed venous saturation

1. Wedged PA catheter is **most common** cause (catheter is in contact with arterialized blood)
2. Low O_2 consumption: cyanide toxicity (no aerobic metabolism), hypothermia
3. High cardiac output: sepsis, burns, left-to-right shunts
4. Mitral regurgitation

Sample questions: None . . . because they usually just ask you to list the factors that increase or decrease the mixed venous saturation, sooooo . . . **MEMORIZE!**

Chapter 86

Cardiac Pacemakers

Consist of

1. A pulse generator
2. Two electrodes: positive electrode is ground, negative electrode is stimulating electrode

Location of electrodes dictates type of pacing

1. Unipolar pacing: ground electrode located far from heart
2. Bipolar pacing: both electrodes are in chamber being paced

Two basic modes of pacing

1. Fixed:
   A. Pacemaker fires whether there is native activity present or not
   B. Carries risk of triggering malignant tachycardia/fibrillation
2. Synchronous:
   A. Pacer is inhibited by native activity
   B. Pacer rate is set lower than average intrinsic rate

Pacemaker mode conversion

1. Is achieved by placing a magnet on top of the pulse generator
2. Is suggested preoperatively to verify pacer function if patient's intrinsic rate is high enough to inhibit pacer activity
3. Conversion of demand pacers to asynchronous mode using an external magnet may cause reprogramming of pacer . . . not evident until magnet removed . . . put it back and call cardiology

All pacers are described by a five-letter code

Pay the most attention to the first three letters:

First letter: indicates chamber being paced (A = atrium, V = ventricle, D = dual)

Second letter: indicates which chamber is being monitored for native electrical activity (A = atrium, V = ventricle, D = dual, O = none . . . pacer is asynchronous)

Third letter: indicates how the pacer responds to native electrical activity (T = pacer is triggered, I = pacer is inhibited, D = dual, O = none)

Fourth letter: indicates functions that can be programmed (P = output only, M = multiprogrammable, C = communicating, O = none)

Fifth letter: indicates what type of antitachycardia function it has
(B = bursts, N = normal, S = scanning, E = external)

Perioperative things that may alter pacer function

1. Hypokalemia (? hyperventilation)
2. Hyperkalemia (? succinylcholine)
3. Positive pressure ventilation (distance between leads and heart can be increased)
4. Lithotripsy (shock waves can inhibit demand pacers)
5. MRI (magnetic field can convert to asynchronous mode)
6. Electrocautery (especially unipolar, can inhibit demand pacer)

Recommendations for electrocautery use in patients with pacemakers

1. Consider converting to asynchronous mode
2. Use bipolar cautery if possible
3. Place grounding pad as far from pulse generator as possible
4. Use lowest current possible
5. Apply current in short bursts
6. Have external converting magnet and defibrillator available

NOTE: If defibrillation is required, be aware that putting paddles over the pulse generator can alter the stimulation threshold and lead to capture failure.

Most common indications for preoperative pacemaker insertion

Especially if patients have syncope

1. Tachy-brady syndrome
2. Sick sinus syndrome
3. AV conduction defects

NOTE: Bifascicular block is *not* an indication, but you should consider establishing central access since there is a chance for progression to complete heart block.

Sample questions

Single best answer

1. A dual-chamber pacemaker that paces and senses both the atria and ventricle which is triggered by atrial activity and inhibited by ventricular activity is correctly labeled
   1. DTI
   2. DDD
   3. DDT
   4. DDI
   5. TDI

A = 1, 2, 3   B = 1, 3   C = 2, 4   D = 4 only   E = all are correct

2. A patient scheduled for surgery has a VVI pacemaker. His preoperative EKG is shown below.

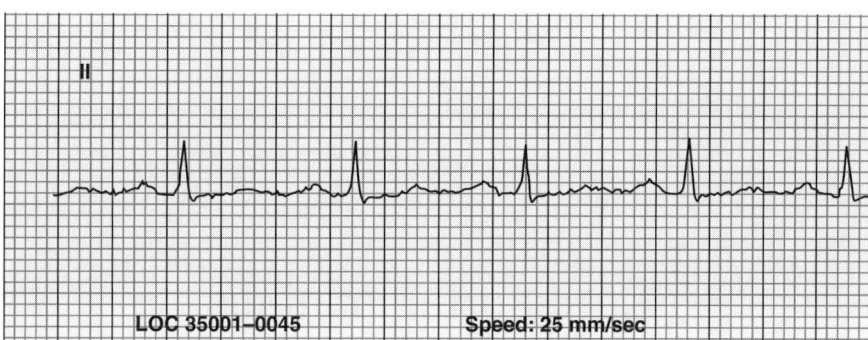

Figure 86–1.

Correct statements include:
1. Atrial activity is inhibiting the pacemaker
2. The pacemaker rate is lower than the intrinsic rate
3. Placing an external magnet over the pulse generator will produce paced beats
4. The ventricular sensing electrode is properly functioning

3. A DDD pacemaker with ventricular leads placed in the right ventricular myocardium
   1. Requires atrial pacing to stimulate ventricular pacing
   2. Will stimulate the ventricle if no intrinsic ventricular activity follows a pacer-induced P wave
   3. Always follows a pacer-induced P wave with a pacer-induced R wave
   4. Will produce left bundle branch block during ventricular pacing

Answers: 1. 2   2. C   3. C

Cardiac Tamponade

Defect: Excessive fluid in the pericardial sac

$\uparrow$ intrapericardial pressure $\rightarrow$ $\begin{cases} \uparrow \text{ central venous pressure} \\ \uparrow \text{ LVEDP} \rightarrow \text{coronary artery compression} \rightarrow \downarrow \text{myocardial perfusion} \\ \downarrow \text{ diastolic filling} \rightarrow \downarrow \text{SV} \rightarrow \downarrow \text{CO} \rightarrow \text{tachycardia, hypotension and acidosis} \end{cases}$

Figure 87–1.

Diagnostic tests

1. ECHO: gold standard
2. CxR: insensitive, no change in cardiac silohuette until ~250 mL of pericardial fluid
3. EKG:
   A. Tachycardia
   B. Decreased voltage
   C. Electrical alternans (on alternate beats, the voltage axis changes)
   D. Pulsus paradoxus (>10 mmHg drop in systolic pressure with spontaneous inspiration)
4. Equalized heart pressures (RAP = RVEDP = PAP = LAP = LVEDP)

Treatment

Pericardiocentesis under local anesthesia if no risk of recurrence or hemodynamically unstable, pericardotomy under local or general if recurring or hemodynamically stable

Anesthetic management

1. Maintain preload (volume resuscitate)
2. Maintain myocardial contractility (beware of volatile agents and other myocardial depressants)
3. Maintain normal to high pulse (maintains CO in the face of a relatively fixed SV, but beware that a pulse too high will drop CO by reducing filling time)
4. Maintain systemic vascular resistance (to sustain coronary and systemic perfusion)
5. Maintain spontaneous ventilation if possible (positive pressure may further decrease venous return). If positive pressure is required, use a fast rate, low tidal volume, low PIP, avoid PEEP)

Helpful drugs

1. Ketamine (increases pulse, SVR and contractility)
2. Pancuronium (increases pulse)
3. Inotropes (maintain SVR, pulse)

Sample questions

A = 1, 2, 3   B = 1, 3   C = 2, 4   D = 4 only   E = all are correct

1. Expected findings in a patient with cardiac tamponade include
   1. Diminished voltage on EKG
   2. Increased central venous pressure with spontaneous inspiration
   3. A greater than expected decrease in systolic blood pressure during spontaneous inspiration
   4. An elevated pulmonary capillary wedge pressure during controlled ventilation

2. A 45-year-old female with systemic lupus erythematosus is to undergo treatment for a recurrent pericardial effusion. Her vital signs include blood pressure 100/52 mmHg, pulse 116, and a CVP of 15 mmHg. After performing a pericardiocentesis under local anesthesia, the most appropriate course of management would include
   1. Pericardotomy under general anesthesia
   2. Serial chest X-rays
   3. Radial artery cannulation
   4. High-dose steroid therapy

Answers: 1. E   2. B

Mitral Stenosis

Defect: Fusion of mitral leaflets and narrowing of mitral orifice following rheumatic fever

Pathophysiology

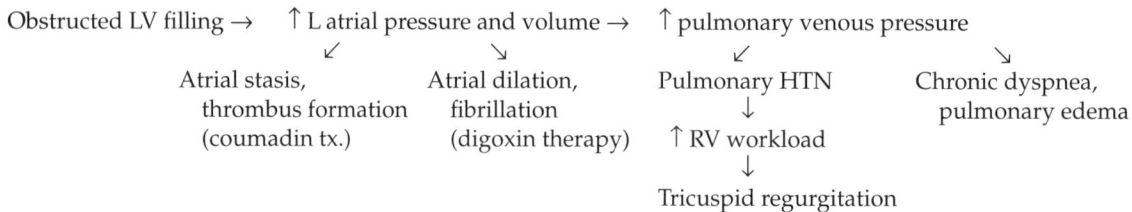

Figure 88.1.

Preoperative management

1. Avoid anticholinergic premedicants (cause tachycardia)
2. Avoid excess sedation (risk of hypoventilation and thus, increased pulmonary vascular resistance)
3. SBE prophylaxis
4. Consider stopping coumadin (not been shown to increase risk of emboli)

Anesthetic management

1. Maintain sinus rythym (atrial kick provides 40% of LV filling)
2. Maintain normal pulse rate (tachycardia drops CO by decreasing filling time, bradycardia drops CO because CO is rate dependent 2° to "fixed" SV)
3. Maintain LV preload and stroke volume (keep LA pressure high while avoiding pulmonary edema. PA catheter can guide you, but remember that PAD isn't an accurate reflection of LVEDP)
4. Prevent further increases in pulmonary vascular resistance (no hypoxia, hypercarbia, acidosis, N_2O)
5. Avoid sudden decreases in SVR (can't raise SV to maintain BP, and tachycardia worsens the picture)

Management of acute-onset atrial fibrillation with mitral stenosis

1. Cardiovert with 25 joules
2. Esmolol or diltiazem for *immediate* rate control
3. Digoxin for *prolonged* rate control (onset is slow)

Sample questions

A = 1, 2, 3   B = 1, 3   C = 2, 4   D = 4 only   E = all are correct

1. Anesthetic premedication and maintenance agents that should be avoided in mitral stenosis include
   1. Ketamine
   2. Pancuronium
   3. Atropine
   4. Nitrous oxide

2. A 42-year-old, 70-kg female with mitral stenosis is in the PACU following laparoscopic cholecystectomy under general anesthesia with nitrous oxide, oxygen, isoflurane, and vecuronium. Blood loss was 50 mL, and she received 2500 mL of Ringer's lactate. She now has bibasilar rales and an $SaO_2 = 91\%$ on a face mask with F_iO_2 0.4. Possible causes of these findings include
   1. Hypoventilation due to residual anesthetic effect
   2. Trendelenburg position intraoperatively
   3. Excessive fluid administration
   4. Nitrous oxide

Answers: 1. E   2. E

CHAPTER 89

Mitral Regurgitation

Defect: Incompetent mitral valve, allowing systolic and diastolic regurgitation of ventricular blood into left atrium. Regurgitant fraction > 0.6 is considered severe.

Two distinct subsets of mitral regurgitation

1. **Acute:**
   A. Due to chordae tendinae rupture following SBE or papillary muscle dysfunction following myocardial infarction
   B. Poorly tolerated
   C. Other valvular defects not usually present
2. **Chronic:**
   A. Rheumatic fever most common cause, may also be 2° to annulus stretching from LVH
   B. Well tolerated for years
   C. Often associated with mitral stenosis

Pathophysiology

1. **Acute**

$$\text{MI or SBE} \rightarrow \text{LV dysfunction}$$
$$\downarrow$$
$$\text{papillary muscle dysfunction or chordae tendinae rupture}$$
$$\downarrow$$
$$\text{acute regurgitation of stroke volume into small, noncompliant left atrium}$$
$$\downarrow$$
$$\text{acute increase in LA pressure} \rightarrow \text{pulmonary congestion} \rightarrow \text{PA hypertension} \rightarrow \text{RV failure}$$

Figure 89–1.

2. **Chronic**

Scarring 2° to rheumatic fever renders valve progressively more incompetent → gradual increase in regurgitant fraction → increase in volume work by LA and LV → atrial dilation with maintenance of normal pressures (atrial fibrillation common) or LVH with variable systolic dysfunction

Factors affecting amount of regurgitation

1. Heart rate: bradycardia increases time available for diastolic regurgitation

2. SVR: ↑ SVR promotes regurgitation, ↓ SVR promotes forward flow
3. Valvular orifice: ↑ size = ↑ regurgitant fraction

Anesthetic management

Goal is to promote forward flow

1. Maintain normal to slightly high pulse
2. Avoid ↑ SVR
3. Avoid myocardial depression (there is always some degree of systolic dysfunction)
4. Consider PA catheter (if MR severe, V waves increase as regurgitant fraction increases)
5. SBE prophylaxis

Sample questions

A = 1, 2, 3   B = 1, 3   C = 2, 4   D = 4 only   E = all are correct

1. Mitral regurgitation
   1. Produces "v" waves on the pulmonary artery wedge tracing
   2. Is less dependent on atrial contraction than mitral stenosis
   3. Produces symptoms more rapidly when accompanied by mitral stenosis
   4. Is usually an isolated valvular defect

2. True statements regarding the use of pulmonary artery catheters in patients with mitral regurgitation include
   1. Nitroprusside reduces the amplitude of the "v" waves
   2. The wedge pressure more accurately reflects left ventricular end-diastolic pressure in acute mitral regurgitation than chronic mitral regurgitation
   3. As the regurgitant fraction increases, the amplitude of the "v" wave increases
   4. A large increase in the regurgitant fraction can occur without elevating left atrial pressure in patients with chronic regurgitation

Answers: **1. A   2. E**

Aortic Stenosis

Defect: Abnormally narrow aortic valve orifice, limiting cardiac output and increasing left ventricular pressure work.

Causes

1. Congenital bicuspid valve (isolated valvular defect)
2. Rheumatic fever (usually associated with mitral valve disease)

Pathophysiology

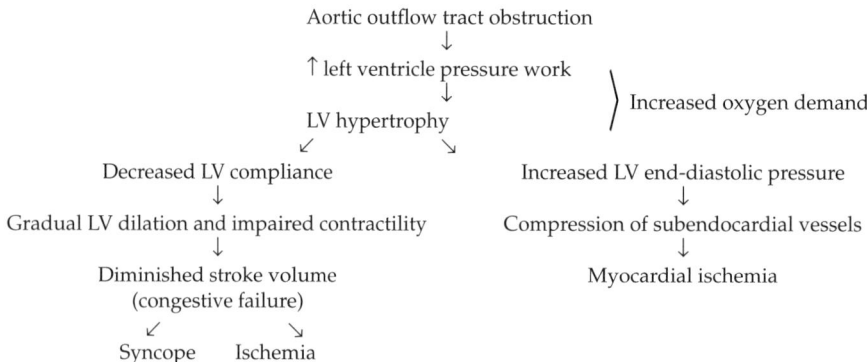

Figure 90–1.

Signs/symptoms

Angina/syncope/LV failure (symptoms take ~20 years to develop)

Anesthetic management

1. Maintain sinus rythm (noncompliant LV dependent on atrial kick for 40% of preload)
2. Maintain normal heart rate (too fast prevents adequate filling, too slow allows overfilling)
3. Maintain intravascular volume (can't maintain falling cardiac output with usual tachycardic response)
4. Avoid acute ↑ or ↓ in SVR (too low decreases coronary perfusion pressure, too high ↑ pressure work of left ventricle)
5. SBE prophylaxis
6. Invasive monitors if AS is severe (transvalvular gradiaent > 50 mmHg, valve area < 1 cm^2)

REMEMBER: Mean PAOP underestimates LVEDP; LVEDP correlates to the PAOP "a" wave.

Theoretical concerns regarding specific anesthetic techniques and drugs

1. Regional: decreased SVR will decrease coronory perfusion pressure
2. Volatile agents: myocardial depression can decrease stroke volume (especially halothane); decreased SA node automaticity causes loss of atrial kick
3. Neuromuscular blockade: histamine release can drop SVR (atracurium); tachycardia impairs LV filling and increases oxygen demand (pancuronium)

Sample questions

A = 1, 2, 3   B = 1, 3   C = 2, 4   D = 4 only   E = all are correct

1. Factors that contribute to decreased coronary artery perfusion in patients with aortic stenosis include
   1. Decreased systemic diastolic pressure
   2. Increased left ventricular diastolic pressure
   3. Tachycardia
   4. Increased systemic vascular resistance

2. A 58-year-old mentally handicapped man with severe aortic stenosis and a history of syncope is scheduled for complete dental extraction under general anesthesia prior to his valve replacement. In the preoperative holding area, he is diaphoretic and complaining of chest pain. His pulse is 135/min, blood pressure is 78/55 mmHg, and the T waves are inverted on leads V4-6 in the EKG. The most appropriate immediate treatment is to administer
   1. Phenylephrine 100 µg IV
   2. Nitroglycerin infusion at 1 µg/kg/min
   3. Midazolam 2 mg IV
   4. Propanolol 1 mg IV
   5. Oxygen therapy and immediate transesophageal echocardiography

Answers: 1. A   2. D

Aortic Regurgitation

Defect: Incompetent aortic valve allows diastolic regurgitation of stroke volume into left ventricle

Two distinct subsets of aortic regurgitation

1. **Acute:**
   A. Follows SBE, trauma, dissecting aneurysm
   B. Nondilated, nonhypertrophied ventricle can't accommodate acute volume overload
   C. Usually requires immediate valve replacement
2. **Chronic:**
   A. Follows rheumatic fever, hypertension
   B. Ventricle accommodates to gradual volume overload
   C. Valve replacement eventually required

Pathophysiology

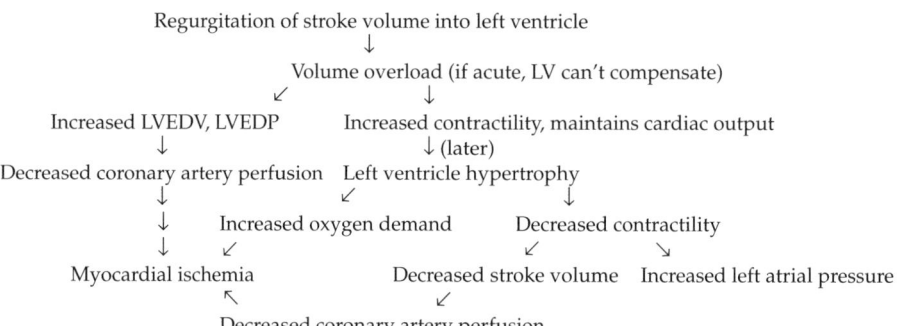

Figure 91–1.

Factors increasing the degree of regurgitation

1. Bradycardia: increases diastolic time available for regurgitation
2. High systemic vascular resistance: discourages forward flow

Anesthetic management

1. Maintain sinus rythm at high normal rates (minimizes time available for regurgitation)
2. Avoid acute increases in SVR (increases regurgitation, precipitates con-

gestive failure. Treat with vasodilator like nitroprusside to decrease afterload)
3. Maintain myocardial contractility
4. SBE prophylaxis

Sample question

Single best answer

1. A 58-year-old female is scheduled for replacement of a severely incompetent aortic valve. In the preoperative holding area, she is diaphoretic and complains of dyspnea, substernal chest pain, and nausea. Her heart rate is 85/min, blood pressure is 140/90 mmHg, SaO_2 is 94% on room air, and there is ST segment depression on leads V4-6 on EKG. The most appropriate immediate therapy is administration of
    1. Digoxin 1.25 mg IV
    2. Nitroglycerin paste 1 inch applied to chest wall
    3. Esmolol 10 mg IV
    4. Furosemide 10 mg IV
    5. Nitroprusside infusion at 1 μg/kg/min

Answer: 1. 5

CHAPTER 92

Idiopathic Hypertrophic Subaortic Stenosis

Defect: Dynamic obstruction of left ventricular outflow tract due to asymmetrical hypertrophy of interventricular septum and displacement of anterior mitral valve leaflet into outflow tract

Factors that increase degree of obstruction

1. Decreased preload
2. Decreased afterload
3. Increased ejection velocity (increased contractility or increased rate)

Pathophysiology

```
                        ↙ LV contraction ↘
Anterior mitral valve leaflet obstructs LV ejection     Asymmetrical septum impedes LV ejection
                        ↘               ↙
                Increased myocardial oxygen consumption
                                ↓
                Left ventricular hypertrophy       → LV failure
                                ↓
                ↑ Left atrial pressure    → Left atrial dilation
```

Figure 92–1.

Signs/symptoms

Angina/syncope/congestive failure/dysrythmias (symptoms mimic aortic stenosis)

Anesthetic management

1. Maintain normal sinus rythym (noncompliant LV is dependent on atrial kick for preload)
2. Avoid decreased preload (ventricular walls encroach on outflow tract at low ventricular volumes)
3. Avoid decreased afterload (fast ejection of volume causes venturi effect, promoting obstruction)
3. Attempt mild myocardial depression

Sample questions

A = 1, 2, 3   B = 1, 3   C = 2, 4   D = 4 only   E = all are correct

1. Appropriate management of a patient with hypertrophic subaortic stenosis includes each of the following EXCEPT
    1. Volatile agents for maintenance of anesthesia
    2. Preferential use of ephedrine versus phenylephrine for management of hypotension
    3. Maintaining normal to slightly high preload
    4. Maintaining normal to slightly high heart rate to promote forward flow past the obstruction

Single best answer

2. In a 65-kg patient with hypertrophic subaortic stenosis, which of the following anesthetic techniques is least likely to cause hemodynamic perturbations during repair of a varicocele?
    1. Thiopental 200 mg, halothane 1.2%, and pancuronium 6.5 mg
    2. Field block with 40 mL 0.5% bupivicaine with 1:200,000 epinephrine
    3. Propofol 130 mg, halothane 1.2%, vecuronium 6.5 mg
    4. Spinal block to T6 with 100 mg lidocaine and epinephrine 1:200,000
    5. Epidural block to T6 with 16 mL lidocaine 2% wihtout epinephrine

Answers: 1. C   2. 3

CHAPTER 93

Thoracic and Abdominal Aneurysms

General goals

1. Minimize further dissection by lowering MAP while maintaining adequate perfusion of brain, myocardium, kidneys
2. Reduce shear forces by reducing heart rate and myocardial contractility

Physiologic effects of applying aortic cross clamp

1. **Proximal effects:** ↑ SVR, MAP, PCWP, PVR, CVP, LVEDP and LVEDV but ↓ cardiac output. Result: dilation of LV and high LVEDP can lead to subendocardial ischemia, acute LV failure, and dysrythmias, especially if prior cardiac dysfunction or coronary artery disease present.
2. **Distal effects:** hypotension resulting in hypoperfusion/ischemia of:
   A. Kidneys (leads to acute renal failure)
   B. Abdominal viscera (leads to intestinal infarction)
   C. Spinal cord (leads to hemiparesis/plegia, due to reduced flow through *anterior* spinal artery). Monitoring SSEPs no help, because they look at *dorsal* columns. Risk is greatest with supraceliac clamping.
   D. Distal extremities (anaerobic metabolism creates lactate load to central circulation when clamp released)

Severity of effects of aortic cross clamp depends on

1. Location of cross clamp: greatest effect seen with clamp supraceliac > suprarenal > infrarenal
2. Presence of collateral circulation (someplace to shunt blood)
3. Preoperative amount of aortic blood flow: severely atherosclerotic patients with reduced aortic flow may not demonstrate much hemodynamic change with cross clamping

Physiologic effects of releasing aortic cross clamp

1. Profound hypotension due to a relative hypovolemia and acute ↓ SVR. *(This is your biggest problem.)*
2. ↑ CVP due to return of venous blood pooled in lower extremities
3. Metabolic acidosis (wash-in of lactate from lower extremities)
4. ↑ end-tidal CO_2 (same as #3)
5. ↓ SvO_2 (due to oxygen-poor blood returning from legs)

Anesthetic management: monitors and what they tell you

1. Arterial line: right radial reflects cerebral perfusion pressure, preferred site for descending thoracic aneurysms, left radial best for ascending. Femoral line reflects renal/visceral perfusion pressures.
2. PA catheter: LVEDV/LVEDP, cardiac output . . . lets you gauge degree of LV load.
3. TEE: early detection of regional wall motion abnormalities is **most sensitive** indicator of myocardial ischemia.
4. Foley catheter: Measurement of urine output is poor predictor of renal failure.

Maneuvers to be done prior to cross clamping

1. Give mannitol (furosemide benefit less well established): pretreatment is more renal-protective than giving after cross clamp is on
2. Prevent HTN and risk of myocardial ischemia by creating relative hypovolemia via underhydration and vasodilators:
   A. **Nitroglycerin:** better prevention of myocardial ischemia than nitroprusside because it decreases preload, leading to decreased LVEDV/LVEDP (LV dilation and elevated LVEDP are biggest causes of ischemia)
   B. **Nitroprusside:** better reduction of MAP than NTG. Best result may be combination of the two drugs.

Maneuvers to be done prior to releasing cross clamp

1. Discontinue vasodilators
2. Gradually volume-load } both prevent hypotension upon clamp release
3. Consider renal dose dopamine if urine output is low

Maneuvers to prevent renal failure

1. Pretreat with mannitol, maybe furosemide
2. Maintain highest MAP that myocardium will tolerate
3. Consider renal dose dopamine

Maneuvers to prevent spinal cord ischemia

1. Maintain highest MAP that myocardium will tolerate
2. Place spinal fluid drain (↓ spinal fluid pressure . . . cord perfusion pressure = MAP − spinal fluid pressure)
3. Place shunt to maintain distal perfusion
4. Consider circulatory arrest or hypothermic cardiopulmonary bypass

Possible nerve injuries during thoracic aneurysms repair

Besides spinal cord ischemia

1. Brachial plexus palsies (kinked due to patient positioning)
2. Recurrent laryngeal nerve (due to proximity to aorta)

Sample questions

Single best answer

1. A 65-year-old man with a history of angina pectoris undergoes resection of an abdominal aortic aneurysm with nitroglycerin infusion to control blood pressure. Prior to cross-clamp removal, the nitroglycerin is discon-

tinued, pulse is 80/min, blood pressure is 120/75 mmHg, pulmonary artery diastolic pressure is 10 mmHg and end-tidal CO_2 is 35 mmHg. Immediately following release of the cross-clamp, blood pressure decreases to 74/45 mmHg, pulmonary artery diastolic pressure decreases to 4 mmHg, and end-tidal CO_2 increases to 50 mmHg. The EKG reveals a heart rate of 135/min, and there is new ST segment depression. The most appropriate first therapy is
1. Increase minute ventilation
2. Put the cross-clamp back on
3. Reinstitute the nitroglycerin infusion
4. Rapid transfusion with two units packed red blood cells on pressure infusors
5. Institute dopamine infusion to maintain renal perfusion and increase blood pressure

2. A 58-year-old, 70-kg man with a history of angina and hypertension treated with propanolol and isosorbide undergoes abdominal aortic aneurysm resection under general anesthesia. Prior to cross-clamping the aorta, blood pressure is 145/85 mmHg, pulse is 65/min, pulmonary artery diastolic pressure is 6 mmHg. Upon placement of the aortic cross-clamp, blood pressure increases to 200/108 mmHg, pulmonary artery diastolic pressure increases to 18 mmHg, and pulse remains 65/min. The EKG reveals ST segment depression in lead V and occasional premature ventricular contractions. Initial therapy should be
1. Administer lidocaine IV
2. Hyperventilate with F_iO_2 1.0
3. Initiate nitroprusside infusion
4. Infuse mannitol 70 g IV
5. Increase volatile agent concentration

Answers: 1. 4   2. 3

Chapter 94

Heparin

Mechanism of action: Forms a complex with antithrombin III, potentiating the inhibitory action of antithrombin III on factor 10 and thrombin

Coagulation tests it prolongs

1. Whole blood clotting time (typically, an activated clotting time or ACT)
2. Activated partial thromboplastin time (APTT)

Factors affecting duration

1. Dose: $t_{1/2}$ is dose dependent
2. Metabolism: cleared by reticuloendothelial system and hepatic heparinase
3. Hypothermia: prolongs clearance

Causes of heparin resistance

1. Antithrombin III deficiency (congenital or acquired)
2. Drug interaction (prior heparin therapy, oral contraceptives, nitroglycerin)
3. Coronary artery disease (how ironic)
4. Old age
5. Pulmonary embolus
6. Hypereosinophilia

Management of heparin resistance

1. Additional doses of heparin
2. Fresh-frozen plasma to restore low antithrombin III levels

Complications of heparin therapy

1. Thrombocytopenia:
    A. A type II allergic reaction
    B. Triad of signs: thrombocytopenia, heparin tachyphylaxis, thrombus formation
    C. Diagnosed by demonstrating in vitro platelet aggregation following heparin administration
    D. Treatment: stop heparin. If cardiopulmonary bypass needed, give Iloprost (short-acting platelet inhibitor)

2. Bleeding
3. Alopecia, osteoporosis (weird and rare things)

Sample questions

A = 1, 2, 3   B = 1, 3   C = 2, 4   D = 4 only   E = all are correct

1. Beneficial effects of preoperative subcutaneous heparin therapy include
   1. Reduced risk of deep venous thrombosis
   2. Inhibition of antithrombin III
   3. Reduced risk of pulomonary embolus
   4. Platelet aggregation

2. Factors causing prolonged duration of heparin effect include
   1. Oral contraceptives
   2. Hepatic dysfunction
   3. Renal dysfunction
   4. Hypothermia

3. Factors causing prolonged activated clotting times include:
   1. Heparin therapy
   2. Hemodilution
   3. Hypothermia
   4. Serine protease inhibitor therapy (Aprotonin)

4. The activated clotting time is a measure of
   1. Platelet function
   2. Fibrinolyis
   3. Isolated coagulation factor deficiencies
   4. Whole-blood clotting

Answers: 1. B   2. C   3. E   4. D

Protamine and Other Things

Mechanism of action of protamine

1. Forms inactive complexes with heparin, terminates heparin effect.
2. Also has intrinsic anticoagulant effect.

Protamine reactions

1. Rash/urticaria
2. Bronchospasm
3. Pulmonary vasoconstriction
4. Reduced systemic vascular resistance, profound hypotension, cardiovascular collapse

Proposed mechanisms of protamine reaction

1. Potentiation of IgE-mediated histamine release
2. Complement activation and thromboxane production

Factors causing increased risk of protamine reaction

1. Prior exposure to protamine
2. Prior exposure to NPH or PZI insulin (the "P" stands for protamine) . . . may have IgE or IgG antibodies. (Isn't it ironic that so many of the patients for CABG are diabetics and may have had NPH before?)
3. Seafood allergy: protamine is derived from salmon semen
4. Male patient s/p vasectomy (violation of blood–testis barrier may cause antibody formation)
5. Rapid injection of protamine

> **PEARL:** This has nothing to do with protamine, but they love to ask about coumadin reversal and emergency surgery. Ways to reverse coumadin effect:

1. Vitamin K: response takes ~24 hr . . . not helpful for emergency surgery
2. Fresh-frozen plasma: response is immediate
3. Infuse concentrates of vitamin K–dependent factors: response is immediate

Sample question

Single best answer

1. A 60-year-old man has coronary artery bypass grafting and aortic valve replacement and is weaning from cardiopulmonary bypass for which he was anticoagulated with 10,000 units of heparin. He has received 5 units whole blood, is on dobutamine 5 µg/kg/min, his pulmonary artery diastolic pressure is 15 mmHg, cardiac output is 4.6 L/min and blood pressure 123/66 mmHg. Protamine 100 mg is administered IV following an activated clotting time of 200 sec. Shortly after the aortic cannula is removed, pulmonary diastolic pressure is 45 mmHg, blood pressure 80/55 mmHg, cardiac output 2.0 L/min. The most appropriate response is
   1. Increase dobutamine to 10 µg/kg/min
   2. Transfuse with two units packed red blood cells
   3. Aspirate central venous port and roll patient to left lateral decubitus postion
   4. Hyperventilate with pure oxygen and administer epinephrine 1 µg/kg/min IV
   5. Administer furosemide 20 mg IV to reduce pulmonary edema

Answer: 1. 4

CHAPTER 96

Cardiopulmonary Bypass

Description of generic circuit: Canulae inserted into superior and inferior vena cavae remove venous blood, routing it to the bypass circuit oxygenator. Oxygenated blood is returned via an arterial cannula to the aorta. Flow is generated by a roller pump.

Flow requirements

1. Are based on body weight and metabolic demands (O_2 consumption, CO_2 production)
2. Limited by:
   A. Tubing diameter
   B. Size of arterial cannula
   C. Speed of pump

Pressure requirements

1. Higher in adults than kids.
2. ≥30 mmHg is probably lowest acceptable pressure.
3. Pressure within tubing is greater than that at the tissue level.

Blood gases during CPB

1. Do not have to be temperature-corrected (i.e., use the alpha-stat method)
2. Attempt normal pH, PO_2, PCO_2
3. Maintain mixed venous PO_2 > 40 mmHg, saturation >60%

The most common complications during or following CPB are hypotension and hypoxemia.

Causes of hypotension during CPB

1. Inadequate circuit volume
2. Inadequate pump rate
3. Vasodilation (due to hypercarbia, anaphylaxis)
4. Anemia

Causes of hypotension after CPB

1. Hypovolemia
2. Myocardial dysfunction
3. Protamine reaction

4. Air embolus
5. Electrolyte disorder (Ca^{++}, Mg^{++})
6. Metabolic acidosis
7. Ischemia
8. Low total peripheral resistance

Causes of hypoxemia during CPB

1. Oxygenator failure
2. Increased O_2 consumption (rewarming, incomplete relaxation)

Causes of hypoxemia after CPB

1. Pulmonary edema
2. Atelectasis
3. Pneumothoax/hemothorax/hydrothorax
4. Vasodilator therapy and inhibition of hypoxic pulmonary vasoconstriction
5. Cell crud in pulmonary capillaries

Sample question

A = 1, 2, 3   B = 1, 3   C = 2, 4   D = 4 only   E = all are correct

1. Despite normovolemia and normal hematocrit following cardiopulmonary bypass, a patient requires defibrillation during weaning from bypass. He returns to ventricular tachycardia. In addition to instituting lidocaine therapy and repeat defibrillation, which of the following should be evaluated?
    1. Core temperature
    2. Serum potassium
    3. Position of pulmonary artery catheter
    4. Serum magnesium

Answer: 1. E

CHAPTER 97

Intraaortic Balloon Pumps

Description: A long, narrow balloon placed in the descending aorta just distal to the left subclavian artery

How it works

1. Inflation is triggered by ventricular diastole, displacing blood from thoracic aorta. Blood displaced **proximally** augments coronary artery perfusion, blood displaced **distally** augments systemic perfusion.
2. Deflation occurs just prior to ventricular diastole, causing an acute afterload reduction and augmenting forward flow of blood (ventricular unloading).

Hemodynamic effects

1. Decreased afterload
2. Decreased LVEDP, LVEDV, and wall tension . . . thus, decreased myocardial O_2 consumption
3. Increased arterial and aortic diastolic pressure . . . thus, increased coronary artery perfusion

Limitations

1. Normal heart rate and rhythm required for optimum function
2. Low-resistance alternate pathways for blood limit effectiveness (aortic regurgitation, aortic collaterals)
3. Can cause "double counting" of pulse obtained from arterial waveforms
4. Not effective in biventricular failure
5. If inflation is done too early, LV ejection is impeded
6. If deflation is done too early, emptying of distal aorta impaired, systemic perfusion compromised

Indications

1. Myocardial contractile dysfunction: cardiogenic shock, myocardial infarction, failure to wean from bypass, contusion)
2. Persistent dysrhythmias
3. LV volume overload lesions (mitral regurgitation, VSD)

97 ■ Intraaortic Balloon Pumps

Sample questions

A = 1, 2, 3   B = 1   C = 2, 4   D = 4 only   E = all are correct

1. Following acute myocardial infarction and emergency coronary artery bypass surgery, a 60-year-old, 70-kg male is unable to wean from bypass. He is currently on dopamine and isoetharine. Hemoglobin 10 g/dL, temperature 34°C, arterial blood gas = pH 7.30, PCO_2 40 mmHg. Maneuvers that may assist weaning from bypass include:
   1. Transfuse with two unit packed red blood cells
   2. Active rewarming
   3. Correction of metabolic acidosis
   4. Institute an intraaortic ballon pump just distal to the innominate artery

2. Expected effects of an intraaortic balloon pump include
   1. Decreased left ventricular afterload
   2. Increased pulmonary venous saturation
   3. Increased coronary artery perfusion
   4. Decreased pulmonary artery PO_2

Answers: 1. A   2. A (# 2 is theoretical, since pump decreases myocardial O_2 consumption)

Mediastinoscopy

Indications

1. Evaluate extent of spread of lung cancer
2. Place atrial pacing wires

Approach

Through a suprasternal incision, direct the scope anterior to the trachea and posterior to the aortic arch into the mediastinum

Contraindications

1. Previous mediastinoscopy (absolute contraindication)
2. Distorted anatomy (tracheal deviation, thoracic aortic aneurysm . . . relative contraindications)
3. Superior vena cava syndrome (engorged vessels . . . increased risk of tearing)
4. Cerebrovascular disease (due to risk of carotid compression)

Anesthetic considerations

May be done with local or general anesthetic

1. Consider neuromuscular blockade (prevents straining and venous engorgement)
2. At risk for air embolus (increased risk if spontaneously ventilating or reverse trendelenburg)
3. At risk for bradycardia (due to aortic arch compression)
4. At risk for vascular compression (usually innominate artery, which becomes the R. subclavian and the R. common carotid . . . R. radial arterial line is sensitive monitor for compression. Be sure to have blood pressure cuff on opposite arm)

Complications

1. Bleeding **(most common)**
2. Pneumothorax
3. Recurrent laryngeal nerve injury
4. Tracheal collapse
5. Phrenic injury
6. Air embolism

7. Chylothorax
8. Esophageal injury

Sample question

Single best answer

1. A 55-year-old male with a diagnosis of right upper-lobe lung cancer is undergoing mediastinoscopy under general anesthesia with vecuronium, isoflurane, air, and oxygen 0.5. A catheter is placed in the right radial artery to monitor blood pressure and the pulse oximeter is placed on the right index finger. Approximately 5 min after insertion of the scope, his pulse drops to 40/min and the arterial waveform disappears. The pulse oximeter begins to steadily decrease and breath sounds are equal bilaterally. After changing the F_iO_2 to 1.0, the most appropriate next step is
   1. Tube thoracostomy to relieve the tension pneumothorax
   2. Check a noninvasive blood pressure on the left arm
   3. Administer atropine 1.0 mg IV
   4. Administer phenylephrine 200 µg IV
   5. Place the patient in the head-down position and flood the surgical field with 0.9% saline solution

Answer: 1. 2

CHAPTER 99

Double-Lumen Tubes

Indications for double-lumen tubes

1. Prevent spillage of pus or blood from diseased lung into healthy lung
2. Unilateral pulmonary lavage
3. Severe unilateral disease or ventilatory dysfunction (like shotgun blast to one lung)

} absolute indications

4. To improve surgical exposure (a relative indication)

How do you decide whether to use a right-sided tube or a left-sided tube?

There are basically three choices:

● Table 99–1

Intubate the Operative Lung	Intubate the Nonoperative Lung	Always Use Left-Sided Tube
Advantages	**Advantages**	**Advantages**
Can see where the tube is, reposition if needed	Avoids risk of dislodging due to surgical manipulation	1. Avoids risk of not ventilating right upper lobe
Disadvantages	**Disadvantages**	2. Relatively easy to place without fiberoptic assistance
1. Surgical handling may dislodge tube	If right mainstem is intubated, you risk not ventilating right upper lobe, because distance from carina to upper lobe takeoff is extremely short (hard to place bronchial cuff between the two points)	3. Is acceptable in most surgical instances
2. Ventilated (dependent) bronchus can collapse under weight of mediastinal structures (poor ventilation)		**Disadvantages**
		None

There are basically two techniques for placing the tube

1. Perform standard laryngoscopy. Insert tip of styletted tube through vocal cords, then rotate 90° toward the desired side. Remove stylet and advance until mild resistance is felt. Inflate both cuffs and confirm placement by one of the methods described below.
2. Intubate as above, stop advancing tube once tracheal cuff is immediately below cords. Insert fiberoptic scope through bronchial lumen. Use scope to guide placement into desired bronchus via "Seldinger" technique. Confirm placement as described below.

Confirmation of tube placement

Again, there are two choices
1. **Fiberoptic method:** Insert fiberoptic bronchoscope through tracheal lumen, viewing bronchial cuff in the mainstem bronchus. Verify lack of herniation of bronchial cuff over carina.
2. **Auscultatory method:** For clarity, all scenarios pertain to a left-sided tube with both cuffs inflated

Step 1: Ventilate through both lumens

Bilateral breath sounds ↓ Tube in trachea, not too deep

Unilateral breath sounds ↓ Tube too deep, both lumens in same bronchus

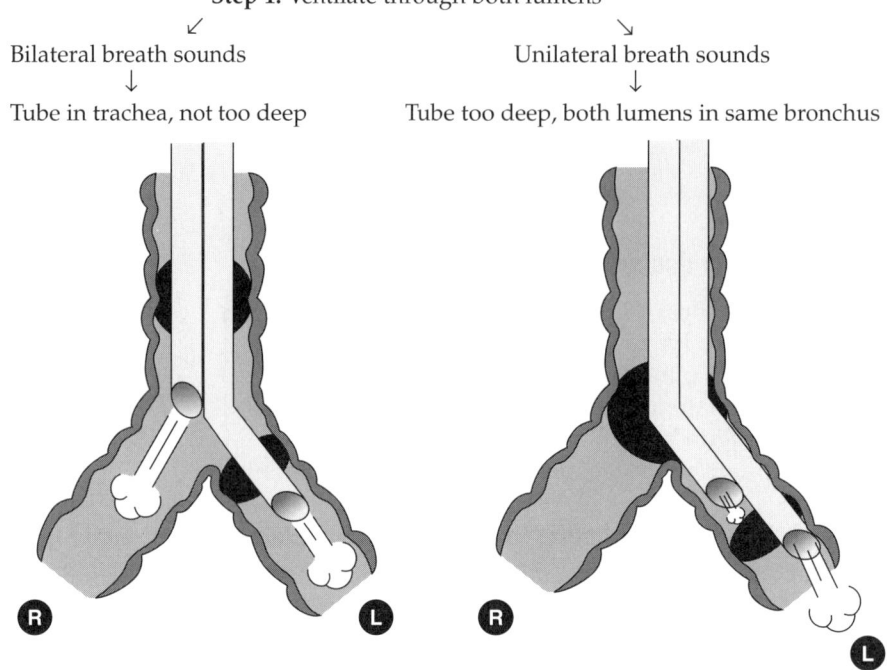

Figure 99–1.   Figure 99–2.

Step 2: Ventilate with tracheal lumen clamped (checks bronchial lumen position)

Breath sounds only on left ↓ Bronchial lumen correctly placed

Breath sounds only on right ↓ Both lumens in right mainstem

Bilateral breath sounds ↓ Tube too high, both lumens in trachea

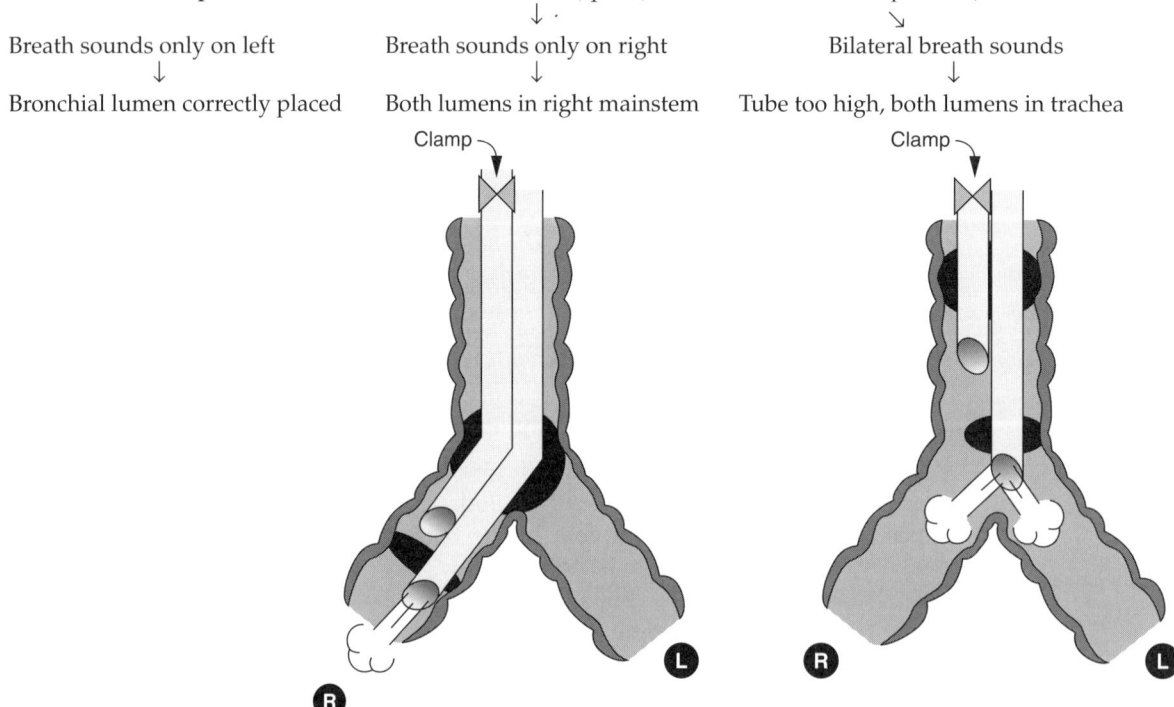

Figure 99–3.   Figure 99–4.

Step 3: Ventilate with bronchial lumen clamped (checks tracheal lumen position)

↙ ↘

Breath sounds on right   Absent or quiet breath sounds, hard to ventilate
↓   ↓
Tracheal lumen correctly placed   Deflate bronchial cuff
↙ ↘
Breath sounds only on left   Breath sounds bilaterally
↓   ↓
Tube too deep, both lumens in left mainstem   Tube too high, bronchial cuff in trachea blocking gas flow from tracheal lumen

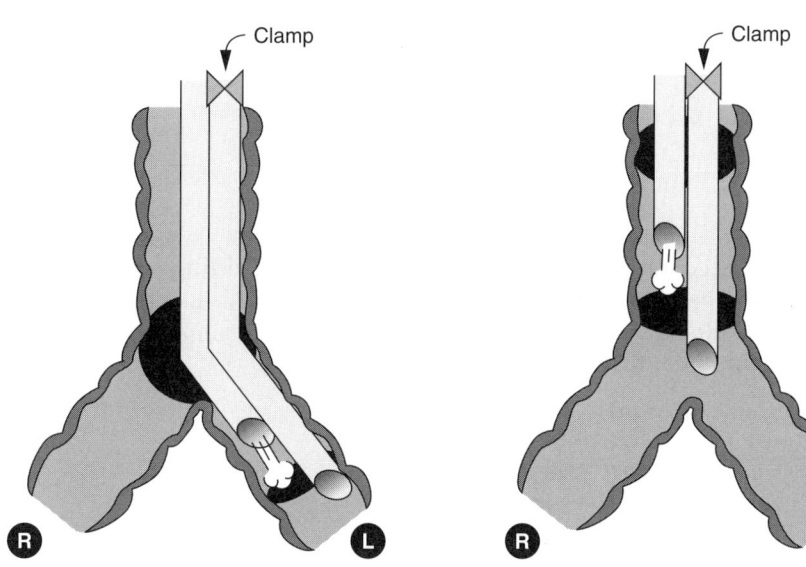

Figure 99–5.   Figure 99–6.

Sample questions

A = 1, 2, 3   B = 1, 3   C = 2, 4   D = 4 only   E = all are correct

1. After insertion of a left-sided double-lumen endotracheal tube and inflation of both cuffs, auscultation with the bronchial lumen clamped reveals absent breath sounds bilaterally and negligible end-tidal CO_2 by capnography. Possible locations of the tube include
   1. Both lumens are in left mainstem bronchus
   2. Both lumens are in the trachea above the carina
   3. Both lumens are in the right mainstem bronchus
   4. Esophageal intubation

2. Regarding the above patient, which findings are consistent with a right mainstem intubation with both lumens?
   1. Deflation of the bronchial cuff produces breath sounds on the right
   2. Unclamping the bronchial lumen reveals breath sounds on the right
   3. Deflation of the tracheal cuff produces absent breath sounds
   4. Ventilation through the bronchial lumen with the tracheal lumen clamped produces breath sounds on the right

Answers: 1. E   2. E

CHAPTER 100

One-Lung Ventilation and Pneumonectomy

Prior to lung resection, you must determine if the remaining lung mass can support the patient postoperatively. Tests of whole lung function are done first. Results that indicate risk of inadequate postoperative pulmonary function include:

1. ABGs: $PaCO_2 > 45$ mmHg on F_iO_2 .21
2. Spirometry: $FEV_1 < 50\%$ of FVC or $< 2L$
   MMV $< 50\%$ predicted
   RV $> 50\%$ of TLC
   DLCO $< 50\%$

If whole lung studies are abnormal, split-function PFTs are indicated. **Poor outcome is predicted by:** estimated postop $FEV_1 < 850$ mL **OR** $>70\%$ total pulmonary blood flow goes to operative lung (postop FEV_1 = preoperative $FEV_1 \div$ contralateral percentage of perfusion)

If split functions are also abnormal, but resection is still desired, try to create the postop condition: Poor outcome is predicted if balloon occlusion of operative main pulmonary artery results in:

Mean PAP > 40 mmHg **OR:** $PaCO_2 > 60$ mmHg **OR:** $PaO_2 < 45$ mmHg

One-lung ventilation is usually carried out in the lateral decubitus position. Pulmonary physiology is different in the upright and in the supine patient. For clarity, when discussing the physiologic changes, we will refer to the lungs as:

1. DL (dependent lung, the one being ventilated)
2. NDL (nondependent lung, the one not being ventilated)

Physiologic parameters of importance in the lateral decubitus position

● Table 100–1

	Pulmonary Blood Flow		Tidal Volume Distribution		Functional Residual Capacity	
	Two-Lung Ventilation	One-Lung Ventilation	Two-Lung Ventilation	One-Lung Ventilation	Two-Lung Ventilation	One-Lung Ventilation
Nondependent lung	40%	20%	60%	0%	70%	↓
Dependent lung	60%	80%	40%	100%	30%	↑

What causes the shift of blood flow during one-lung ventilation?

1. Gravity (most important)
2. Hypoxic pulmonary vasoconstriction (HPV) (hypoxia in NDL → vasoconstriction → ↑ pulmonary vascular resistance → blood is redirected to DL)

What are causes of hypoxia unique to one-lung ventilation?

1. Lack of HPV in NDL (allows continued perfusion of unventilated lung . . . ↓↓ V/Q ratio i.e., huge shunt)
2. Reduced FRC in DL (2° to compression → ↓↓ V/Q ratio)
3. HPV in DL (compression or absorption atelectasis occurs → areas of hypoxia → HPV → redirect blood back to NDL)
4. Malposition of tube (usually obstructing a lobar bronchus, creating a bigger shunt)

Factors inhibiting HPV

1. Both ↑ or ↓ pulmonary vascular resistance
2. Both ↑ or ↓ PvO_2
3. Vasodilators (nitroprusside)
4. Hypocarbia (although hypercarbia does *NOT* augment HPV)
5. Respiratory alkalosis (although acidosis does *NOT* augment HPV)
6. Volatile agents

Management of one-lung ventilation

1. Maintain two-lung ventilation as long as possible
2. High F_iO_2 (titrating in ~20% air may reduce absorption atelectasis)
3. Large tidal volumes (10–15 cc/kg)
   A. Advantage: maintains FRC in DL
   B. Disadvantage: high PIPs will ↑ PVR and redirect blood to NDL
4. Avoid hypocarbia (inhibits HPV in NDL) and hypercarbia (↑ PVR in DL, redirects blood to NDL)

Management of hypoxia during one-lung ventilation

After you confirm position of tube

1. **First:** CPAP 5–10 cm H_2O to NDL (oxygenates that portion of cardiac output still perfusing the NDL)
2. **Next:** add PEEP 5–10 cmH_2O to DL (increases FRC but beware: the ↑ PVR can shunt blood to NDL)
3. **If still hypoxic:** reexpand NDL with F_iO_2 1.0 and positive pressure
4. **If *still* hypoxic:** ligate pulmonary artery of NDL (is only an option during pneumonectomy)

If you survive the double-lumen tube gauntlet, you'll need to know how to manage postthoracotomy pain: (none of these methods has been proven superior to the others; may also be used to manage rib fractures)

1. Epidural local or narcotics (thoracic placement allows lesser volumes of each, lumbar placement prevents sympathectomy from local, see section on epidural anesthesia for list of complications)
2. Intercostal nerve block (requires ~3 mL 0.5% bupivicaine per nerve, limited duration necessitates repeat injection or adjuvant therapy, carries risk of pneumothorax, toxicity and inadvertant spinal)

3. Cryoanalgesia (often requires supplementation, otherwise low incidence of complications)
4. Interpleural analgesia (local anesthesia through catheter or chest tube)

Sample questions

A = 1, 2, 3   B = 1, 3   C = 2, 4   D = 4 only   E = all are correct

1. Ventilation: perfusion mismatch during one-lung ventilation in the lateral decubitus postion is worsened by
   1. Hypoxic pulmonary vasoconstriction in the nondependent lung
   2. Hypoxic pulmonary vasoconstriction in the dependent lung
   3. Functional residual capacity greater than 20 cc/kg
   4. Nitroprusside

2. During one-lung ventilation via a left-sided double-lumen endotracheal tube for a right-sided pneumonectomy, the surgeon complains that the operative lung is partially reinflated. Possible causes of this include
   1. Continued diffusion of carbon dioxide into the lung
   2. Right mainstem placement of the endotracheal tube
   3. Inadequate seal around the bronchial cuff
   4. Inadequate seal around the tracheal cuff

Answers: 1. C   2. B

Chapter 101

Cardiopulmonary Resuscitation

Goal of CPR: To maintain perfusion to brain and heart

Priorities of CPR

1. Airway: open airway, remove foreign bodies
2. Breathing: determine presence/absence of spontaneous breaths, ventilate if needed
3. Circulation: administer fluids, drugs, and compressions as needed

How do chest compressions create "forward flow" of blood? Via a combination of:

1. The "cardiac pump" theory: a "pumping" action of left ventricle is created by mechanical compression between the sternum and the vertebral bodies.
2. The "thoracic pump" theory: chest compressions raise the intrathoracic pressure. Venous valves provide resistance to backward flow into the venous system, encouraging blood to flow into peripheral arterial system. The heart provides no pumping action based on this theory.

What kind of acid–base disturbances do you usually see during CPR?

1. Usually a combined respiratory and metabolic acidosis
2. In first few minutes, acidosis is chiefly respiratory . . . manage with hyperventilation and F_iO_2 1.0
3. Beware that ABGs underestimate the degree of hypercarbia because of the large venoarterial CO_2 gradient that develops.

How does THAT happen, you ask? CPR doesn't create adequate forward flow to return all venous blood to the heart and lungs, so the venous side accumulates CO_2. Samples of arterial blood represent blood that managed to perfuse the lungs and have its CO_2 removed.

When you get that blood gas result, fight the temptation to give bicarb

Why? Because, bicarb rapidly dissociates to form CO_2, which enters the already acidotic cells much faster than hydrogen can exit them, thereby worsening intracellular acidosis.

Other side effects of HCO_3^- administration during CPR

1. Increased CO_2 production (requires increased minute ventilation)
2. Oxyhemoglobin curve shifts to the left (acute serum alkalosis), worsening tissue oxygenation
3. Hypernatremia (remember, it's *sodium* bicarbonate)
4. Hyperosmolality (you're injecting solute without solution)

Indications for HCO_3^- during CPR

1. Prolonged resuscitations
2. If patient had premorbid metabolic acidosis
3. Treatment for hyperkalemia

Resuscitative drugs and their doses

Atropine: 0.5–1 mg IV Q5min to a total dose of 2 mg
Epinephrine: 1 mg IV 1:10,000 Q5min
Lidocaine: 1 mg/kg IV, then 0.5 mg/kg Q5–10min to a total dose of 3 mg/kg
Bretylium: 5 mg/kg IV, then 10 mg/kg Q5–10min to a total dose of 30 mg/kg
$NaHCO_3$: 1 meq/kg or 0.3 meq × deficit × weight in kg, repeat half the dose Q10min
Calcium: 100–200 mg IV

Besides doing the ABCs and giving drugs, you may also have to defibrillate the patient. Successful defibrillation depends on low thoracic impedence.

Factors that increase thoracic impedence

1. Poor paddle contact (bad positioning, inadequate pressure, inadequate gel)
2. Inappropriate paddle size
3. Prolonged time between shocks (rapidly delivered shocks lower impedence)
4. Increased air space (pneumothorax, full lungs)

CPR algorithms

I've included the most commonly asked CPR algorithms for your memorizing convenience:

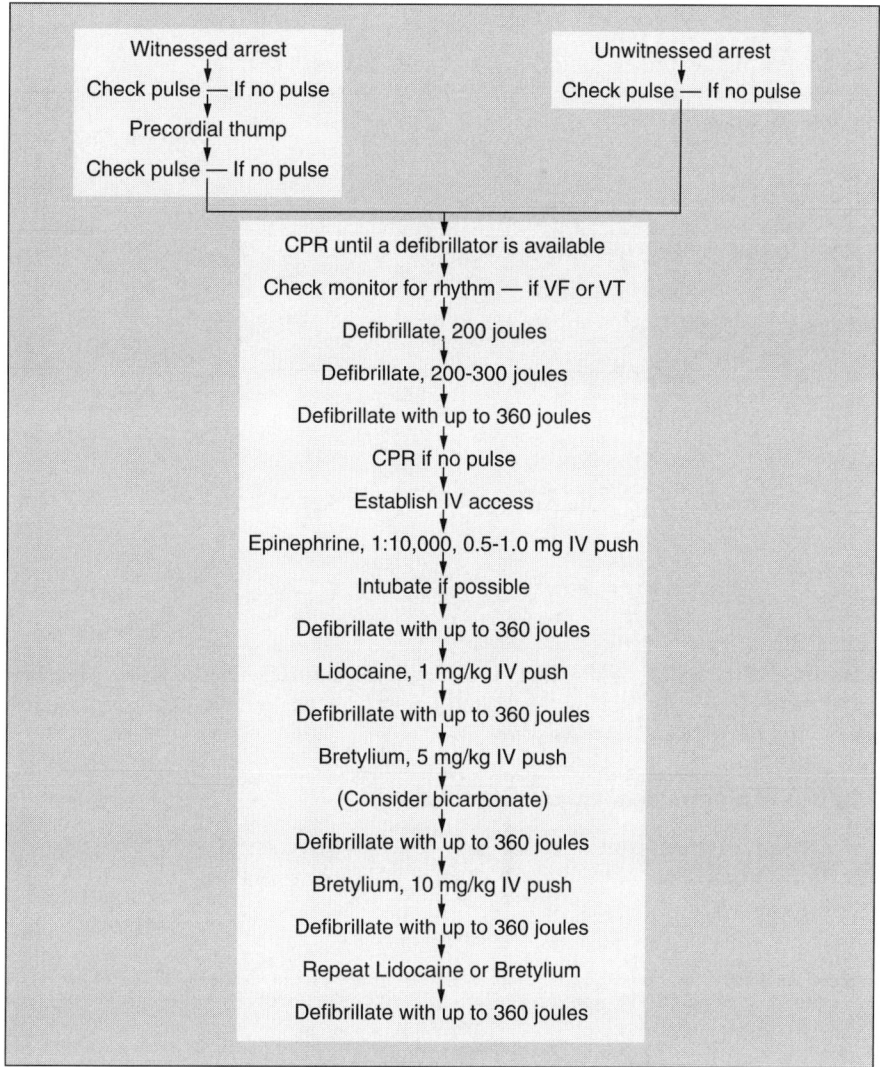

Figure 101–1. ACLS Algorithm for Ventricular Tachycardia/Ventricular Fibrillation. Data from Textbook of Advanced Cardiac Life Support, 1994. Copyright American Heart Association.

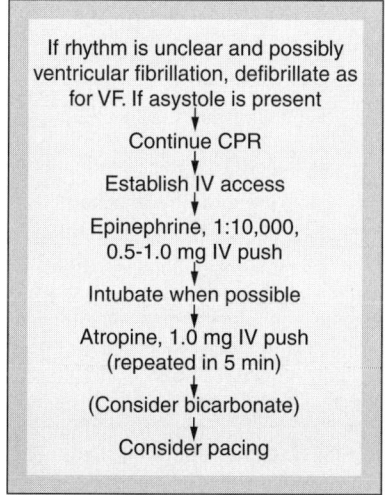

Figure 101–2. ACLS Algorithm for Asystole. Data from Textbook of Advanced Cardiac Life Support, 1994. Copyright American Heart Association.

Causes of intraoperative asystole

1. Oculocardiac reflex
2. Mesenteric traction reflex
3. Hypoxemia
4. Hyperkalemia
5. Succinylcholine

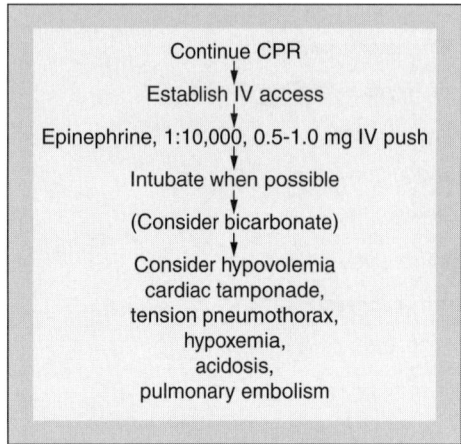

Figure 101–3. **ACLS Algorithm for Electromechanical Dissociation (Pulseless Electrical Activity).** Data from Textbook of Advanced Cardiac Life Support, 1994. Copyright American Heart Association.

Causes of electromechanical dissociation

1. Tension pneumothorax
2. Tamponade
3. Pulmonary embolus
4. Hypovolemia
5. Hypoxemia
6. Acidosis

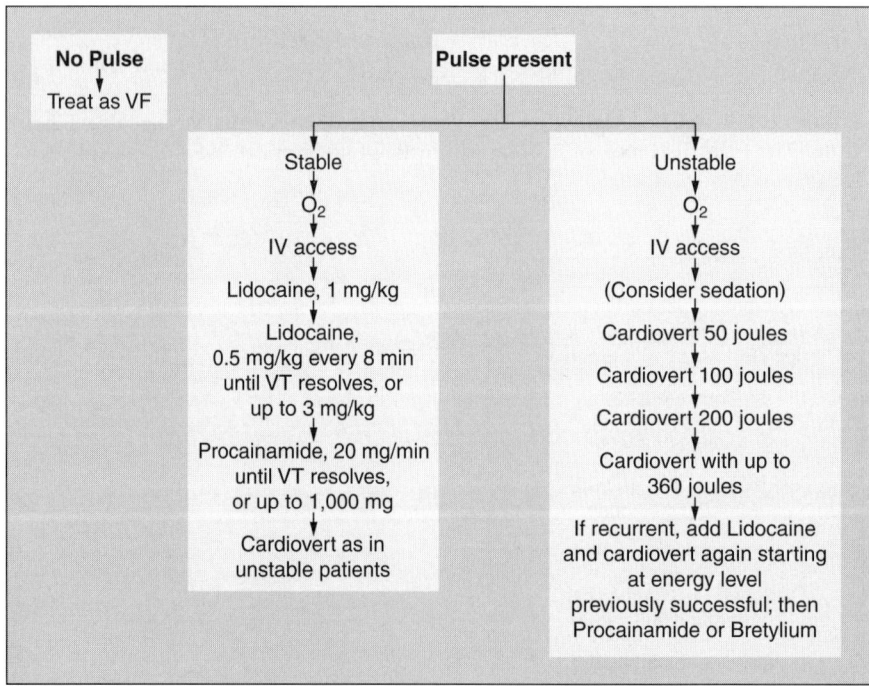

Figure 101–4. **ACLS Algorithm for Supraventricular Tachycardia.** Data from Textbook of Advanced Cardiac Life Support, 1994. Copyright American Heart Association.

Most common causes of supraventricular tachycardia

1. Reentry phenomena: normal QRS width, WPW most common, treat with adenosine 6 mg IV, then 12 mg IV
2. Accessory pathways: wide QRS, treat with Lidocaine or Procainamide
3. Hypoxia/hypercarbia/theophylline toxicity

Types of supraventricular tachyardia

1. Atrial fibrillation
2. Atrial flutter
3. Junctional tachycardia
4. Multifocal atrial tachycardia
5. Reentry rythyms (WPW)

Sample questions

Single best answer

1. While weaning from cardiopulmonary bypass, a 60-year-old man develops supraventricular tachycardia at 180/min. Blood pressure is 65/40 mmHg, wedge pressure is 8 mmHg, oxygen saturation is 97%. The most appropriate action is
   1. Return to bypass
   2. Cardioversion
   3. Carotid massage
   4. Administer esmolol 20 mg IV
   5. Administer verapamil 10 mg IV

2. A 24-year-old driver sustains blunt trauma to the chest and abdomen. Shortly after arrival to the emergency room, the EKG monitor shows a junctional rythm at 55/min, there is no palpable pulse and the pulse oximeter is not tracking. The most appropriate first step is
   1. Tube thoracostomy
   2. Epinephrine 1 mg 1:10,000 IV
   3. Pericardiocentesis
   4. Transfuse two units packed red blood cells
   5. Atropine 0.5 mg IV

Answers: 1. 2   2. 2

SECTION 8

Transfusion Therapy

Chapter 102

Transfusion Therapy

Compatability testing

1. ABO, Rh typing:
   A. ABO incompatability is most common cause of serious transfusion reactions (99.8%)
   B. Rh (D) incompatability is next most common
2. Antibody screening: combine patient's serum with commercial preparation of red blood cells containing known antigens and watch for reaction
3. Cross-matching: donor cells are mixed with patient's serum. Three phases:
   A. Immediate phase (partial cross) takes 5 min: detects M, N, P, Lewis incompatability
   B. Incubation phase: detects antibodies in Rh system
   C. Antiglobulin phase: detects incomplete antibodies in Rh, Kell, Kidd, and Duffy

Efficacy of testing

1. ABO, Rh typing: provides 99.8% safety
2. Screen: increases safety to 99.94%
3. Cross-match: increases safety to 99.95%

If the need for emergency transfusion prohibits a complete cross-match, what type blood would be the best choice?

1. If time permits: type-specific, partially cross-matched (detects ABO, Rh, M, N, P, Lewis incompatability)
2. If less time allowed: type-specific, uncross-matched (risk of reaction 1:1000 if no prior transfusions)
3. If no time allowed: type O, Rh negative, uncross-matched (packed cells preferred to whole blood, because there is less donor plasma and therefore, less chance of antibody exposure)

Transfusion after emergency O-negative transfusion

If patient recieved > **2 units** O negative, you must continue with O negative, because he may have received enough anti-A or anti-B antibodies in the O negative serum to hemolyze his own type blood cells. Continued transfusion with O negative causes minimal lysis of his own cells, as they are gradually being replaced by O negative cells.

Storage of blood

● Table 102–1

Preservative	CPD	CPDA-1	Adsol	Nutrice
Contents	Citrate	Citrate	Mannitol	Citrate
	Phosphate	Phosphate	NaCl	Phosphate
	Dextrose	Dextrose	Glucose	Glucose
		Adenine	Adenine	Adenine
				NaCl
Shelf life	21 days	35 days	42 days	42 days

Function of the preservatives

Citrate: anticoagulant, binds calcium
Phosphate: buffer
Dextrose: energy source, allows glycolysis and maintenance of cellular ATP levels
Adenine: allows cells to resynthesize ATP
Mannitol: maintains osmolality of solution and cells

Alternate methods of storing blood

1. Frozen storage
    A. Long-term (years) storage of extremely rare blood types
    B. Lower incidence of transfusion reaction than traditional storage
    C. Maintains normal 2,3, DPG levels (normal oxygen carrying capacity)
    D. Same hepatitis risk as traditional storage
2. Heparin storage
    A. *Not* a preservative (lacks energy source like glucose)
    B. Extremely short (24–48 hr) shelf life, as heparin quickly loses anticoagulant effect

Characteristics of banked blood

1. Low level of 2,3 DPG (high affinity for O_2, thus, decreased unloading to tissues)
2. Low levels factor V, VIII (not clinically relevant since such low levels are needed for normal coagulation)
3. Platelet poor (essentially all gone by 24 hr of storage, leads to dilutional thrombocytopenia)
4. Hyperkalemic, hyponatremic serum due to stimulation of $Na^+ \cdot K^+$ pump
5. Acidotic serum (high H^+ and PCO_2)
6. Hct ~70%
7. Increased free hemoglobin due to lysis
8. Cold (stored at 4°C)

Clinical consequences of massive transfusion with banked blood

1. Dilutional thrombocytopenia
2. Disseminated intravascular coagulation (more likely due to low-flow states)
3. Hyperkalemia (rarely significant)
4. Microaggregate infusion leading to ARDS (not proven)
5. Metabolic alkalosis (citrate generates HCO_3^-)

6. Hypocalcemia and hypotension (citrate binds calcium)
7. Hypothermia

Characteristics of cell saver blood as compared to banked blood

1. 2,3 DPG levels normal
2. Coagulation factors absent (removed during cell washing)
3. Platelet poor (removed during cell washing)
4. K+ and Na+ within normal limits
5. Alkalotic serum
6. Hct ~60%
7. Increased free hemoglobin and cellular debris (especially if suction apparatus set > 200 mmHg)
8. Anticoagulated with heparin or citrate
9. Can contain fat, bone chips, leukocytes, cellular debris
10. Short shelf life (24 hr), but same RBC circulating half-life once they are transfused

Contraindications to use of intraoperative cell saver

1. Ongoing coagulopathy: salvage removes platelets and coagulation factors, requires anticoagulant
2. Pheochromocytoma resection: washing doesn't remove catecholamines
3. Tumor resection: postulated dissemination of tumor cells (never proven)
4. Surgical field contamination by: intestinal contents, betadine, neomycin, topical anticoagulants (Surgicel, Avitene), methylmethacrylate

Sample questions

A = 1, 2, 3   B = 1, 3   C = 2, 4   D = 4 only   E = all are correct

1. Compared to banked blood, cell saver blood
   1. Has a lower serum potassium
   2. Has a higher P_{50}
   3. Has the same circulating half-life
   4. Has a higher concentration of factors V and VIII

2. Possible complications of transfusion with cell saver blood include
   1. Fat embolus
   2. Infusion of microaggregates
   3. Dilutional thrombocytopenia
   4. Air embolus

3. Disregarding Rh status, a patient with blood type AB can receive
   1. AB whole blood
   2. Type A whole blood
   3. Type B packed cells
   4. Type O whole blood

Single best answer

A 20-year-old man is undergoing exploratory laparotomy following a motor vehicle accident. He has received two units of O-negative blood. The blood bank informs you that he is type A, Rh-positive, antibody screen negative and that the sample volume was insufficient for cross-match. The

patient's vital signs are blood pressure 80/45 mmHg, pulse 120, and his hemoglobin after two units of packed red cells is 8.3 gm/dL. You should
1. Continue transfusing with O-negative whole blood
2. Continue transfusing with O-negative packed red cells
3. Transfuse with type-specific, screened, uncross-matched whole blood
4. Transfuse with type-specific, screened, uncross-matched packed red cells
5. Infuse colloid and send another sample to the blood bank

Answers: 1. A   2. A   3. B   4. 4

CHAPTER 103

Transfusion Reactions

● Table 103–1

	Hemolytic Reactions		Non-Hemolytic Reactions	
	Immediate	Delayed	Febrile	Allergic
Cause	ABO incompatability (usually human error) IgM antibody vs. red blood cell antigen	**Rh, Kidd,** Kell, Duffy, Lewis incompatability Amnestic response in sensitized patient (prior transfusion, pregnancy)	**Most common reaction** Etiology unknown	Foreign proteins
Signs and symptoms	Seen under anesthesia **Hemoglobinuria** Hypotension Coagulopathy Flushing Masked by anesthesia Fever Chills Nausea Chest pain	**Anemia** Jaundice Hemoglobinuria Renal dysfunction (rare)	Fever Chills Nausea Headache Dry cough	Pruritis Urticaria
Presentation	Immediate, because of complement binding	Up to 2 weeks after transfusion	Immediate	Immediate
Diagnostic tests	1. ↓ serum haptoglobin 2. ↑ free hemoglobin in serum and urine 3. ↑ bilirubin	Same as immediate reaction	Direct antiglobulin test rules out antibody binding to red cell antigen	
Treatment	Stop transfusion (mannitol lasix, dopamine, fluids), alkalinize urine, support hemodynamics	Symptomatic support	Antipyretics; may continue transfusion	Antihistamines; continue transfusion

Blood Component Therapy

Blood component administration by anesthesiologists is most often required following massive transfusion.

Features of posttransfusion coagulopathy

1. Dilutional thrombocytopenia (treat with platelet transfusion)
2. Low levels of factors V and VIII (treat with fresh-frozen plasma)
3. Disseminated intravascular coagulation (treat with vitamin K, laboratory-guided component therapy)

Indications for platelet transfusion

Single unit raises platelet count by ~10,000 platelets/m^3)
1. Thrombocytopenia (except immune thrombocytopenia purpura)
2. Nonfunctional platelets

Indications for fresh-frozen plasma

Contains all factors except platelets).[1]
1. Isolated factor deficiency as documented by laboratory evidence (factors **V, VIII,** II, VII, IX, X, XI)
2. Reversal of warfarin effect
3. Antithrombin III deficiency
4. Massive blood transfusion (if factors V and VIII are <25% of normal)
5. Thrombotic thrombocytopenia purpura
6. Treatment of immunodeficiencies
7. Numbers 1 and 4 require a concurrent PT and PTT > 1.5 times normal values

Indications for cryoprecipitate

Contains fibrinogen, factor VIII, von Willebrand factor, and fibronectin.
1. Hemophilia A
2. Factor VIII deficiency
3. Von Willebrand's disease
4. Hypofibrinogenemia

Indications for DDAVP

Not a blood component, but on the boards nonetheless
1. Von Willebrand's disease
2. Mild cases of hemophilia A

Common perioperative coagulation tests

• Table 104–1

Test	Coagulation Parameter Measured	Differential Diagnosis of Prolonged Coagulation
Bleeding time	Platelet function	Thrombocytopenia Platelet dysfunction von Willebrand's disease Drug effect (see list below)
Prothrombin time (PT)	Extrinsic pathway	Coumadin therapy Liver disease (vitamin K deficiency) DIC Low prothrombin, fibrinigen ASA, NSAIDs
Partial thromboplastin time (PTT)	Intrinsic pathway	Heparin therapy Hemophilia A Christmas disease

Drugs that prolong bleeding time

Aspirin
NSAIDs
Ketorolac
Antihistamines
Tricyclic antidepressants
Local anesthetics (lidocaine, cocaine)

α-blockers
β-blockers
Penicillin
Xanthines
Phosphodieterase inhibitors

Sample questions

A = 1, 2, 3   B = 1, 3   C = 2, 4   D = 4 only   E = all are correct

1. Platelet transfusion
   1. Raises the platelet count by 10,000 platelets/m^3 for each unit transfused
   2. With ABO-incompatible platelets can produce sensitization to the Rh antigen
   3. Is not indicated in immune thromocytopenic purpura
   4. Is contraindicated in uremia

2. Fresh-frozen plasma
   1. Poses the same infection risk as packed red blood cells
   2. Is frozen at –70°C
   3. Will reverse the effect of coumadin
   4. Contains the same concentration of factor VIII as cryoprecipitate

Answers: 1. A   2. B

Reference

1. NIH Consensus Conference. Fresh frozen plasma: indications and risks. JAMA 253: 551, 1985.

Intraoperative Fluid Therapy

Water is life. Adult males are 55% water by weight, females are slightly less. Distribution of water in the body:

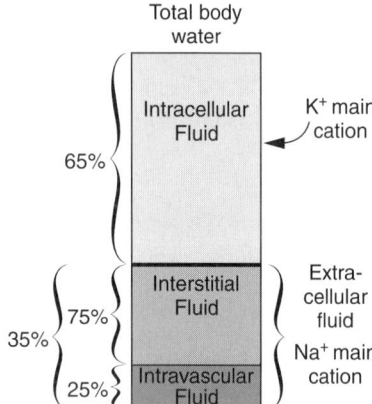

Figure 105–1.

> **NOTE:** that there is flux of water and particles between *all* compartments.

Composition of the various compartments

1. Intracellular compartment: water/osmotically active particles/chief cation is K^+
2. Extracellular compartment:
   A. Interstitial fluid: isotonic fluid/communicates with ICF space, intravascular fluid space, and with slow exchange spaces like intraluminal or cavitary fluid space
   B. Intravascular fluid: isotonic fluid/chief cation is Na^+/composed of 45% erythrocytes and 55% plasma. Erythrocytes exert no oncotic pressure. Plasma is mostly H_2O and is highly oncotic, due mainly to albumin

Intraoperative fluid loss

Most surgical fluid loss is from the extracellular space; specifically, the intravascular space (blood). This is compensated for by shifting interstitial fluid and extravascular proteins to intravascular space. Thus, now there are three spaces that are somewhat depleted: vascular, interstitial, and the space previously occupied by extravascular proteins. Crystalloid, which has low oncotic effect, will readily refill these three spaces, which is why you must replace each 1 mL of blood loss with 3 mL of crystalloid. Colloid, which is highly oncotic, remains in the vascular space much longer, and replacement is 1:1. Bear in mind that: **Volume replacement also refills the extracellular fluid space!**

Guidelines for replacement of intraoperative fluid loss

1. Maintenance: 4-2-1 rule, using isotonic fluid
2. Third space loss: ~3 mL/kg/hr of isotonic fluid for minor surgical exposure
   ~6 mL/kg/hr of isotonic fluid for moderate surgical exposure
   ~9 mL/kg/hr of isotonic fluid for major surgical exposure
3. Blood loss: 3 mL crystalloid per 1 mL blood loss
   OR: 1 mL colloid or blood per 1 mL blood loss

Crystalloid versus Colloid: "To give or not to give?". That is the $64,000 question.

- Table 105–1

	Crystalloid	Colloid
Effect of plasma osmolality?	Reduces	Maintains
Volume for blood replacement	3:1	1:1
Vital risk?	No	No (Albumin is pasteurized, Hetastarch and Dextran are synthetic
Risk of allergic reaction?	No	Yes (Dextran > Albumin > Hetastarch)
Produces coagulopathy?	No	Yes (Dextran, Hetastarch)
Risk of pulmonary edema	More likely	Less likely
Increases O_2 carrying capacity?	No	No

Fun facts about Hetastarch

1. Synthetic
2. Provides better increase in osmotic pressure than equal volume albumin
3. Renal excretion
4. Side effects: inhibit platelet function, elevated amylase, low risk of anaphylaxis

Fun facts about Dextran

1. Synthetic
2. Comes in two weights: Dextran 40 (low molecular weight) and Dextran 70 (high molecular weight)
3. Renal excretion (renal failure increases plasma half-life, large particles can cause obstruction and acute renal failure)
4. Side effects:
   A. Inhibits platelet function and reduces factor VIII
   B. Elevated liver enzymes (SGOT, SGPT)
   C. RBC agglutination
   D. Anaphylaxis
   E. Factitious hyperglycemia

105 ■ Intraoperative Fluid Therapy

Sample questions

A = 1, 2, 3   B = 1, 3   C = 2, 4   D = 4 only   E = all are correct

1. A 24-year-old male pedestrian is struck by a car, sustaining multiple fractures and a liver laceration. During intraoperative rescusitation with type-specific uncross-matched packed red blood cells, lactated Ringer's, 5% albumin, and hetastarch, his blood pressure acutely drops from 110/59 mmHg to 60/35 mmHg. The end-tidal capnograph reveals pronounced upsloping during exhalation and peak airway pressures have increased from 30 cmH$_2$O to 55 cmH$_2$O. Possible causes include:
    1. ABO-Rh incompatability
    2. Albumin allergy
    3. Hetastarch allergy
    4. Tension pneumothorax

2. During early resuscitation of a patient who fell 30 feet
    1. Albumin or blood are better early volume expanders than lactated Ringer's
    2. Hetastarch is preferred to albumin because there is no risk of allergic reaction
    3. Dextran is comparable to crystalloid in that it does not effect coagulation
    4. Dextran produces the greatest increase in oncotic pressure

Answers: 1. E   2. D

Chapter 106

Von Willebrand's Disease

There are three classes of von Willebrand's disease

Type 1: **most common,** autosomal dominant, low *levels* of factor VIII:vWf and factor VIII:C
Type 2: autosomal dominant, *functional* abnormality of factor VIII:vWf
Type 3: autosomal recessive, defective synthesis of factor VIII

The role of factor VIII

Factor VIII complex consists of two parts:

1. Factor VIII: von Willebrand factor, needed for normal platelet function
2. Factor VIII:C, part of the intrinsic coagulation pathway

Coagulation studies

Platelet count: normal
Bleeding time: elevated, because vWf is necessary for normal platelet aggregation
PTT: elevated, because of decreased levels of factor VIII:C

Perioperative management

Transfuse with:

1. **cryoprecipitate (best)**
2. FFP
3. factor VIII concentrate? **NO, because it lacks von Willebrand factor**

When do you transfuse? Peak levels of factor VIII:C obtained at 48 hr (so transfuse the night before surgery). **BUT:** factor VIII:vWf half-life only ~6 hr (transfuse again immediately preop for normal platelets)

Intraoperative management

DDAVP: promotes release of factor VIII:C (dose: 0.3 mg/kg IV)

Sample question

A = 1, 2, 3   B = 1, 3   C = 2, 4   D = 4 only   E = all are correct

1. A 13-year-old, 50-kg male is scheduled for an emergency appendectomy. He has a history of gingival bleeding after brushing his teeth in the past,

but no history of hemarthrosis and has never undergone surgery. Coagulation studies reveal an elevated partial thromboplastin time and bleeding time. Appropriate measures to ready him for surgery include
1. Transfusion with cryoprecipitate
2. Administer DDAVP 15 mg IV
3. Transfusion with fresh-frozen plasma
4. Transfuse with factor VIII concentrate

Answer: 1. A

CHAPTER 107

Hemophilia A and Hemophilia B (Christmas disease)

- Table 107–1

	Hemophilia A	Hemophilia B
Defect	X-linked	X-linked
	Defective/deficient factor VIII:C	Defective/deficient factor IX
Patient population	Males only	Males only
Clinical presentation	Deep tissue bleeding	Same as hemophilia A
	Hemarthrosis	
	Hematuria	
	Central nervous system bleeding	
Coagulation profile	Bleeding time: normal	Bleeding time: normal
	PT: normal	PT: normal
	PTT: prolonged	PTT: prolonged
Treatment	Factor VIII concentrate	Factor IX concentrate
	Dose: 50 units/kg	Dosage regimen same as factor VIII
	Vol. of distribution: 100 mL/kg	
	Serum concentration: 0.5 U/mL	
	Result: 50% of normal activity	

Sample questions

A = 1, 2, 3   B = 1, 3   C = 2, 4   D = 4 only   E = all are correct

1. A 15-year-old, 50-kg male with hemophilia A is scheduled for an appendectomy. His partial thromboplastin time is 160 sec, and both his bleeding time and prothrombin time are normal. By laboratory assay, he has less than 3% factor VIII activity. True statements regarding his preoperative preparation include:
   1. He needs to have at least 30% of normal factor VIII activity
   2. He should receive 2800 units of factor VIII concentrate
   3. The serum half-life of factor VIII concentrate is 12 hr
   4. Correction to 30% factor VIII activity will result in a normal PTT

2. Possible treatments for hemophilia A include
   1. Cryoprecipitate
   2. Fresh-frozen plasma
   3. Factor VIII concentrate
   4. Desmopressin

Answers: 1. A   2. E

CHAPTER 108

Sickle Cell Anemia

Defect: Patients are homozygous recessive for the gene that produces HbS, an abnormal hemoglobin that deforms upon deoxygenation

Effect of deformation

Precipitation of hemoglobin within the RBC, leading to:

1. Chronic hemolysis (anemia, hyperbilirubinemia, jaundice, and cholelithiasis)
2. Vasocclusive crises ("sludging" of blood and end-organ infarction)

End organ effects of sickling

1. Pulmonary infarction (leads to recurrent infection, cor pulmonale)
2. Renal infarction (leads to impaired concentrating ability, renal failure)
3. Liver damage (cirrhosis)
4. Cerebrovascular accident
5. Bone ischemia (aseptic femoral necrosis, aplastic crisis)

Factors that predispose to sickling

1. $PaO_2 < 40$ mmHg
2. Acidosis
3. Hypothermia
4. Dehydration
5. Polycythemia (Hb > 8.5 g/dL)

Preoperative preparation includes

1. Simple transfusion or exchange transfusion to achieve concentration of HbA ≥ 50%, HbS ≤ 40%
2. Adequate hydration (fluids at 1.5 times usual maintenance levels)
3. Correction of existing infections

Sample questions

A = 1, 2, 3   B = 1, 3   C = 2, 4   D = 4 only   E = all are correct

1. Expected findings in a patient with sickle cell disease include
    1. An alveolar-arterial oxygen difference > 8 mmHg
    2. Urine specific gravity < 1.010

3. Serum hemoglobin < 10 g/dL
4. A P_{50} > 27 mmHg

2. A 15-year-old, 50-kg boy with sickle cell disease is scheduled for total hip arthroplasty due to femoral head necrosis. He is otherwise asymptomatic, but has a history of multiple transfusions and bone pain crises. Management should include
    1. Exchange transfusion to decrease the hemoglobin S concentration to at least 40%
    2. Preoperative transfusion to achieve a hemoglobin level of at least 10 g/dL
    3. Intraoperative maintenance intravenous fluids at least 1.5 times usual amounts
    4. Maintaining an operating room temperature of 72°F

Answers: 1. E 2. B

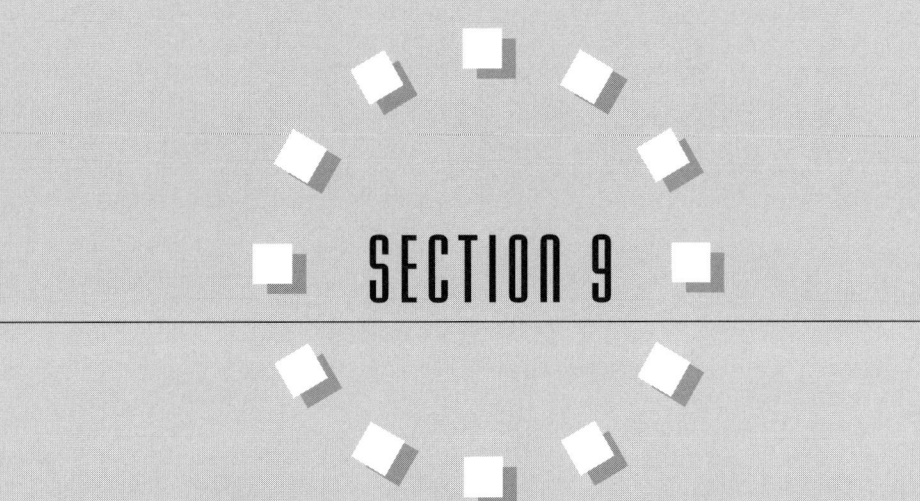

SECTION 9

Neuroanesthesia

Chapter 109

Cerebral Blood Flow and Metabolism

Basic facts: The brain receives ~15% of the cardiac output and is responsible for ~20% of our oxygen consumption

Factors that influence cerebral blood flow

1. **Cerebral metabolic rate (CMR):** directly proportional to CBF

Factors that increase CMR	Factors that decrease CMR
Seizures	Sleep
Any increase in mental activity	Coma
Hyperthermia	Aging
	Hypothermia
	All anesthetics except ketamine
	Vasoactive drugs

2. **Myogenic factors (autoregulation):** Cerebral arterioles vasodilate/constrict in response to changes in mean arterial pressure, keeping CBF constant at mean arterial pressures between 50 and 150 mmHg. At pressures above or below this, CBF is directly proportional to the arterial pressure. Hypertension shifts these values upward.

3. **$PaCO_2$ and pH:** CBF and $PaCO_2$ are linearly related. CBF increases by ~2 mL/100g/min for each 1-mmHg increase in $PaCO_2$. However, CO_2 is not a direct cerebral vasodilator, so how does it exert its effect?

$\uparrow PaCO_2 \rightarrow$ diffuses across blood–brain barrier into interstitium
$\rightarrow$ reacts with H_2O to form H^+ and HCO_3^- $\rightarrow$ interstitial pH decreases
$\rightarrow$ vasodilation and increased cerebral blood flow

CAVEAT: The vasoactive effects of CO_2 are greatest within "normal" physiologic parameters (20–80 mmHg) and are short-lived (normalization of CSF pH occurs within ~8 hr). Also, remember that while the BBB is highly permeable to CO_2, it is impermeable to hydrogen ions; therefore, respiratory acidosis renders rapid changes in CSF pH while metabolic acidosis has minimal effect.

What happens to the patient who is hyperventilated and then later allowed to have a normal $PaCO_2$?

Hyperventilate → lowered $PaCO_2$ → efflux (over several hours) of HCO_3^- from CSF normalizes CSF pH → acute return to normal $PaCO_2$ → unopposed high concentration of H^+ in CSF → severe CSF acidosis → increased CBF → increased ICP

What happens to the hypercarbic, head-injured patient when he's intubated and his $PaCO_2$ is acutely lowered?

Hypercarbia → influx (over several hours) of HCO_3^- into CSF normalizes CSF pH → intubate and induce an acute decrease in $PaCO_2$ → unopposed high concentration of HCO_3^- in CSF → severe CSF alkalosis → decreasedCBF → ischemia

4. **PaO_2**
   <60 mmHg = profound vasodilation
   >60 and <300 mmHg, CBF is constant
   >300mmHg = mild decrease of CBF
5. **Temperature:** hyperthermia raises both CMR and CBF. Hypothermia decreases the CMR, thereby reducing CBF (and will cause further reductions even beyond the isoelectric point on EEG, in contrast to anesthetic agents).
6. **Autonomic factors:** adrenergic, cholinergic, and serotonergic systems all play a poorly defined role. Increased sympathetic tone shifts MAP:CBF curve to right (as in hypertension).

Effects of anesthetic agents on CBF and $CMRO_2$

1. Volatile agents:
   A. ↑ CBF (all cause acute cerebral vasodilation, CBF normalizes over several hours). Halothane >> ethrane > isoflurane, desflurane, sevoflurane.
   B. Nitrous oxide: profound ↑ CBF if used alone or with volatile agents, minimal effect if used with intravenous agents.
   C. ↓ $CMRO_2$ (uncoupling of metabolic link to CBF) isoflurane = ethrane > halothane. Dose-dependent effect, and only halothane continues to decrease $CMRO_2$ beyond the point of isoelectricity on EKG.
2. Intravenous agents:
   A. Autoregulation and CO_2 responsiveness are preserved.
   B. All cause ↓ $CMRO_2$, and thus, ↓ CBF (exception is ketamine, which *increases* both)
   C. Barbiturates, propofol: greatest ↓ CBF, $CMRO_2$
   D. Benzodiazepines, etomidate-intermediate effect (flumazenil ↑'s $CMRO_2$, and CBF if benzodiazepine on board, no effect if sole agent)
   E. Narcotics: minimal effect (alfentanil is least)

Sample questions

A = 1, 2, 3   B = 1, 3   C = 2, 4   D = 4 only   E = all are correct

1. Carbon dioxide
   1. Readily diffuses across the blood–brain barrier
   2. Is a direct cerebral vasodilator
   3. Is linearly related to cerebral blood flow
   4. Manipulation to low arterial partial pressures reduces cerebral blood

flow for as long as the CO_2 level is reduced

2. Cerebral blood flow is reduced by
   1. Hypothermia
   2. PaO_2 greater than 300 mmHg
   3. $PaCO_2$ less than 28 mmHg
   4. Nitrous oxide

3. Which of the following anesthetic combinations will increase cerebral blood flow?
   1. Nitrous oxide 70% and oxygen 30%
   2. Nitrous oxide 70%, oxygen 30%, propofol 200 µg/kg/min
   3. Nitrous oxide 70%, oxygen 29%, isoflurane 1%
   4. Thiopental 5 mg/kg, fentanyl 0.5 µg/kg/hr, air

Answers: 1. B   2. E   3. B

CHAPTER 110

Closed Head Injury and Increased Intracranial Pressure

Closed head injury is a common cause of increased intracranial pressure, often accompanied by neurologic insult, the severity of which is assessed by the Glasgow Coma Scale.

- Table 110–1

Response	Score
Eye opening	
Spontaneous	4
To speech	3
To pain	2
None	1
Best motor response	
Obeys	6
Localizes	5
Withdraws (flexion)	4
Abnormal flexion	3
Extensor response	2
	1
Verbal response	
Oriented	5
Confused conversation	4
Inappropriate words	3
Incomprehensible sounds	2
None	1

Limitations of the Glasgow coma scale

1. Can underestimate unilateral focal motor deficits (convention dictates that you score the best side)
2. Eye opening may be limited by facial trauma
3. Endotracheal intubation limits verbal response
4. Doesn't evaluate brainstem reflexes

Mechanism of increased intracranial pressure in closed head injury

Anything that increases the volume of the intracranial contents will raise the intracranial pressure. The cranial vault contains:

1. Brain (solid tissue and intracellular water)
2. The cerebral blood volume (CBV)
3. The cerebrospinal fluid volume (CSF)

Head injuries increase intracranial pressure by causing:

1. Cerebral edema (increased volume of brain tissue)
2. Increased cerebral blood volume (due to impaired autoregulation)
3. Obstructive hydrocephalus (2° to cerebral edema)
4. Bleeding (extrinsic mass effect)

Compensation for the increase in intracranial volume is attempted by displacing CSF to extracranial locations, but efficacy is limited. As ICP increases, cerebral perfusion declines, resulting in ischemia.

How are ICP and cerebral perfusion related?

Cerebral perfusion pressure = mean arterial pressure − intracranial pressure

Cerebral perfusion can be altered by the following:

- **Table 110–2**

Increased CPP	Decreased CPP
↑ mean arterial pressure > 150 mmHg	↓ mean arterial pressure < 50 mmHg
Impaired autoregulation	Impaired autoregulation
↓ volume of brain tissue	↑ volume of brain tissue
↓ cerebral blood volume	↑ cerebral blood volume
↓ cerebrospinal fluid volume	↑ cerebrospinal fluid volume (hydrocephalus)

The following table summarizes the common mechanisms by which the volume of the intracranial contents is increased (not just in head injury) and includes the most common therapeutic maneuvers for treating each disorder, thereby reducing intracranial pressure and improving cerebral perfusion.

- **Table 110–3**

Intracranial Components	Etiology of Volume Increase	Therapy
Brain	Cerebral edema	Fluid restriction
		Diuresis (mannitol, lasix)
		Hyperventilation
		Steroids
		Hypothermia
		Stabilize blood pressure
	Tumor/hematoma	Surgery
Cerebral blood volume	Cerebral vasodilation	Hyperventilation
		Barbiturates (cerebral vasoconstrictors)
	Hypertension	Stabilize blood pressure
	Coughing/straining	Neuromuscular relaxants
	Impaired venous drainage	Elevate head of bed
Cerebrospinal fluid	Impaired drainage	Shunt
		Acetazolamide
		Mannitol

Mechanisms of cerebral protection with barbiturates

1. ↓ $CMRO_2$ (until EKG isoelectric point is reached/thiopental > methohexital)

2. Cerebral vasoconstriction → ↓ CBV → ↓ ICP → ↑ CPP (thiopental > methohexital)
3. Raise seizure threshold

Indications for barbiturate coma

Reduces ICP but doesn't significantly affect mortality.

1. Global ischemia following cardiac arrest? No change in outcome.
2. Regional ischemia following stroke? No change in outcome.
3. Initial therapy following head injury? No change in outcome.

Anesthetic management of the patient with a closed head injury

Management consists chiefly of maintaining cerebral perfusion pressure by:

1. Supporting blood pressure (fluid resuscitation)
2. Lowering ICP

Preoperatively

1. Fluid resuscitation (hypertonic crystalloid best/blood PRN/avoid glucose-containing solutions)
2. Intubate (if GCS < 8 for airway protection/suspect C-spine injury)
3. Hyperventilate ($PaCO_2$ ~ 25 torr) and avoid hypoxia (hypercarbia and hypoxia increase cerebral blood flow and thus, ICP)
4. Mannitol/furosemide (reduce brain water volume and thus, ICP)
5. Look for EKG changes associated with increased ICP: **bradycardia,** Q and U waves, ST segment depression, T wave inversion, prolonged QT interval
6. Avoid premedication (hypoventilation may increase ICP)

Induction

1. Have patient hyperventilate if awake and not intubated (reduces CBV)
2. Thiopental/etomidate/propofol/lidocaine at induction (all reduce CBV)
3. Narcotics preintubation (blunts response to laryngoscopy)

Maintenance

1. Limit volatile agents (cerebrovasodilators)
2. Limit fluids as tolerated by blood pressure (minimizes edema and CBV)
3. Hyperventilate
4. Additional mannitol PRN

If all your efforts fail, then you'd better know the criteria for brain death:[1]

● Table 110–4

Criteria for Determination of Brain Death	Clinical Tests of Brain Death
Absent cerebral and brainstem function	Cerebral unresponsiveness
Well-defined irreversible etiology	Absent pupillary, corneal, and oculocephalic/oculovestibular reflexes
Persistent absence of all brain function after observation and/or treatment	Absent cough reflex with deep tracheal suctioning
Hypothermia, drug intoxication, metabolic encephalopathy, and shock excluded	No increase in heart rate in response to IV administration of atropine (2 mg)
	No respiratory efforts on apnea testing ($PaCO_2$ > 60 mmHg)
	Electrocerebral silence documented by electroencephalography

Sample questions

A = 1, 2, 3   B = 1, 3   C = 2, 4   D = 4 only   E = all are correct

1. A 65-year-old man with colon cancer and brain metatases is to undergo an exploratory laparotomy for bowel obstruction. Preinduction vital signs are heart rate 70 beats/min, blood pressure 140/88 mmHg. Rapid sequence induction is performed with thiopental 4 mg/kg and succinylcholine 1.5 mg/kg. During laryngoscopy, his blood pressure increases to 210/125 mmHg and his heart rate decreases to 40 beats/min. Appropriate measures at this time include
   1. Administer additional IV thiopental
   2. Administer IV lidocaine
   3. Terminate laryngoscopy and hyperventilate through cricoid pressure
   4. Administer atropine

2. Bradycardia during craniotomy following closed head injury may be due to
   1. Surgical retraction on brain structures
   2. Autonomic hyperactivity
   3. Elevated intracranial pressure
   4. Electrolyte disorders

Single best answer

3. A 30-year-old male presents to the emergency room following a car accident. He had loss of conciousness at the scene. On examination, he opens his eyes to painful stimuli, withdraws his foot from pain, and is groaning and grunting. His Glasgow coma score is
   1. 5
   2. 6
   3. 7
   4. 8
   5. 9

Answers: 1. A   2. E   3. 4

Reference

1. Darby JM, Grenvik A, Stuart SA. Approach to management of the heartbeating "brain dead" organ donor. JAMA 261(15): 2222, 1989.

CHAPTER 111

SIADH versus Diabetes Insipidus versus Fluoride Nephrotoxicity

• Table 111-1

	SIADH	Diabetes Insipidus	Fluoride Nephrotoxicity
Defect	Secretion of vasopressin despite low serum osmolality	Lack of vasopressin or primary renal dysfunction	Damage to renal medulla
Causes	Head trauma Liver disease Cardiac disease Renal disease Adrenal insufficiency Thyroid disease	If defect is lack of vasopressin: Head trauma Pituitary disease Sarcoidosis	Volatile agent metabolites
		Polyuria Polydipsia	Polyuria
Diagnostic criteria	Hyponatremia < 130 mEq/L	Hypernatremia	Hypernatremia
	Hypo-osmolality < 270 mOsm/L	Hyperosmolality > 320 mOsm	Hyperosmolality > 320 mOsm/L
	Urine sodium > 20 mEq/L	Urine-specific gravity < 1.010 in the presence of hypertonic serum	Urine-specific gravity ↑ 1.010
	↓BUN, creatinine, uric acid, and albumin	Responds to vasopressin	↑BUN, creatinine Resistant to vasopressin
	Concentrated urine in the presence of hypertonic serum		
Treatment	Water restriction	Replace H_2O, electrolytes DDAVP 5 units SQ Q4–6 hr Thiazide diuretics Chlorpropamide (causes release of vasopressin)	

Sample question

A = 1, 2, 3   B = 1, 3   C = 2, 4   D = 4 only   E = all are correct

1. A 25-year-old man has undergone an exploratory laparotomy and emergency nephrectomy following a motor vehicle accident. General anesthesia with thiopental, vecuronium, and isoflurane was used, estimated blood loss ~750 mL, and he received 3500 mL crystalloid. He was combative at induction, and is slow to awaken postoperatively and remains intubated. The PACU nurses reports that his urine output has been > 10mL/kg for the first hour and is very dilute, vital signs are pulse 105 bpm, blood pressure 92/65. Serum electrolytes are Na+ 150 mEq/L, BUN 10, serum osmolality 325 mOsm/L. Appropriate therapeutic measures include
   1. Fluid restriction
   2. Administer vasopressin
   3. Transfuse with packed red cells
   4. Hyperventilate to $PaCO_2$ ~25 mmHg

Answer: 1. C

Cerebral Aneurysm Clipping

Presentation: Spontaneous rupture with subarachnoid hemorrhage (SAH)

Factors predisposing to spontaneous rupture

1. Size ≥ 10mm diameter (most common)
2. Hypertension

Signs/symptoms of SAH

Severe headache with/without loss of conciousness and a wide range of neurologic deficits including:

1. Isolated cranial nerve palsies
2. Altered mental status (confusion, stupor, coma, seizures)
3. Motor dysfunction (hemiparesis, decerebrate posturing)
4. EKG changes: Q and U waves, inverted T waves, prolonged QT interval, ST segment elevation; all thought to be due to increased catecholamines

Neurologic changes are due to

1. Elevated ICP (mass effect of blood)
2. Cerebral ischemia (immediate vasospasm at aneurysm site)

Complications following SAH

1. **Vasospasm:**
   A. Peak incidence ~ 7 days after SAH
   B. Treatment:
      1. Nimodipine (calcium channel blocker, prevents vasoconstriction)
      2. Maintain cerebral perfusion pressure by:
         a. Lowering ICP: mannitol, remove CSF via ventriculostomy
         b. Raising MAP—volume loading, vasopressors
         c. Altered viscosity of blood (mild anemia)
2. **Rebleeding:**
   A. Peak incidence within 24 hr. May occur up to 2 weeks after SAH
   B. Prevention: bedrest and sedation/antihypertensives/antifibrinolytics
   C. Treatment: clipping (early vs. late surgical intervention has same morbidity)
3. **Hydrocephalus:** relatively uncommon

Cerebral aneurysm preoperative evaluation

1. Evaluate neurologic status: facilitates immediate postop evaluation for presence of new deficits
2. Evaluate volume status: especially if h/o CHF or intentional volume expansion to treat vasospasm
3. Electrolytes: high risk of hyponatremia, with or without SIADH
4. EKG: may have coexisting coronary artery disease. Not all EKG changes are due to head injury!

Intraoperative monitors

1. Arterial line (zero and place at level of head)
2. CVP or Swan (especially if h/o CHF, myocardial infarction, hypertension)

Induction

1. Rupture is biggest risk
2. Establish *deep* anesthesia prior to laryngoscopy
3. Have antihypertensives, beta-blockers immediately available

Maintenance

Goals are to prevent rupture and aid surgical exposure via:

1. Decreased brain volume (mannitol, hyperventilate, CSF drainage, barbiturates)
2. Deliberate hypotension (**nitroprusside**, nitroglycerine, isoflurane, trimethephan)

> **NOTE:** Beware of pupillary dilation from trimethephan . . . don't confuse it with a new neurologic deficit.

Emergence

Goals are rapid emergence (early detection of neurologic deficit) and smooth hemodynamics (prevents rebleeding).

What if it ruptures?

1. At induction:
   A. Give additional thiopental (lowers $CMRO_2$)
   B. Lower blood pressure slightly (decreases bleeding a little, but you have to maintain cerebral perfusion pressure in the face of acutely increased ICP)
   C. Hyperventilate (lowers ICP and arterial inflow)
2. Intraoperatively:
   A. Give blood
   B. Lower blood pressure to ~40–50 mmHg until surgeon gets control of bleeding (reduces bleeding)
   C. Unilateral/bilateral carotid compression (minimizes bleeding)

Sample questions

A = 1, 2, 3   B = 1, 3   C = 2, 4   D = 4 only   E = all are correct

1. Factors predisposing cerebral aneurysms to rupture include
   1. Age of the patient
   2. Location of the aneuysm

3. Male gender
4. Size greater then 10 mm diameter

2. Management of cerebral vasospasm following subarachnoid hemorrhage includes
    1. Inducing hypervolemia
    2. Elevating the head of the bed
    3. Calcium channel blockers
    4. Hypocarbia

Answers: 1. D   2. A

Carotid Endarterectomy

Indications

1. Ulcerated atherosclerotic plaques in carotid artery
2. Recurrent transcient ischemic attacks
3. Carotid artery lumen reduction > 80%

Surgical technique

Dissect and cross-clamp common carotid artery

1. If no evidence of cerebral ischemia developing, proceed with or without shunt.
2. If signs of cerebral ischemia develop, unclamp, then either place shunt or raise mean arterial pressure before replacing cross-clamp (shunt may still be necessary).

Preop evaluation

1. CNS: check existing deficits/ability to reproduce TIAs with changes in head position
2. Cardiovascular: hypertension/coronary artery disease/renal dysfunction 2° to hypertension

Anesthetic goals

1. Maintain blood pressure within patient's normal range. This will let you avoid:
   A. Cerebral ischemia (perfusion pressure too low). **HINT:** the safest way to raise blood pressure in these patients is to lighten anesthesia, not artificially raise it with phenylephrine.
   B. Cerebral edema (2° to blood pressure too high in a brain with impaired autoregulation)
   C. Myocardial ischemia (2° to wall tension and afterload too high)
2. Rapid awakening (allow early neurologic evaluation)

• Table 113-1

Regional Anesthesia for CEA	General Anesthesia for CEA
Technique	Technique
Deep, superficial cervical plexus blocks	Thiopental—some cerebral protection
	Isoflurane—least ischemic risk
	Maintain normocarbia
Morbidity/mortality	Morbidity/mortality
5% chance of stroke	Equal to regional
Advantages	Advantages
Can monitor cerebral function by talking to patient	Agents *may* offer cerebral protection
Disadvantages	Disadvantages
Increased carotid sinus reactivity with surgical manipulation	Need additional monitors to assess cerebral function and cerebral blood flow
No cerebral protection from anesthetic drugs	

Methods for monitoring cerebral blood flow (ischemia) and cerebral function:

1. SSEP: hard to interpret, easily affected by anesthetic drugs.
2. EEG: detects regional ischemia, hard to interpret/affected by drugs, temp, $PaCO_2$/typical EKG changes during carotid cross-clamping are decreased amplitude or increased amplitude with decreased frequency.
3. Stump pressure: simple measurement of carotid pressure distal to clamp, is a reflection of the pressure in circle of Willis. Pressure > 60 mmHg = adequate cerebral perfusion pressure/false negatives are possible.

Postoperative complications

1. Hypertension (**most common**/leads to cerebral edema, myocardial ischemia): treat with nipride or hydralazine
2. Hypotension (leads to cerebral ischemia): treat with fluid bolus, phenylephrine, local infiltration of carotid sinus
3. Carotid body dysfunction (patient won't hyperventilate in response to hypoxia)
4. Hematoma formation with airway compromise
5. Myocardial infarction/stroke

Sample questions

Single best answer

1. Prior to placing the cross-clamp during carotid endarterectomy, the patient's pulse drops from 85 to 50 bpm and the blood pressure drops from 147/88 to 100/56 mmHg. This physiologic change
    1. Can be prevented by local infiltration of lidocaine at the surgical site
    2. Is due to carotid body stimulation
    3. Can be reversed with atropine
    4. Is best treated with a fluid bolus

2. Carotid artery stump pressure will be increased with
    1. Administration of barbiturates
    2. Administration of halothane
    3. Hypocarbia
    4. Hypoxia

Answers: 1. 2 (If you answered "1," I gotcha . . . this is a favorite trick on the boards)   2. 2

CHAPTER 114

Anesthetic Effects on EEG

Types of EEG waveforms

1. Delta: 0–4 Hz, seen in normal sleep, deep anesthesia, brain tumors, hypoxia, metabolic encephalopathy
2. Theta: 4–8 Hz, sleep and anesthesia in adults, common with hyperventilation in children
3. Alpha: 8–13 Hz, resting alert adult with closed eyes, abolished if startled or eyes opened.
4. Beta: 13–30 Hz, concentration (like when doing arithmetic), light anesthesia, frontal lobe origin in the presence of benzodiazepines or barbiturates

The normal awake EEG consists of

Chiefly beta activity with small amounts of delta and theta.

Progression of EEG changes with anesthesia

Induction → ↓ alpha waves and ↑ beta waves (excitation) → deeper plane → theta and delta predominate → deeper still → burst supression → deeper → isoelectricity

Or to say it another way:

Increased frequency (light anesthesia) → decreased frequency, increased amplitude → decreased frequency, decreased amplitude → isoelectricity (profound anesthesia)

Which anesthetics follow this progression?

1. Barbiturates (with progressively larger doses)
2. Etomidate (with progressively larger doses)
3. Inhalational agents (with progressively larger doses)

Exceptions

1. Ketamine: only produces increased frequency
2. Nitrous oxide: only produces increased frequency
3. Opioids: decrease frequency, increase amplitude

Physiologic variables that alter EEG

1. Hypoxia (same progression as with barbiturates, with increasing degrees of hypoxia)
2. Hypercarbia (same as hypoxia)
3. Temperature (same as hypoxia, excluding the stage of increased frequency)

Burst suppression: what is it and what causes it?

It is: periods of electrical silence alternating with low frequency, high amplitude waves. It is caused by:
1. High-dose etomidate and barbiturates
2. High concentrations of isoflurane
3. Severe hypothermia (as in cardiopulmonary bypass)
4. Cerebral hypoxia

Sample question

A = 1, 2, 3   B = 1, 3   C = 2, 4   D = 4 only   E = all are correct

1. True statements regarding EEG intraoperative monitoring include
   1. Mild hypoventilation produces increased beta waves
   2. Hypothermia will continue to decrease the cerebral metabolic rate even beyond the point of EEG isoelectricity
   3. Clonus associated with etomidate is not accompanied by EEG activity
   4. The predominant wave of the normal sleep state is delta

Answer: 1. E

Sensory Evoked Potentials

Technique: Intermittent application of low-voltage stimulation to a peripheral nerve and measurement the resultant electrical activity along the pathway to the cerebral cortex

Uses

Any operative procedure with the potential to damage neural tissue via direct trauma or through compromise of the blood supply

Categories of potentials

1. Near field: the recording electrode is close to the neural generator (i.e., scalp and cerebral cortex) and the position of the electrode greatly influences wave morphology.
2. Far field: the recording electrode is distant from the neural generator (i.e., scalp and brainstem) and the position of the electrode has no effect on wave morphology.

What part of the waveforms are we interested in?

1. Latency (time from stimulus to response): increased latency = ischemia
2. Amplitude (the degree of deflection of the wave): decreased amplitude = ischemia; increased amplitude = excitation

There are three commonly used types of sensory evoked potentials

1. **Brainstem auditory evoked potentials**
   Stimulus: clicking noises in the ear
   Parameter measured: integrity of the auditory pathway
   Indications: procedures involving auditory pathway, posterior fossa, or brainstem
   Advantages: easy to perform, reliable, not prone to electrical interference
   Disadvantages: won't work if patient is deaf in the ear to be monitored. Technique most easily affected by anesthetic drugs
2. **Visual evoked potentials**
   Stimulus: flashes of light applied to one eye
   Parameter measured: visual nerves and cortex
   Indications: procedures involving any visual structures
   Advantages: most resistant to interference by anesthetic drugs
   Disadvantages: very unreliable, technically difficult to perform
3. **Somatosensory evoked potentials**

Stimulus: low-voltage stimulation of large sensory nerve (posterior tibial or median)

Parameter measured: integrity of dorsal column sensory tracts from peripheral nerve to sensory cortex

Indications: procedures involving structures near spinal cord

Disadvantages: prone to electrical and anesthetic drug interference. Does not directly monitor motor tracts, therefore, profound motor injury can occur in the presence of a normal SSEP.

How is it possible to have normal SSEPs and wind up with motor deficits?

Because the majority of the blood supply to the motor tracts is from the anterior spinal artery, while the sensory tracts are supplied by the posterior spinal arteries. Therefore, the supply to the motor tracts can be greatly impaired without rendering an abnormal SSEP.

SSEP pathway

Stimulate large fiber sensory nerve → dorsal root ganglion
→ ipsilateral dorsal column nuclei → medial lemniscus
→ crosses to contralateral thalamus → frontoparietal sensorimotor cortex

Anesthetics and their effects on the various SSEPs

1. SSEP: ↑ latency and ↓ amplitude with all volatile agents and all IV agents (barbiturates, narcotics, benzodiazepines, propofol). Exceptions:
   A. Nitrous oxide: no effect on latency
   B. Etomidate: ↑ latency AND amplitude
   C. Ketamine: no effect on latency, ↑ amplitude
2. BAEP: ↑ latency and ↓ amplitude with all volatile agents, etomidate. Exceptions:
   A. Nitrous oxide: no effect on latency
   B. Barbiturates: no effect on amplitude
3. VEP: ↑ latency and ↓ amplitude with all volatile agents. Exceptions: halothane: no effect on amplitude

Physiologic factors that can alter evoked potentials

1. Hypotension (MAP < 50 mmHg)
2. Hypoxia
3. Anemia
4. Hyperthermia

All cause a decrease in amplitude only

5. Hypothermia: ↑ latency, ↓ amplitude

Sample questions

A = 1, 2, 3   B = 1, 3   C = 2, 4   D = 4 only   E = all are correct

1. A 14-year-old girl is undergoing Harrington rod placement for correction of idiopathic scoliosis. Anesthetic management includes a nitroprusside infusion, vecuronium, 30% oxygen, isoflurane at 0.75% end-tidal, and a fentanyl infusion at 2 µg/kg/hr. Vital signs are BP 78/45, pulse 85, temperature 36.8°C, hematocrit 33%. As the surgeon is reducing the angle of the spinal curvature, the SSEP waveform reveals a decrease in amplitude and increased latency. After informing the surgeon, which of the following are appropriate measures to take?
   1. Fluid bolus of 10 mL/kg of lactated Ringer's

2. Discontinue the nitroprusside infusion
3. Increase the fraction of inspired oxygen
4. Transfuse with packed red blood cells

Single best answer

2. All of the following will produce an decrease in amplitude and an increase in latency of the SSEP waveform except:
   1. Thiopental
   2. Etomidate
   3. Isoflurane
   4. Propofol
   5. Midazolam

Answers: 1. A   2. 2

Chapter 116

Spinal Cord Transection

Mechanisms

1. Trauma: **most common,** males > females, usually cervical spine (specifically, C7)
2. Atraumatic: multiple sclerosis (most common), rheumatoid arthritis, Down's syndrome

Symptoms are dependent on

1. Acuity
2. Level of transection
    A. **>C4:** death likely, due to diaphragmatic failure
    B. **>T6:** hypoventilation and hypoxia (always), autonomic hyperreflexia (after spinal reflexes regained)
    C. **>T10:** autonomic hyperreflexia is **rare**

- Table 116–1

Clinical Parameter	Acute Spinal Cord Injury ("spinal shock," lasts 1–3 weeks)	Chronic Spinal Cord Injury
Motor function	Flaccid paralysis	Spastic paralysis
Sensory function	Absent	Absent
Cord reflexes	Absent	Present
Temperature regulation	Absent	Impaired
Cardiovascular system	Hypotension (loss of sympathetic tone, hypovolemia, left ventricular dysfunction) Bradycardia EKG signs of ischemia	Autonomic hyperreflexia
Pulmonary system	Hypoxia/hypoventilation (if diaphragm or intercostals involved)	Hypoxia/hypoventilation (same as acute)

Complications of spinal cord injury

1. **Acute:**
    A. Pulmonary aspiration (impaired ability to clear secretions)
    B. Pneumonia (as above and alveolar hypoventilation)
    C. Hypoxia
    D. Pulmonary embolus

E. Pulmonary edema (requires agressive volume resuscitation, and left ventricle may fail due to loss of sympathetic ability to increase contractility)
2. **Chronic:**
   A. Autonomic hyperreflexia (see below)
   B. Recurrent pulmonary and urologic infections
   C. Altered thermoregulation

What it this thing called autonomic hyperreflexia?

It's stimulated by:

1. Surgery
2. Distention of viscus (bladder, rectum)

Pathophysiology

Stimulation below the level of transection ⇒ Sensory impulses enter cord ⇒
Reflex sympathetic outflow without normal inhibition from higher centers ⇒
Generalized vasoconstriction below the level of transection ⇒
Increased blood pressure ⇒ Carotid sinus stimulation ⇒ Bradycardia
⇓
Vasodilation above transection, may not offset effects of vasoconstriction

Figure 116–1.

• **Table 116–2**

Signs	Symptoms
Acute, profound hypertension	Central nervous system disturbances Headache/blurred vision/cerebral and subarachnoid hemorrhage/retinal hemorrhage/seizures Cardiovascular disturbances Bradycardia/pulmonary edema 2° to left ventricular failure
Acute, profound bradycardia	Loss of conciousness
Vasodilation above transection	Nasal stuffiness/cutaneous flushing
Dysrythymias	Loss of conciousness

Treatment of autonomic hyperreflexia

Central-acting antihypertensives don't work.

1. Ganglionic blockers (trimethephan)
2. Alpha-blockers (prazosin, phentolamine)
3. Directs vasodilators (sodium nitroprusside)
4. General anesthesia
5. Spinal anesthesia (epidural is ineffective, especially for urologic cases, because of sacral sparing)

Anesthetic management for spinal cord injuries

• **Table 116-3**

Acute Spinal Cord Injury	Chronic Spinal Cord Injury
Assume C-spine injury	PREVENT AUTONOMIC HYPERREFLEXIA!
Liberal fluid administration	(mostly by providing adequate anesthesia)
Intubate/ventilate (full stomach precautions)	If hyperreflexia occurs:
	Have nipride infusion ready
Aggressive warming measures	Pick from above list of treatments
If relaxant needed	SUCCINYLCHOLINE CONTRAINDICATED!
Pancuronium: vagolytic effect desirable	(risk of hyperkalemia if injury 4 days–6 months old)
Succinylcholine: unlikely to cause hyperkalemia in first few hours after injury	Aggressive warming measures
	Beware of hypercalcemia (2° to bone resorption)

Sample questions

A = 1, 2, 3   B = 1, 3   C = 2, 4   D = 4 only   E = all are correct

1. Acceptable methods of intubating the trachea immediately following cervical spine injury include
   1. Topical anesthesia and fiberoptic intubation
   2. Rapid-sequence intubation with in-line traction of the cervical spine
   3. Topical anesthesia and light wand intubation
   4. Induction of general anesthesia followed by placement of a laryngeal mask airway

2. A 24-year-old paraplegic male is scheduled for cystoscopy. His spinal cord injury occurred 2 years ago and his sensory function is intact above the nipples with intact motor function of the upper extremities. The surgeon declines your assistance and proceeds to perform the procedure utilizing local anesthetic jelly on the cystoscope. As the surgeon is filling the bladder, the patient becomes acutely hypertensive with a blood pressure of 190/100 and his pulse drops from 88 to 45 bpm. Appropriate measures at this time include
   1. Initiate a nitroprusside infusion
   2. Atropine 0.4 mg IV
   3. Rapid-sequence induction of general anesthesia with thiopental and rocuronium bromide
   4. Induce general anesthesia with thiopental and support the airway with bag-mask ventilation

3. Common electrolyte abnormalities seen in patients with chronic spinal cord injuries include
   1. Hyponatremia
   2. Hyperkalemia
   3. Hypomagnesemia
   4. Hypercalcemia

4. A 25-year-old, 65-kg male paraplegic whose injury was at the level of the sixth thoracic vertbrae 4 months ago is scheduled to undergo an exploratory laparotomy for a small-bowel obstruction. Rapid-sequence in-

duction is initiated with thiopental 300 mg and succinylcholine 100 mg. Immediately after administration of the induction agents, the EKG monitor shows widening of the QRS complex and elevation of the T-waves. True statements regarding this phenomenon include
1. Induction with 250 mg thiopental and 50 mg succinylcholine would not produce this effect
2. d-Tubocurare 3 mg IV 3 min before induction will prevent this response
3. He would be unlikely to have this response if his injury were below T10
4. He would be less likely to exhibit this response 12 months from now

Answers: 1. B 2. B 3. D 4. D

Chapter 117

Electroconvulsive Therapy

Indications

1. Severe depression not responsive to pharmacologic intervention
2. Coexisting medical conditions precluding use of standard antidepressants
3. Acute schizophrenia (sometimes)

Physiologic effects of ECT seizures

Which are generalized tonic-clonic seizures

1. Cardiovascular: initial parasympathetic stimulation (bradycardia, hypotension) followed by sympathetic stimulation (tachycardia, tachydysrythymias, hypertension); must not have recent myocardial infarction
2. Cerebral: Increased $CMRO_2$, therefore will also have increased CBF and ICP (must not have intracranial mass lesion or recent stroke)
3. Increased intraocular pressure
4. Increased intragastric pressure (must be NPO)

Interactions of common psychotropic medications and anesthetic adjunctive agents

1. Monoamine oxidase inhibitors
   A. Action: inhibit breakdown of norepinephrine, dopamine, serotonin (central, peripheral)
   B. Interactions: indirect-acting sympathomimetics may precipitate hypertensive crisis; direct-acting sympathomimetics less likely to produce hypertensive crisis; meperidine may precipitate severe (potentially fatal) excitation reactions
2. Tricyclic antidepressants
   A. Action: block reuptake of norepinephrine, serotonin, dopamine (central, peripheral)
   B. Interactions: direct-acting sympathomimetics may precipitate hypertensive crisis anticholinergic side effects are common, so best to use noncentrally acting anticholinergics
3. Lithium
   A. Action: affects release of dopamine, norepinephrine, and distribution of ions
   B. Interactions: prolongs neuromuscular blockade (succinylcholine, pancuronium); more memory loss and confusion after ECT than in nonlithium patients

Anesthetic drugs that lower siezure threshold

1. Etomidate
2. Enflurane
3. Methohexital
4. Ketamine
5. Laudanosine (atracurium metabolite)

Sample question

A = 1, 2, 3   B = 1, 3   C = 2, 4   D = 4 only   E = all are correct

1. Absolute contraindications to electroconvulsive therapy include
   1. Intracranial mass lesion
   2. Pheochromocytoma
   3. Myocardial infarction within the last 3 months
   4. Cerebrovascular accident within the last 3 months

Answer: **1. E**

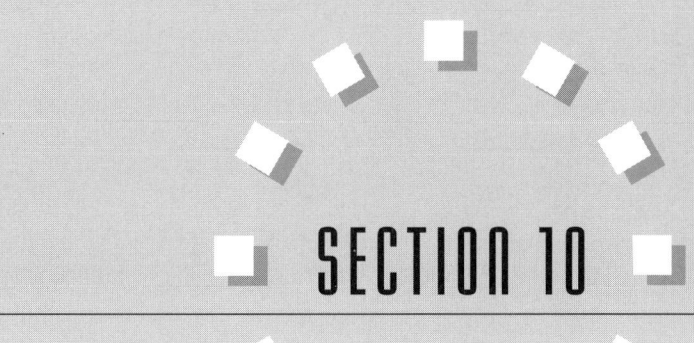

SECTION 10

Anesthesia Equipment

CHAPTER 118

Gas Cylinders

(Tank you very much . . .)

Characteristics of the common medical gases when stored in "E" cylinders (the size we use)

• Table 118–1

	Nitrous Oxide	Oxygen	Carbon Dioxide	Air	Helium
Physical state	Liquid	Gas	Liquid	Gas	Gas
Liters when tank full	1600	660	1600	625	500
psig when full	745	2200	840	2000	1600
Molecular weight	44	32			
Critical temperature	36.5°C	–118°C			

Key points

1. Both *liquids* have 1600 L when full, and the psig is equal to their vapor pressure.
2. All *gases* have ~600 L and are stored under high pressure.
3. Cylinders containing nonliquified gas undergo a steady decline in pressure as the tank empties. The pressure of cylinders containing liquified gas remains equal to the vapor pressure of the gas until all agent is in the gaseous phase, then the pressure declines as gas is released.
4. All tanks decrease in weight as they empty, regardless of physical state (liquid or gas).

Importance of critical temperature

Critical temperature is the temperature at which a liquid becomes a gas and cannot be kept in the liquid phase, no matter how much pressure is applied to the liquid phase. Compare the CT° of oxygen with that of nitrous oxide: the CT° of oxygen is so far below room temperature that it must be stored in E cylinders as a gas. Nitrous oxide is still in liquid phase at room temperature because it hasn't reached CT° yet.

Importance of filling density

All tanks must be kept below safe pressure limits. Since nonliquid gases will have increased pressure when heated, their filling is limited to a pressure not to exceed 10% greater than the service pressure. In contrast, liquified gases won't increase their pressure when heated. Thus, filling volume is based on the filling density, which is the ratio of the weight of a tank filled with gas vs. the weight of the amount of water it takes to fill the tank.

Required permanent tank markings include

1. Type of material tank is made of
2. Service pressure in psi (highest normal working pressure)
3. Date of last pressure test
4. Serial number
5. Manufacturer's symbol

Additional markings you may see

☆: can be retested in 10 years instead of the usual 5-year test period
✚: cylinder can be filled to 10% over service pressure
"SPUN" or "PLUG": refers to manner in which tank was closed

How to calculate the time remaining in an oxygen "E" cylinder at a given flowrate

1. **The hard way:** First, you have to remember that a full tank = 2200 psi and 660 L. Then you have to do all this math: Example tank has 1200 psi at 4 L/min. Thus:
   1. $1200 \div 2200 = 55\%$ full.
   2. $660\ L \times 0.55 = 363\ L$
   3. $363\ L \div 4\ L/min = 90$ minutes left
2. **The easy way:** (psig × 0.28) ÷ flowrate in L/min = minutes remaining in tank. So, for example tank:

   $(1200 \times 0.28) \div 4\ L/min = 84$ minutes remaining in tank

   (It's a fudge, but it works.)

Calculating time remaining in a nitrous oxide tank

1. **If there's still liquid in the tank (psig = 745),** weigh the tank. The weight of the empty tank is stamped on the tank (remember?). Then, you have to know that *at room temperature,* each gram molecular weight of N_2O (44 g) will produce 0.5 L of gas. So:
   1. Actual tank weight – empty tank weight in grams
   2. Weight from step 1 ÷ 44
   3. Product of step 2 × 0.5 = liters of N_2O in tank
   4. Liters of N_2O ÷ flowrate in L/min = minutes remaining
2. **At the *exact moment* that all liquid N_2O becomes gas,** you can use Boyle's law $P_1V_1 = P_2V_2$

   $P_1 = 745$ psi, the vapor pressure of N_2O
   $V_1 = 5$ liters, the volume of a nitrous tank
   $P_2 = 14.8$ psi, the atmospheric pressure

   So:
   $(745 \times 5) \div 14.8 = 253$ L of N_2O, then divide by flowrate to get the remaining time

And when tank pressure start to fall

Example: gauge reads 500 psi: (500 psi ÷ 745 psi) × 253 L = 169 L

Sample questions

Single best answer

1. A nitrous oxide cylinder that is cold to the touch and has a pressure gauge registering zero is removed from an anesthesia machine and stored in a room at 21°C. Four hours later the guage registers 745 psi. The most likely explanation of this is
    1. There was some liquid remaining in the tank when it was stored
    2. The gas in the tank has expanded upon warming and exerts a measurable pressure
    3. There was some oxygen mixed in with the nitrous oxide
    4. The pressure gauge is broken
    5. The operating room temperature was too cold to allow normal gauge function

2. Nitrous oxide is stored in cylinders as a liquid as opposed to oxygen, which is stored as a gas because compared with oxygen nitrous oxide
    1. Tanks cannot withstand as high a pressure as oxygen tanks do
    2. Is flammable when stored as a gas
    3. Has a higher critical temperature
    4. Occupies fewer liters per gram molecular weight
    5. Has a higher molecular weight

Answers: 1. 1   2. 3

Explanation of question #1: As liquid converts to gas, it cools. If a tank cools during gas release, it means there's still some liquid in the tank. When you stop releasing gas, the remaining liquid converts to gas and the tank pressure goes back to normal.

CHAPTER 119

Oxygen Therapy

Nonpositive pressure oxygen therapy devices can be classified two ways

1. Low-flow systems: O_2 flowrate is too low to meet patients' inspiratory requirements, so entrainment of room air is necessary. Anything changing amount of entrainment can alter F_iO_2
2. High-flow systems: O_2 flowrate meets patients' inspiratory flowrate needs. F_iO_2 is determined by controlling the amount of room air entrained by employing the Venturi principle. Venturi principle states that at a given flowrate, as a gas flows through an outlet tube with a side port for entrainment of room air, the amount of room air entrained is determined by the size of the side port.

Examples of low-flow systems

1. Nasal cannula
2. Simple oxygen mask
3. Simple oxygen mask with reservoir bag

Determinants of F_iO_2 in low-flow systems

1. Size of oxygen reservoir (for cannula, reservoir is nasopharynx)
2. O_2 flowrate ($\uparrow$ flow = $\uparrow F_iO_2$)
3. Respiratory rate (slow rate = $\uparrow F_iO_2$)
4. Inspiratory flowrate ($\uparrow$ flowrate = $\uparrow$ entrainment = $\downarrow F_iO_2$)
5. Tidal volume ($\uparrow V_T = \downarrow F_iO_2$)

Example of high-flow systems

1. Venturi mask (maximum F_iO_2 0.4)
2. Face shield with high-volume nebulizer and large-bore tubing

Approximate F_iO_2 attained with a nasal cannula

L/Min	F_iO_2
1	.24
2	.28
3	.32
4	.36
5	.40

Sample questions

A = 1, 2, 3   B = 1, 3   C = 2, 4   D = 4 only   E = all are correct

1. Besides the delivery rate set on the oxygen flowmeter, the F_iO_2 achieved with nasal prongs depends on
   1. Tidal volume
   2. Nasopharyngeal volume
   3. Respiratory rate
   4. Use of a low-volume humidifier

Single best answer

2. A patient with a respiratory rate of 15/min is wearing an aerosol mask connected via corrugated tubing to a cool nebulizer set at F_iO_2 0.4 and 8 L/min. The best way to increase the F_iO_2 is
   1. Change to a Venturi mask
   2. Add positive end-expiratory pressure
   3. Increase the flowrate to 10 L/min
   4. Change to a heated nebulizer
   5. Add sections of corrugated tubing to the expiratory side of mask

Answers: 1. A   2. 5

Flowmeters

Design

1. A hollow glass tube with an inner diameter that is smaller at the bottom than the top
2. Contains a "float" of some type (ball, bobbin, etc.)
3. Flow is measured at the **center** of a ball float, and at the **top** of a bobbin float
4. Calibrated for a specific gas (flowmeters are not interchangeable among gases)

Function

Gas entering the bottom of the flowmeter creates pressure and makes the bobbin rise. This creates a space between the bobbin and the inside of the flowmeter through which gas flows. This space increases as you ascend this gradually widening tube (thus the term: variable orifice). As the orifice widens, more flow is required to create enough pressure to keep the bobbin afloat.

Factors affecting gas flow

Temperature
Atmospheric pressure (if hyperbaric, flow delivered is < float indicates and vice versa)
Pressure drop across bobbin
Length of bobbin
Radius of tube (effect depends on flowrate)
Viscosity of gas (only a factor for low flowrates, which create laminar flow)
Density of gas (only a factor for high flowrates, which create turbulent flow)

At low flowrates

Flow is *laminar*, explained by Poiselle's law:

$$\text{Flow} = \frac{\pi p r^4}{8 v \ell}$$

Note: Radius is to 4th power, and flow is inversely related to viscosity.

At high flowrates

Flow is *turbulent,* because:

Flow ∝ r2 ∝ p ∝ length ∝ 1/square root of density

Note: Radius is squared, and flow is inversely related to density.

Safety features of flowmeters on anesthesia machines

	Oxygen	Nitrous oxide
Control knob:	large, fluted	small, not fluted
Color:	green	blue
Position:	closest to common gas outlet	upstream from oxygen

Oxygen flowmeter malfunction

Problem	Result
Tube outlet is blocked	Tube will rupture or begin to leak
Dirt inside tube	Orifice is narrowed; flow is less than float indicates
Back pressure	Pushes float down; flow is greater than float indicates
Leak	Lower concentration of oxygen in final mixture

Sample questions

A = 1, 2, 3   B = 1, 3   C = 2, 4   D = 4 only   E = all are correct

1. True statements regarding medical gas flowmeters include
   1. For a given flowmeter at low flow, gases of similar viscosities will deliver similar amounts of gas.
   2. At low flows, flow is inversely related to the length of the flowmeter.
   3. For a given flowmeter at high flow, gases of similar densities will deliver similar amounts of gas
   4. At high flows, flow is directly proportional to the length of the flowmeter

2. Malfunctions of a flowmeter resulting in greater than expected flow include
   1. Back pressure from the patient circuit
   2. Using the flowmeter at an altitude higher than that at which the flowmeter was calibrated
   3. Use of a gas with a lower density than the flowmeter is designed for
   4. Dirt particles within the flowmeter

Single best answer

3. If there is a leak in the air flowmeter, which of the following positions of the oxygen flowmeter is most likely to deliver a hypoxic mixture?

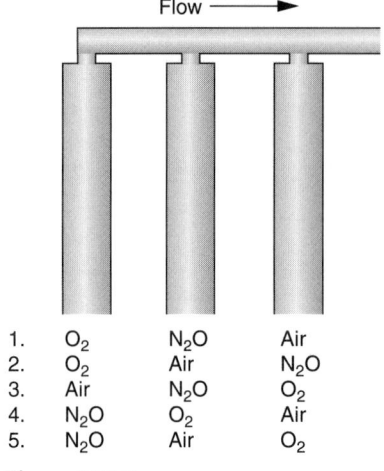

1. O_2 N_2O Air
2. O_2 Air N_2O
3. Air N_2O O_2
4. N_2O O_2 Air
5. N_2O Air O_2

Figure 120–1.

Answers: 1. B   2. B   3. 2

Chapter 121

Vaporizers

Generic design

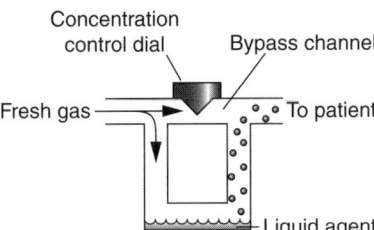

Figure 121–1.

General principles of vaporizer function

1. Vaporizers are agent specific with regard to vapor pressure, specific heat, and thermal conductivity.
2. The concentration dial controls the proportion of gas entering and by-passing the vaporizing chamber.
3. Ease of vaporization depends on the vapor pressure (VP) of the agent (the partial pressure at which liquid agent reaches equilibrium with gaseous state).

> **NOTE:** Vapor pressure is determined by only two things: (1) temperature ($\uparrow T° = \uparrow VP$, but is nonlinear), (2) physical characteristics of the liquid.

Translated, this means that a vaporizer designed for an agent with a low VP (hard to vaporize) will direct a relatively larger flow through the vaporizing chamber for a given concentration than will a vaporizer with an agent of high VP.

Factors affecting vaporizer output

1. **Temperature:**
$$\uparrow T° = \uparrow VP = \uparrow \text{output}$$

Evaporation causes cooling, which reduces VP and impedes further vaporization. Vaporizers are made of substances with high specific heat and high thermal conductivity, both of which reduce cooling.

2. **Carrier gas:**
   A. N_2O is more soluble than oxygen, so when added as a carrier gas, some of it dissolves into the liquid agent and vaporizer output is reduced because there's less gas available to "carry" vapor.
   B. If N_2O is removed from the carrier gas mixture, a transient increase in vaporizer output occurs as nitrous comes out of solution, creating more carrier gas.
3. **Flow rate of carrier gas:**
   A. At low flows, output < dial setting because agents are dense and there's insufficient forward flow to push out vaporized agent.
   B. At high flows, output < dial setting because flow is too fast to allow complete saturation of carrier gas.
4. **The pumping effect:** caused by intermittent back pressure during positive pressure ventilation or use of the oxygen flush valve. **Effect is more pronounced with:**
   A. Low flow rates
   B. Low concentration settings
   C. Low liquid level in vaporizer
   D. Wide, fast swings in circuit pressure

   How it works: Gas gets compressed in vaporizer by back pressure. When pressure is released, vapor escapes out normal exit as well as through bypass chamber, causing increased output.

5. **Altitude:** at high altitude, atmospheric pressure is reduced. The partial pressure of the agent is a bigger fraction of atmospheric (e.g., halothane at sea level = 240/760 ≈ 33%. On Mt. McKinley, 240/500 ≈ 50%). Thus at high altitudes, you'll deliver more than the dial says. The converse is true at low altitudes (under the sea).

Vaporizer hazards

1. Tipping (not cows): liquid agent enters bypass chamber, ↑↑↑ output. What do you do? Set dial at low concentration and run at high flows for ~ 1/2 hour.
2. Overfilling: same result as tipping.
3. Leaks: note that vaporizer must be turned on to detect leak. If machine has check valves: must do negative pressure test to detect leak. If machine lacks check valves: routine positive pressure check will detect leak.
4. Fill vaporizer with wrong agent: if an agent that evaporates easily (high VP) is put into a vaporizer intended for an agent with a low VP, it will be exposed to an inappropriately high fresh gas flow and you'll deliver more agent than the dial indicates. If the agents have similar vapor pressures, it's still possible to overdose by putting a more potent agent than intended in the vaporizer.

In case you don't know vapor pressures

Halothane, isoflurane	~240 mmHg
Enflurane	~180 mmHg
Desflurane	~660 mmHg
Sevoflurane	~160 mmHg
Methoxyflurane	~25 mmHg

Graphically, you can remember it this way

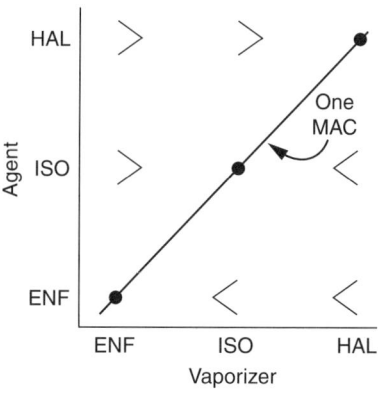

Anything above the line = over dose
Anything below the line = underdose

Figure 121–2.

Sample questions

A = 1, 2, 3   B = 1, 3   C = 2, 4   D = 4 only   E = all are correct

1. The vaporizer filling errors posing a risk of overdose include
   1. Halothane in an enflurane vaporizer
   2. Sevoflurane in a methoxyflurane vaporizer
   3. Desflurane in a sevoflurane vaporizer
   4. Isoflurane in a halothane vaporizer

2. Vapor pressure of an inhalational anesthetic is increased if
   1. Humidity is reduced
   2. Atmospheric pressure is increased
   3. The size of vaporizing chamber is reduced
   4. Temperature is increased

3. A free-standing vaporizer tips over, and liquid agent spills out. Before using this vaporizer, you should
   1. Send it back to the manufacturer to be serviced
   2. Let the vaporizer run at a low concentration setting for half an hour
   3. Do nothing special
   4. Empty the remaining liquid agent out and refill the chamber with fresh agent
   5. Mount it on a more stable stand

Answers: 1. E   2. D   3. B

CHAPTER 122

The Dreaded Copper Kettle

Here's what it looks like

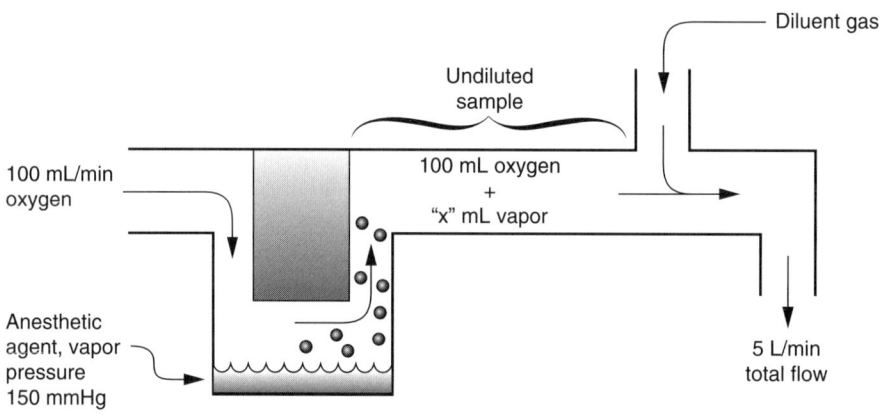

Figure 122–1.

The typical scenario you'll be given

There is a flow of 100 mL/min oxygen through the vaporizing chamber. Vapor pressure of the volatile agent is 150 mmHg. Total flow to the patient is 5 L/min.

Questions they will ask you

1. What is the final concentration of volatile agent delivered to the patient?
2. What is the total volume of gas exiting the vaporizing chamber? (No, it's not 100 mL.)
3. How much diluent gas must be added to the system to achieve a total flow of 5 L/min?

How it works

To calculate the *final* concentration of agent, you must first know the *starting* concentration (i.e., the concentration in an undiluted sample, or: *"What percent of atmospheric pressure does the agent occupy?"*). That's easy math: 150 mmHg ÷ 760 mmHg = 20%. So in our example, the bracketed area labeled "Undiluted sample" is 20% agent. That means the remaining 80% of undiluted sample is our 100 mL of oxygen. So what's the total volume of gas exiting the vaporizing chamber? . . . well, you need to know how many mL of agent you picked up. Again, it's simple math:

$$\frac{\text{"x" mL of agent}}{20\% \text{ of sample}} \times \frac{100 \text{ mL oxygen}}{80\% \text{ of sample}}$$

Solving for x, you see that x = 25 mL of agent, So a *total* of 125 mL of gas exits the vaporizer. Then, to find the final concentration simply divide mL of agent by mL of total flow:

$$\frac{25 \text{ mL agent}}{5000 \text{ mL total}} = 0.005 \times 100 = 0.5\% \text{ final concentration of agent}$$

Sample questions: We just did one.

The Desflurane Vaporizer

General design

1. Separate circuits for fresh gas and vapor
2. Vapor chamber is electrically heated (39°C), creating a constant reservoir of vapor pressurized to two atmospheres absolute

Design of the fresh gas circuit

1. Prior to reaching patient, flow is directed through a fixed restrictor, creating back pressure
2. Back pressure pushes against a pressure transducer that is interfaced with the pressure regulator of the vapor circuit

Design of the vapor circuit

Prior to delivery to the patient, vapor passes through, in order:

1. Shut-off valve (only open when vaporizer is warmed up and concentration dial is turned on)
2. Pressure regulator (interfaces with fresh gas circuit and maintains pressure in vapor circuit = pressure in fresh gas circuit)

> **NOTE:** Pressure in circuit = working pressure of vaporizer. Working pressure is constant at a fixed flow rate. As fresh gas flow increases, working pressure increases linearly.

Factors affecting output

1. Carrier gas composition: just as other variable bypass vaporizers, when carrier gas of 100% oxygen is diluted with nitrous oxide or air, the output decreases.
2. Altitude: at high altitudes, there is no internal effect because vaporizer operates at absolute pressures. However, once vapor enters ambient atmosphere, the volume percent of vapor is reduced. To maintain the same concentration, the dial setting must be increased.

Sample questions

A = 1, 2, 3   B = 1, 3   C = 2, 4   D = 4 only   E = all are correct

1. At constant fresh gas flow, as the concentration setting is increased on a desflurane vaporizer
   1. The back pressure created by fresh gas flow is increased
   2. Output of vapor in mL/min is increased
   3. The shut-off valve is opened more
   4. The concentration delivered to the patient increases

2. At a constant dial setting, as the fresh gas flow is increased on a desflurane vaporizer
   1. The temperature of the vaporizing chamber is increased to offset cooling due to evaporation
   2. Working pressure is increased
   3. The fresh gas flow restrictor widens
   4. Output of vapor in mL/min is increased

Single best answer

3. The vaporizing chamber of desflurane is heated
   1. To prevent excessive cooling due to rapid vaporization
   2. To create adequate working pressure
   3. To create a reservoir of vapor
   4. To prevent condensate from forming within the chamber
   5. Because of the low vapor pressure of desflurane

Answers: 1. C   2. C   3. 3

CHAPTER 124

The Anesthesia Machine

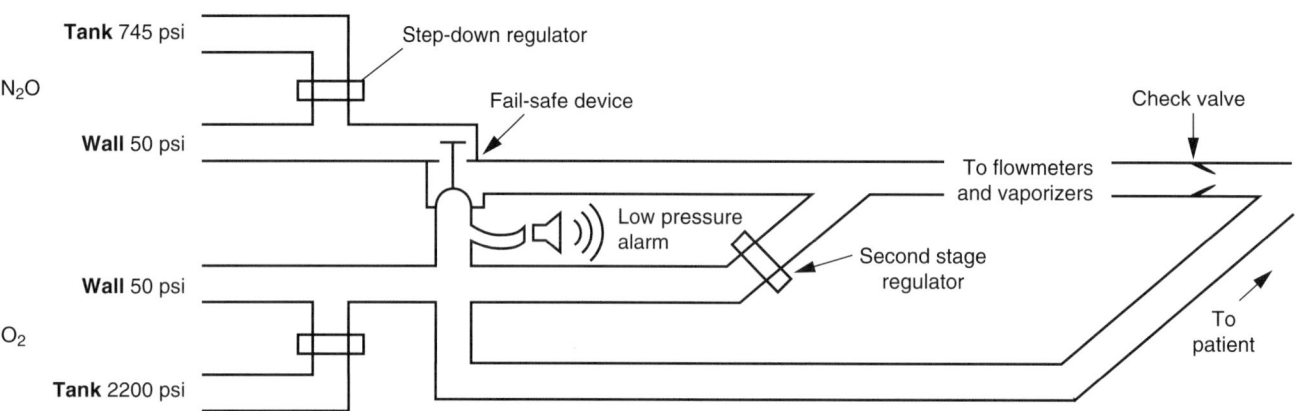

Figure 124–1.

Detailed explanations of the inner workings are available in all the major anesthesia texts. The goal here is to focus on those topics they love to ask.

1. Machine preferentially takes flow from 50-psi wall source vs. down-regulated 45-psi tank source.
2. Second-stage regulators are optional, but help maintain delivery of constant pressure to flowmeters, despite fluctuations in system pressure.
3. Check valves prevent reverse flow into vaporizers (which causes "pumping effect"), but are not present in all machines.
4. The oxygen flush valve enters the patient circuit beyond flowmeters and check valve, creating potential to deliver high pressure (50-psi) oxygen directly to patient!!!

Machine features that help prevent delivery of hypoxic gas mixtures

1. **Oxygen supply pressure alarm:** will alarm if supply pressure is < ~30 psi
2. **"Fail-safe" valve:**
    A. Requires a certain threshold pressure of oxygen (~20 psi) against the piston valve to open the channel and allow flow of N_2O.
    B. Closure of channel can be:
        1. All-or-none: if pressure > 20 psi, channel is completely open.
        2. Graduated: as oxygen pressure falls, so does N_2O, and flow follows proportionately.

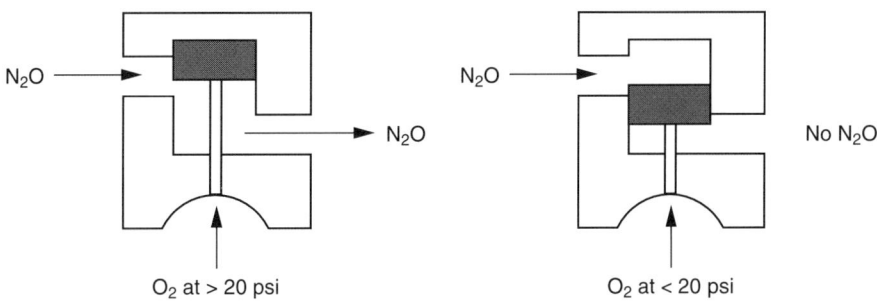

Figure 124–2.   Figure 124–3.

3. **Second-stage regulator:** maintains O_2 flowmeter output as long as at least ~12 psi is in the system.

> **NOTE:** Fail-safe device cuts off N_2O flow when O_2 pressure < 30 psi.

4. **Mechanical linking of N_2O and O_2 flowmeters:** On Ohmeda machines, both the N_2O and O_2 flowmeters have uniquely sized sprockets connected by a chain. The N_2O sprocket is larger. As the N_2O knob is turned up, it mechanically turns up the O_2 flowmeter, maintaining a 3:1 ratio. As the O_2 flowmeter is turned down, it pulls the N_2O knob along, but because the N_2O knob is bigger, it reaches its end point (off) sooner. Minimum allowed F_iO_2 is 25%.
5. **Pressure linking of the N_2O and O_2 flowmeters:** Drager flowmeters are linked with a valve similar to the fail-safe device. Back pressure from the O_2 flowmeter is exerted on a slave valve, forcing the piston into the open position to allow N_2O flow. Conversely, as N_2O flows are turned up, the N_2O flowmeter exerts back pressure on the slave valve, closing the flow channel.
6. **Physical arrangement of the flowmeters:** O_2 is always located downstream, closest to the patient (see Chapter 120, Flowmeters).

Anesthesia machine check

1. **For delivery of $F_iO_2 > .21$:** the O_2 analyzer is the only monitor downstream from flowmeters
2. **The positive pressure test:**
   A. Function: tests integrity of low-pressure circuit (from flowmeter to the patient), except in machines with check valves
   B. How: With the pop-off valve closed and the patient Y-connector occluded, flows are set at 5 L/min until the reservoir bag just fills. Flows are reduced until pressure gauge reads ≤ 20 cmH$_2$O. Squeezing the bag at this point will ↑ pressure to ~50 cmH$_2$O if the system is intact, but will ↓ pressure if there's a big leak.
   C. Disadvantages: won't detect small leaks; doesn't check integrity of flowmeters or vaporizers in machine with check valves
3. **The negative pressure test:**
   A. Function: tests integrity of flowmeters and vaporizers in machine with check valves.
   B. How: After connecting the machine to pipeline sources and opening flowmeters, create a no-flow state by turning off the machine and closing vaporizers. Attach a suction bulb to the common gas outlet and pump bulb until collapsed. If there is a leak in the flowmeters, the negative pressure of the bulb draws in room air and the bulb re-

fills. Repeat the test with each of the vaporizers turned on. Integrity of the circle system is still checked with positive pressure test.

Sample questions

A = 1, 2, 3   B = 1, 3   C = 2, 4   D = 4 only   E = all are correct

1. Standard low-pressure alarms on an anesthesia machine will detect
   1. A cracked nitrous oxide flowmeter
   2. "Swapped" connection of nitrous oxide and oxygen supply lines
   3. A poorly seated carbon dioxide absorber
   4. A leak in the oxygen supply line

2. A positive pressure test will detect a leak in the
   1. Circle system of a machine without check valves
   2. Circle system of a machine with check valves
   3. Flowmeters of a machine without check valves
   4. Flowmeters of a machine with check valves

3. During controlled ventilation, activating the oxygen flush valve
   1. During inspiration creates high pressures that cannot be vented
   2. Delivers pure oxygen to the patient
   3. During exhalation creates high pressures that can be vented out the scavenger spill valve
   4. Will temporarily disable the low oxygen supply pressure alarm

Answers: 1. D   2. A   3. A

CHAPTER 125

Mapleson Breathing Circuits

(All classified as semi-closed)

Factors affecting amount of rebreathing with Mapleson D and Bain circuits

1. Fresh gas flow rate (high flow = less rebreathing)
2. Respiratory rate (slow rate = more time to remove alveolar gas from circuit = less rebreathing)
3. Tidal volume (large tidal volume = more alveolar gas exhaled = more rebreathing)

Advantages of Bain circuit

Compact, portable, easy scavenging, exhaled gases warm the inhaled gases

Disadvantages of Bain circuit

Risk of disconnect or kinking of inner hose

How to detect a leak of the inner hose of a Bain circuit

Occlude the patient end of the circuit. Inflate reservoir with high flows. Release patient end. IF INTACT: high flow creates a Venturi effect, causing reservoir to deflate. IF NOT INTACT: no Venturi effect created, FGF enters exhalation limb and reservoir stays full.

See Table 125–1 on page 326.

Table 125-1.

Mapleson classification	A	B	C	D	Bain (modified "D")
What it looks like	(diagram: FGF, Pop-off, Patient)	(diagram: FGF, Pop-off, Patient)	(diagram: FGF, Pop-off, Patient)	(diagram: Pop-off, FGF, Patient)	(diagram: Pop-off, FGF, Patient)
Function during spontaneous ventilation	DG meets FGF in corrugated tube, AG is forced out pop-off. Next breath is DG and FGF mixture. High FGF ↑'s venting of DG	FGF mixes with DG and AG. All 3 gases are vented. Next breath is FGF and a small fraction AG	Function is same as Mapleson B, but inspired gas has a higher fraction of AG due to short reservoir tubing	Preferentially vents DG and AG, because FGF pushes it down tube and away from patient. Next breath is mostly FGF, small amount of DG and AG	Same as Mapleson D
Flow for no rebreathing (spontaneous)	= MV	> 2 × MV	> 2 × MV	> 2 × MV	Same as Mapleson D
Function during controlled ventilation	Tightened pop-off allows positive pressure ventilation. AG is rebreathed before pressure causes venting.	Functions the same as during spontaneous ventilation	Functions the same as during spontaneous ventilation	Positive pressure forces DG and AG out, so minimal rebreathing occurs	Same as Mapleson D
Flow for no rebreathing (controlled)	> 20 L / min	> 2 × MV	> 2 × MV	Kids: ~ 300 mL/kg/min Adults: ~ 70 mL/kg/min	Same as Mapleson D
Efficiency of function	Best circuit for spontaneous ventilation, worst circuit for controlled ventilation	Worst circuit for spontaneous ventilation		Best circuit for controlled ventilation	

Note: for Mapleson D and Bain circuits, flows for maintaining normocarbia with spontaneous ventilation are less than flows to prevent rebreathing.
Flowrates: 100 mL/kg/min for adults, 200 mL/kg/min for kids
For brevity: DG = deadspace gas, AG = alveolar gas, FGF = fresh gas flow, MV = minute ventilation

Sample questions

A = 1, 2, 3   B = 1, 3   C = 2, 4   D = 4 only   E = all are correct

1. The proper use of the breathing circuit shown

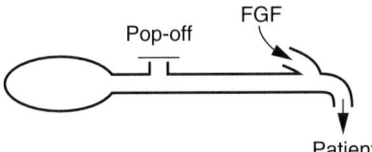

Figure 125–1.

   1. Requires flows two times larger than the exhaled minute ventilation to prevent rebreathing during spontaneous ventilation
   2. Requires flows two times larger than the exhaled minute volume to maintain normocarbia during spontaneous ventilation
   3. Requires flows less than twice the exhaled minute ventilation to maintain normocarbia during spontaneous ventilation
   4. Is the most efficient circuit for spontaneous ventilation

2. Characteristics of the Bain circuit include
   1. More efficient function in children than adults
   2. Preferentially forces fresh gas through pop-off valve
   3. Fresh gas flows equal to minute ventilation prevent rebreathing during spontaneous ventilation
   4. Partial rebreathing of alveolar gas

Single best answer

2. A 20-kg child is spontaneously breathing sevoflurane, nitrous oxide, and oxygen through a Bain circuit with a fresh gas flow of 3000 mL/min and a respiratory rate of 15/min. Arterial blood gases reveal a $PaCO_2$ of 60 mmHg and PaO_2 of 75 mmHg. All of the following are false **except**
   1. Fresh gas flow should be at least doubled
   2. There is a left-to-right shunt at the atrial level
   3. This flow rate would not prevent rebreathing in a Mapleson A circuit
   4. A Mapleson D at this flowrate would not demonstrate rebreathing
   5. The patient is exhibiting early signs of malignant hyperthermia

Answers: 1. B   2. D   3. 1

References

1. Bain JA, Spoerel WE. A streamlined anesthetic system. Can Anaesth Soc J 19: 426–435, 1972.
2. Mapleson WW. The elimination of rebreathing in various semiclosed anaesthetic systems. Br J Anaesth 26: 323–332, 1954.
3. Willis BA, Pender JW, Mapleson WW. Rebreathing in a T-piece: volunteer and theoretical studies of the Jackson-Rees modification of Ayre's T-piece during spontaneous respiration. Br J Anaesth 47: 1239–1246, 1975.

Chapter 126

The Circle System

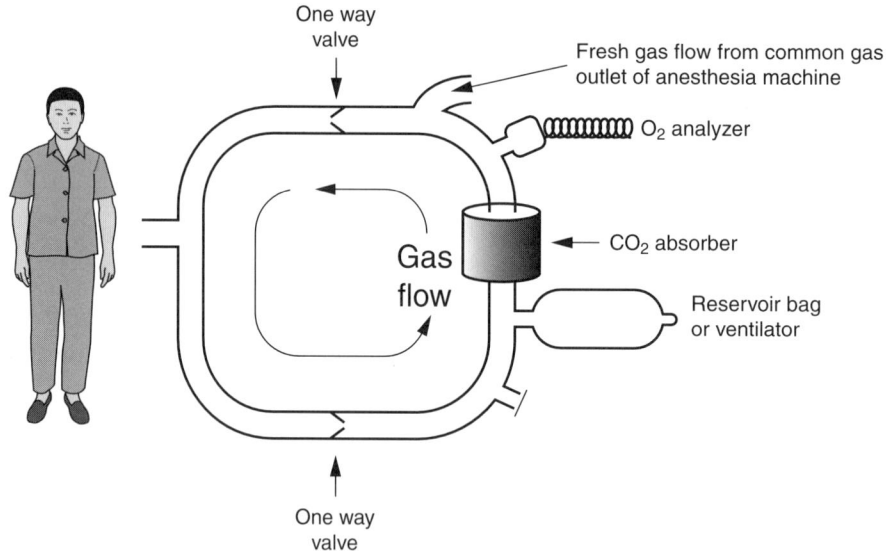

Figure 126–1.

> **NOTE:** The only deadspace in the circle system is at the "Y"

Advantages to this location of the CO_2 absorber

1. Upstream form gas inlet, so no dust enters circuit.
2. Positive pressure easily overcomes resistance created by absorber.
3. "Back-filling" during exhalation creates large reservoir of fresh gas for next breath.
4. Avoids creating PEEP, which can happen when located on expiratory limb.

Alternate locations of the O_2 analyzer and their disadvantages

1. **At the patient "Y":** gives accurate F_iO_2, but increases deadspace.
2. **On expiratory limb:** will read falsely low if running low fresh gas flows.

Alternate locations for the fresh gas inlet and their disadvantages

1. **Patient side of the inspiratory valve:** allows continuous flow, wastes gas, and causes inaccurate measurement of exhaled volume.
2. **Patient side of the expiratory valve:** washes alveolar gas from expiratory limb into lungs (rebreathing), blows dust from CO_2 absorber into lungs, and being upstream from pop-off valve allows loss of delivered tidal volume during positive pressure ventilation.

Alternate locations of the one-way valves

At patient "Y": absorbent life is prolonged, because expansion of corrugated tubing during positive pressure ventilation will dilute CO_2.

Malfunction of the one-way valves

Rebreathing occurs with both incompetent inspiratory and expiratory valves.

Example of the capnographs

Notice that shape looks normal, but it never returns to zero.

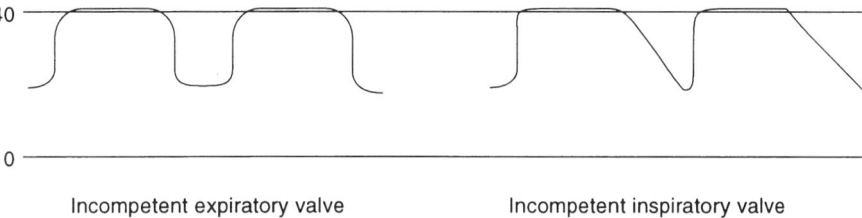

Incompetent expiratory valve   Incompetent inspiratory valve

Figure 126–2.

Incompetent inspiratory valve

More slurred in inspiration. Also, although Figure 126–2 doesn't depict it, the inspiratory phase returns closer to baseline than with expiratory valve malfunction.

Alternate locations of the pop-off valve and the disadvantages

1. **Inspiratory limb between patient and one-way valve:** allows escape of fresh gas during positive pressure ventilation; allows alveolar gas to enter inspiratory limb during exhalation, creating rebreathing.
2. **Expiratory limb between patient and one-way valve:** releases tidal volume delivered under positive pressure.

Alternate locations of the reservoir bag and the disadvantages

Between patient and either of the one-way valves: create a reservoir of exhaled gas, causes rebreathing.

Function of oxygen analyzer in the circuit

1. It's the *only* monitor of low-pressure system integrity downstream from flowmeters.
2. Consumes oxygen molecules . . . may be important during closed-circuit anesthesia.

3. Three basic types of analyzers:
   A. Polarographic ⎱ Require O_2 diffusion across a permeable membrane,
   B. Galvanic cell ⎰ then reduce (consume) O_2 during measurement
   C. Paramagnetic: no diffusion needed, analysis is based on response of a reference gas and the sample gas to a rapidly changing magnetic field

Sample questions

A = 1, 2, 3   B = 1, 3   C = 2, 4   D = 4 only   E = all are correct

1. In a patient spontaneously breathing through a circle system, inspired PCO_2 will be increased by
   1. Incompetent one-way valve on the inhalation limb
   2. Pop-off valve located on inhalation limb between patient and one-way valve
   3. Incompetent one-way valve on the exhalation limb
   4. Morphine 0.2 mg/kg

2. Deadspace in a circle system is contained in the
   1. Expiratory limb
   2. Carbon dioxide absorber
   3. Expiratory unidirectional valve
   4. Y-connector

3. The pop-off valve is
   1. Most efficient during spontaneous breathing when placed at the Y-connector
   2. Dependent on back pressure to function correctly
   3. Most efficient during controlled ventilation when placed on the expiratory limb between the patient and the CO_2 absorber
   4. Will vent excess gas when it reaches the pressure set on the peak inspiratory pressure limit knob on the anesthesia machine

4. During spontaneous ventilation with a circle system, rebreathing of carbon dioxide will occur with
   1. Incorrect adjustment of the pop-off valve
   2. Large tidal volumes
   3. Low fresh gas flow
   4. An incompetent expiratory valve

Answers: 1. A   2. D   3. B   4. E

CHAPTER 127

Closed-Circuit Anesthesia

Definition: In a circle system, the use of fresh gas flows that exactly equal uptake of oxygen and anesthetic agents, resulting in no venting of gas through the pop-off valve

Equipment

1. Flowmeter: accurate down to 100 mL/min
2. Gas monitors:
   A. Oxygen analyzer
   B. Anesthetic agent analyzer: sidestream analyzers aspirate gas from the system, so volume is maintained by returning sample to circuit or by increasing fresh gas flow
3. Bellows that ascends during exhalation
   A. Allows early detection of leaks, but note that excess negative pressure from scavenger gives false appearance of "full" bellows.
   B. Descending bellows will fill despite a leak due to gravtiy and will entrain air or driving gas, diluting anesthetic concentration.
4. Leak-free system (no uncuffed endotracheal tubes . . .)

Induction using low flows is slow because

1. Nitrogen washout into the breathing circuit dilutes concentration of anesthetic agent.
2. Anesthetic washin is slow (effect on induction speed is greater with soluble agents than insoluble).

Advantages to closed-circuit anesthesia

1. Less pollution
2. Uses less gas/agent
4. Conserves heat/humidity
3. Conserves absorbent

Beware that some pretty noxious things can accumulate in the closed circuit

1. Carbon dioxide (especially if absorber is exhausted or one-way valves malfunction)
2. Carbon monoxide (due to breakdown of hemoglobin)
3. Nitrogen

4. Hydrogen
5. Methane
6. Acetone
7. And for drunks: ethanol will accumulate, because it's eliminated by lungs

Sample questions

A = 1, 2, 3   B = 1, 3   C = 2, 4   D = 4 only   E = all are correct

1. Causes of an ascending bellows exceeding previous exhaled volumes include
   1. Decreased oxygen consumption
   2. Negative pressure transmitted from the scavenger system
   3. Fresh gas flows too high
   4. High concentration set on the vaporizer

Single best answer

2. Causes of an ascending bellows not returning to previously achieved volumes include all EXCEPT:
   1. Gas sampling using a sidestream gas analyzer
   2. Use of a polarographic oxygen analyzer
   3. Hyperthermia
   4. Increased uptake of nitrous oxide
   5. Use of a scavenger with a passive gas removal assembly

Answers: 1. A   2. 5

CHAPTER 128

CO_2 Absorbers

Two principal absorbants used

1. Soda lime
2. Baralyme

- **Table 128–1**

	Soda Lime	Baralyme
Contents	Calcium hydroxide (~80%) Water Sodium hydroxide (catalyst) Potassium hydroxide (activator)	Calcium hydroxide (~80%) Water Barium hydroxide (catalyst)
Additives	Silica	No silica
pH indicator	Ethyl violet (fluorescent light can deactivate)	Ethyl violet (fluorescent light can deactivate)
Color change	White → blue/purple	Pink → blue/gray
End-products or reaction	Water Heat Calcium carbonate Sodium carbonate Potassium carbonate Sodium hydroxide Potassium hydroxide	Water Heat Calcium carbonate Barium carbonate

Factors that increase absorption

1. Large surface area (small granules increase surface area, but also increase resistance to flow)
2. Soft granules (softness predisposes to dust formation, though)

Factors that decrease absorption

1. Channeling (because of resistive forces, gas flows past same granules repeatedly, decreasing the effective surface area)
2. Hard granules (silica confers hardness, but decreases dust formation)

Incompatibilities of soda lime

When used in the presence of the anesthetic agent trichloroethylene, it makes:

1. Carbon monoxide
2. Phosgene (a pulmonary toxin)
3. Dichloroacetylene (a neurotoxin)

Sample questions

Single best answer

1. Which of the following is NOT an end product of the reaction of carbon dioxide with soda lime?
    1. Calcium carbonate
    2. Sodium hydroxide
    3. Calcium hydroxide
    4. Potassium hydroxide
    5. Sodium carbonate

2. All of the following statements regarding soda lime are true EXCEPT
    1. Maximum absorbence is 26 L of carbon dioxide gas per 100 g of soda lime
    2. The silica additive reduces the effective absorbence
    3. The granules change to a purplish color when their pH drops below 10.3
    4. The granules change color when the critical temperature is reached
    5. While unstable in sevoflurane, there are no toxic by-products

Answers: 1. 3   2. 4

Chapter 129

Scavenging Systems

I know you hate them, but you gotta know them! Remember: the scavenging system is in continuity with the patient breathing system, so badness in the scavenger can cause harm to your patient and your wallet.

The system has five parts

1. **Gas collecting assembly:** receives excess gas vented from:
   A. Pop-off valve
   B. Ventilator relief valve
2. **Transfer tubing:** worst place to have an occlusion, because there's nowhere to vent excess pressure
3. **Scavenging interface:**
   A. Protects the breathing circuit from excess positive and negative pressure via relief valves or holes
   B. Designated as open (has holes that are open to atmosphere) or closed (has valves)
   C. ALL interfaces must have positive pressure reliefs, regardless of the type of disposal system
   D. Interfaces with active disposal systems also require a negative pressure relief
4. **Gas disposal tubing**
5. **Disposal assembly** (2 types)
   A. Active disposal
      1. Gas is removed by vacuum
      2. Can create excess negative pressure in the breathing circuit
      3. Dictates the need for a negative pressure relief
   B. Passive disposal: gas is removed by bulk flow

Summary of scavenger interface characteristics

- Table 129–1

Interface Type	Disposal	Pressure Reliefs Needed	Valves Present?
Open	Active	+ and −	No
Closed	Active	+ and −	Yes
Closed	Passive	+	Yes

Fine points about OPEN interfaces

1. Require no valves because the holes allow equilibration of pressures with the atmosphere.
2. MUST be used with an active disposal (to prevent spillage of waste gas).
3. Should have a reservoir to store waste gas in until it can be eliminated.
4. Efficiency depends on:
   A. Vacuum flowrate ≥ minute volume of waste gas (or else spillage occurs)
   B. Reservoir > volume of a single breath (or else spillage)
   C. Low turbulence (or else spillage)

Hazards of scavenging systems

1. Transmission of excess positive pressure to patient breathing circuit
   A. Usually due to obstruction (kinks, running over hoses with machine, misconnections)
   B. Worst place for obstruction is upstream from interface (nowhere to vent waste gas)
2. Transmission of excess negative pressure to patient breathing circuit
   A. Only seen when active disposal system in use
   B. Caused by obstruction of the negative pressure relief or by vacuum rate too high
   C. Results in patient circuit collapse (by sucking all the gas from the circuit) or excess positive pressure (pulls the pop-off valve closed and they can't vent exhaled gas)

Sample questions

Single best answer

1. Following induction of general anesthesia with endotracheal intubation and spontaneous ventilation on F_iO_2 0.3 and no PEEP, a patient has a tidal volume = 800 cc, rate = 14. After you place the patient in Tredelenburg, the manometer on the ventilator shows a continuous pressure of 20 cmH$_2$O, exhaled tidal volume = 200 cc, respiratory rate = 20. Breath sounds are equal bilaterally with a shortened inspiratory phase. The most likely reason for this is
   1. Endobronchial intubation
   2. The manometer is not calibrated correctly
   3. Pulmonary embolus
   4. A mucus plug in the endotracheal tube
   5. There is an obstruction between the patient and the scavenging interface

A = 1, 2, 3   B = 1, 3   C = 2, 4   D = 4 only   E = all are correct

2. The effectiveness of a closed scavenging interface with an active disposal system depends on
   1. The in-flow rate of waste gas
   2. The volume of the reservoir
   3. The vacuum flowrate
   4. The absence of turbulent flow

Answers: 1. 5   2. A

Chapter 130

Anesthesia Ventilators

Mode of ventilation: Volume preset, controlled ventilation

Termination of inhalation is

1. Time-cycled (preset time in which to deliver VT)
2. And might also be pressure limited (if peak inspiratory pressure exceeds a predetermined limit, the remainder of VT is "dumped" to atmosphere)

Determinants of inspiratory time

1. Set tidal volume
2. Inspiratory flow rate
3. Respiratory rate

Bellows classification

Determined by the direction of movement during exhalation

1. Descending type: rarely used because it delays detection of leaks. Driving gas continues to push bellows up during inspiration, and gravity allows descent during which entrainment of driving gas or room air occurs
2. Ascending type: most common because lack of ascent allows early leak detection

Function of generic ventilator with ascending bellows

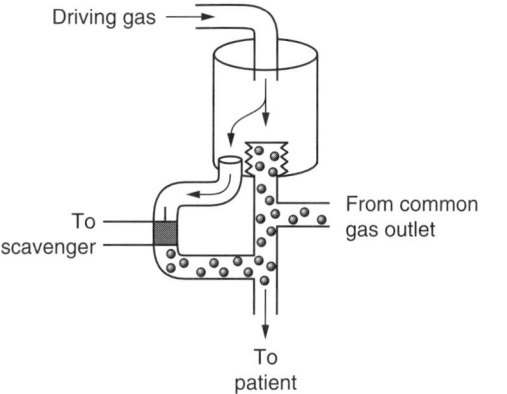

Figure 130–1.

Inhalation, during which the driving gas
1. Forces bellows to deliver contained V_T to patient
2. Closes the scavenger system spill valve, preventing loss of V_T

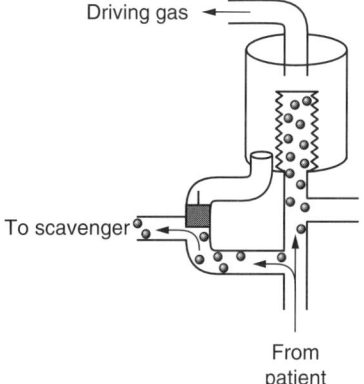

Figure 130–2.

Exhalation, during which the driving gas
1. Exits the bellows housing, allowing:
   A. Filling of the bellows with fresh gas and exhaled gas
   B. Opening of the scavenger spill valve

Common malfunctions of anesthesia ventilators

1. Leaks/disconnects
2. Hole in the bellows
3. No-flow states
4. Excessive positive pressure
5. Excessive negative pressure

Potential sources of leaks/disconnects

Focusing on areas distal to common gas outlet

1. Any and all connection sites (patient Y-connector *most common* site for disconnect)
2. Loose or cracked bellows housing
3. Incompetent scavenger system spill valve
4. Incompetent pop-off valve

Detection of leaks/disconnects

1. $ETCO_2$ **most sensitive** monitor besides human observation
2. Adjustable pressure threshold monitor: should set it to alarm at pressure more than 5 cmH_2O below peak inspiratory pressures. Setting the limit too low may not detect a partial disconnect
3. Respiratory volume monitor: measures exhaled minute volume or VT; set high and low values just above and just below the measured volume

Effects of a hole in the bellows

1. Hyperventilation/barotrauma due to delivery of high pressure driving gas
2. Altered F_iO_2: can ↑ or ↓, depending on the composition of the driving gas
3. Failure of ascending bellows to refill completely
4. Entrainment of room air or driving gas if bellows is descending type

Causes of no-flow states

1. Complete disconnect ⎫
2. Misconnection of ventilator hose to nongas source ⎬ Low pressure alarm will sound
3. Kink/obstruction of endotracheal tube/corrugated tubing ⎫
4. Insertion of ball-type PEEP valve in inspiratory limb ⎬ High pressure alarm will sound

Causes of excessive positive pressure

1. Oxygen flush during inhalation (because scavenger spill valve is closed)
2. Obstructed scavenger system: spill valve stuck closed or kinked hose proximal to reservoir
3. Ventilator stuck in inspiratory mode
4. Hole in bellows (driving gas is under high pressure)

Causes of excessive negative pressure pressure

1. Excessive suction on scavenger assembly
2. Rapid descent of hanging bellows (exacerbated with low flows)

Sample questions

A = 1, 2, 3   B = 1, 3   C = 2, 4   D = 4 only   E = all are correct

1. On a standard anesthesia machine, if the ventilator fails during exhalation after the bellows is filled:
   1. The patient will receive a higher-than-expected oxygen concentration with the next breath
   2. The low threshold pressure alarm will sound
   3. The respiratory volume monitor will only measure that volume due to continuous flowmeter function
   4. The apnea alarm will sound

2. Excessive suction through the scavenger assembly can cause
   1. A higher F_iO_2 than expected if driving gas is pure oxygen
   2. Excessive positive pressure in the patient circuit
   3. A reduction in $PaCO_2$
   4. Excessive negative pressure in the patient circuit

3. Failure of the low-pressure alarm to detect a leak can occur if
   1. There is constant end-expiratory pressure
   2. An uncuffed endotracheal tube is used
   3. A leak occurs in the flowmeters
   4. The alarm set point is higher than the peak inspiratory pressure

4. During pressure-limited ventilation with 3 L/min N_2O and 2 L/min O_2 and a rate of 30/min, the connection at the patient Y-connector loosens, but does not completely disconnect. This should cause
   1. Decreased inspiratory time
   2. Decreased breath sounds
   3. Decreased tidal volume
   4. Decreased peak inspiratory pressures

Answers: 1. D   2. C (choice 2 is right because suction can draw the spill valve closed, blocking exit of gas from circuit)   3. B   4. B

Chapter 131

Mechanical Ventilation

Two basic modes of positive pressure ventilation

1. Volume ventilation: most common for adults
2. Pressure control ventilation: usually neonates

General features of volume ventilation

Clinician sets:

1. Tidal volume to be delivered (V_T)
2. Rate
3. Inspiratory time

Independent variables

1. Actual tidal volume received:
   A. If the circuit is compliant, part of V_T is compressed in circuit and never delivered to patient
   B. If lung compliance is ↓, pressure limit may be reached before all V_T is delivered
2. Peak inspiratory pressure (PIP):
   A. If lung compliance ↓ or airway resistance ↑, the peak inspiratory pressure will go as high as necessary to deliver the preset V_T (risk of barotrauma)
   B. Barotrauma is prevented by:
      1. Setting a pressure limit for the PIP, beyond which any remaining volume is "dumped"
      2. Lengthening the inspiratory time to allow slower delivery of V_T, creating less pressure in airway

Modes of volume ventilation and their features

1. **Control:** ventilator cycles at fixed intervals; no flow is available for spontaneous ventilation
2. **Assist/control:** low backup rate delivers control mode ventilation. Patient can also trigger additional positive pressure breaths by creating negative pressure in circuit
3. **IMV:** controls mode ventilation with the addition of *continuous* gas flow for spontaneous ventilation
4. **SIMV:** assists/controls ventilation with the addition of gas flow *available on demand* for spontaneous ventilation. Patient gets a breath in 1 of 3

ways: (1) spontaneous breath; (2) triggers a mechanical breath; (3) control breath (trigger not needed)

Modes of pressure ventilation and their features

1. **Pressure control:** Clinician sets:
   A. Fixed peak inspiratory pressure
   B. Rate
   C. Inspiratory time (inverse I:E ratio easy to achieve)

   Independent variables: Tidal volume, which is a function of:
   A. Flowrate and I_{time} (VT = mL/sec ÷ inspiratory time)
   B. System compliance (↑ circuit compliance = loss of V_T to circuit, ↓ lung compliance = less volume delivered per unit of pressure)
2. **Pressure support:**
   A. Clinician sets: peak inspiratory pressure
   B. Operation: patient respiratory effort opens a demand valve, allowing delivery of high flow of gas until the preselected pressure is met. As patient effort begins to decline, flow shuts off.

You may ask "How does this differ from SIMV?

1. Low driving pressure (as pressure increases, looks more and more like SIMV)
2. VT determined by how long patient draws in gas

Cardiopulmonary effects of all modes of positive pressure ventilation

1. Hypotension:
   A. ↓ venous return → ↓ cardiac output . . . responds to intravascular volume expansion
   B. Also, catecholamine levels that are high during stress of hypoxia or hypercarbia will recede, followed by hypotension
2. Increased deadspace ventilation (↑ V/Q ratio): distribution of pulmonary blood flow is always gravity dependent, but distribution of ventilation depends on lung compliance and resistance of airways, both of which are more "mechanical ventilation friendly" in the nondependent (less perfused) lung regions

NOTE: V_T during spontaneous ventilation is 6–7 mL/kg, V_T during mechanical ventilation is 10–15 mL/kg to offset effect of ↑ V_D.

What is the difference between PEEP and CPAP?

1. PEEP: refers to continuous positive airway pressure applied during mechanical ventilation
2. CPAP: refers to continuous positive airway pressure applied during spontaneous ventilation

What's the benefit of adding PEEP or CPAP?

1. Increased FRC: by increasing alveolar size (volume), we improve V/Q matching. Before PEEP, alveoli are collapsed and V/Q approaches zero (huge shunt). With PEEP, alveoli are open and V/Q approaches one (no shunt, no deadspace).
2. Reduce pulmonary edema: gravity forces interstitial lung water to migrate away from hilum and away from lymphatic system. By distending

alveoli, PEEP/CPAP limit the space available for lung water, forcing it to move toward hilum.
3. Decreased left ventricular afterload (**Huh?!?**) Theoretically, of course. Afterload is, among other things, a result of the transmural pressure of the aorta. If extravascular pressure is increased with PEEP, the net result is a reduction in transmural pressure and a reduction in afterload. HOWEVER, the reduction in venous return probably outweighs this effect.

What are the detrimental effects of CPAP/PEEP?

1. Increased deadspace ventilation ($\uparrow$ V/Q ratio). $\uparrow P_A \rightarrow$ compression of pulmonary arterioles/venules $\rightarrow$ reduced pulmonary blood flow $\rightarrow \uparrow V_D$. This effect is compounded by:
   A. Positive pressure ventilation
   B. Nonhomogenous lung pathology (nondiseased alveoli get overdistended, additive to the deadspace already present in diseased alveoli)
2. Decreased cardiac output
   1. $\downarrow$ venous return $\rightarrow \downarrow$ stroke volume $\rightarrow \downarrow$ cardiac output
   2. $\uparrow$ pulmonary vascular resistance $\rightarrow \downarrow$ RV ejection fraction $\rightarrow \uparrow$ RV end-diastolic volume $\rightarrow$ interventricular septum shifts, encroaching on LV $\rightarrow \downarrow$ LV filling $\rightarrow \downarrow$ cardiac output
3. Barotrauma: "pneumo-anything"
4. Decreased renal blood flow, GFR, and UOP

High-frequency jet ventilation (an alternate mode of ventilation)

How it works: a jet cannula is inserted in the endotracheal tube lumen. Gas is pulsed under high pressure (<50 psi) at rapid rates (60–300/min). Venturi effect at the distal end of the cannula entrains gases from ETT. Distribution of ventilation depends on *resistance of airways,* not compliance of lungs. Is more at efficient oxygenation than CO_2 removal.

Sample questions

A = 1, 2, 3   B = 1, 3   C = 2, 4   D = 4 only   E = all are correct

1. Positive end-expiratory pressure
   1. Increases right ventricular afterload
   2. Decreases left ventricular afterload
   3. Decreases the ratio of pulmonary shunt to cardiac output
   4. Reduces the arterial to alveolar carbon dioxide gradient

2. In a patient with a minute ventilation of 5 L/min, the ratio of deadspace ventilation to tidal volume increases with
   1. Administration of IM atropine
   2. Mechanical ventilation
   3. Application of positive end-expiratory pressure
   4. A change in respiratory rate from 10/min to 20/min, holding minute ventilation constant

3. During controlled, volume-preset mechanical ventilation, peak inspiratory pressure will increase with
   1. Pulmonary edema
   2. Shortening the inspiratory time
   3. Secretions in the endotracheal tube
   4. Administration of neostigmine

4. During pressure support ventilation, a reduction of the inspiratory pressure
   1. Increases work of breathing
   2. Reduces tidal volume
   3. Reduces mean airway pressure
   4. Reduces the rate of gas flow to the patient

5. An 80-kg patient with a large left-sided pleural effusion is mechanically ventilated with a tidal volume of 700 mL, rate of 10/min and 5 cmH$_2$O positive end expiratory pressure. Iatrogenic causes of a low PaO$_2$ include
   1. Sodium nitroprusside infusion
   2. Inadequate tidal volume
   3. Nitroglycerin infusion
   4. Positive end-expiratory pressure

Answers: 1. A 2. E 3. E 4. B 5. E

Perioperative Hypoxia

Causes of intraoperative hypoxia

1. V/Q mismatch: see Chapter 6, Pulmonary Physiology
2. Hypoventilation: drug effect if spontaneous ventilation, inadequate V_T if mechanical ventilation, secretions, bronchospasm, mainstem, or esophageal intubation
3. Inadequate F_iO_2: wrong supply gas, disconnection, hole in bellows or flowmeter
4. Impaired diffusion: pulmonary edema, pulmonary fibrosis
5. Right-to-left shunt
6. Aspiration
7. Pneumothorax
8. $\downarrow O_2$ carrying capacity

Causes of early postoperative hypoxia

1. Diffusion hypoxia: N_2O rapidly exits blood and enters alveolus, displacing O_2 and causing hypoxia. More likely to occur if patient is breathing room air.
2. Hypoventilation: residual volatile agent or neuromuscular blockade, narcotic effect, "splinting"
3. V/Q mismatch
4. $\uparrow O_2$ consumption as the patient rewarms or shivers
5. Hypercarbia: similar to nitrous effect . . . CO_2 displaces O_2 from alveolus

Signs of perioperative hypoxia

1. Tachycardia (progresses to bradycardia)
2. Hypertension (progresses to hypotension)
3. Dark blood in the surgical field
4. Decreased pulse oximeter reading
5. Agitation in the awake patient
6. Cyanosis

Causes of postoperative respiratory distress

1. Inadequate reversal of neuromuscular blockade (or "recurarization" after antibiotics)
2. Laryngospasm, bronchospasm
3. Decreased O_2-carrying capacity
4. Vocal cord dysfunction: nerve palsy or mechanical trauma to cords
5. Airway edema or hematoma

Sample questions

Single best answer

1. Following a general anesthetic, a patient with a history of angina is combative upon arrival to the recovery room. Pulse 130/min, blood pressure 160/98 mmHg, hemoglobin 9.3 gm/dL and there is 2-mm ST segment depression on the EKG. The most appropriate first therapy is
   1. Administer fentanyl
   2. Initiate nitroglycerin infusion
   3. Administer labetolol
   4. Administer oxygen F_iO_2 0.4 by face mask
   5. Transfuse with two units packed red blood cells

   A = 1, 2, 3   B = 1, 3   C = 2, 4   D = 4 only   E = all are correct

2. After open cholecystectomy, a 70-kg patient receives 4 mg neostigmine and 1 mg atropine following train of four with one twitch, is extubated from N_2O/O_2 70/30%, and sent to recovery. Arterial blood gases on face mask 0.3 F_iO_2 are pH 7.30, $PaCO_2$ 49 torr, PaO_2 79 torr. Possible causes of hypoxia include
   1. Right lower lobe atelectasis
   2. Diffusion of nitrous oxide into alveoli
   3. Incomplete reversal of neuromuscular blockade
   4. Hypercarbia

Answers: 1. 4   2. E

CHAPTER 133

Intraoperative Hypercarbia and Hypocarbia

Causes of hypercarbia

1. Increased CO_2 production: fever, malignant hyperthermia, thyroid storm
2. Decreased CO_2 removal: hypoventilation, impaired diffusion and rebreathing 2° to exhausted CO_2 absorber, incompetent valves or increased deadspace
3. Exogenous CO_2: gas supply error, administration of HCO_3^- or carbonic anhydrase inhibitor, insufflation of abdomen with CO_2

Physiologic effects of hypercarbia

1. Tachycardia
2. Hypertension
3. Catecholamine release: dysrythmias
4. Direct depression of myocardium and vascular smooth muscle tone: ↓ contractility and SVR
5. Pulmonary vasoconstriction
6. Hypoxia (an alveolus full of CO_2 has no room for O_2)
7. Shift of oxyhemoglobin curve to right (improved delivery to tissues . . . helps offset the hypoxia)
8. Cerebral vasodilation: ↑ CBF and ICP, increased frequency on EEG
9. Hyperkalemia: due to shifting of hydrogen ions into cells in response to acidosis . . . may increase dysrthymias

Causes of hypocarbia

1. ↑ removal: hyperventilation is most common cause
2. ↓ production: hypothermia and reduced metabolic rate

Physiologic effects of hypocarbia

1. ↓ cardiac output: decreased contractility of myocardium due to ↑ pH → ↓ ionized calcium as well as reduced sympathetic stimulation of myocardium
2. Shift oxyhemoglobin curve to left: impairs tissue oxygenation
3. ↑ O_2 consumption: hypercarbia uncouples oxidative phosphorylation
4. Inhibition of hypoxic pulmonary vasoconstriction: may worsen V/Q mismatch
5. Bronchospasm

6. ↑ excretion of HCO_3^-: depletes body stores of CO_2, predisposing to apnea
7. Cerebral vasoconstriction: ↓ CBF and ICP, slowing of EEG
8. Hypokalemia: due to shifting of hydrogen ions out of cells in response to alkalosis

Sample question
Single best answer

1. A 6-year-old, 25-kg child is undergoing inguinal hernia repair under general anesthesia and spontaneous ventilation with N_2O 2 L/min, O_2 1 L/min, and halothane 1.2% expired. As the surgeon infiltrates the surgical site with 8 mL 0.25% bupivicaine with epinephrine 1:200,000, the EKG converts to bigeminy. Initial treatment should be
   1. Decrease the halothane concentration
   2. Increase the fresh gas flows
   3. Initiate positive pressure ventilation at a rate of 25/min
   4. Reduce the bupivicaine concentration
   5. Reduce the epinephrine concentration

Answer: 1. 3

CHAPTER 134

Pulse Oximetry

Purpose: Provides a noninvasive, continuous means of assessing arterial oxygen saturation

Design

Two light-emitting diodes with different wavelengths (660 nm and 940 nm) and a photoreceptor

How does it work?

There are two species of hemoglobin in normal blood: deoxygenated (Hb) and oxygenated (O_2Hb). Deoxygenated hemoglobin preferentially (but not exclusively) absorbs light at 660 nm, while oxygenated hemoglobin preferentially absorbs light at 940 nm. Both wavelengths are transmitted through a vascular bed, and the percentages of O_2Hb and Hb are calculated from the ratio of light "received" by the photoreceptor. The result is displayed as the SaO_2.

How does the machine differentiate absorption by arterial hemoglobin from absorption by all other tissues?

Arterial pulsations change the length of the light path, thereby altering the amount of light absorbed (the Lambert-Beer law). By emitting rapid pulsations of light, the photoreceptor can detect differences in the amount of light absorbed during arterial pulsations versus that absorbed by venous blood and tissue. It then only considers the light absorbed during arterial pulsations when calculating the saturation.

Factors producing spurious readings

● Table 134–1

Falsely High Readings	Falsely Low Readings	Suspected of Interference
Ambient light Carboxyhemoglobin Methemoglobin Anemia	Diminished pulsatile flow (hypothermia, hypoperfusion, vasoactive drugs) Movement Tissue thickness Pigments (methylene blue, indigo carmine, indocyanine green, nail polish, melanin)	(effect unknown) Sulfhemoglobin Cyanomethemoglobin

> **CAVEAT:** Carboxyhemoglobin will always produce a falsely high saturation because it absorbs light at ~940 nm, the same as oxyhemoglobin. However, methemoglobin has greater absorption than both oxyhemoglobin and deoxyhemoglobin at 940 nm, and absorption equal to deoxyhemoglobin at 660 nm. Therefore, at a saturation > 85%, the pulse oximeter underestimates the true value; at saturations < 85%, it overestimates the true value.

Factors not affecting accuracy

1. Fetal hemoglobin
2. Sickle hemoglobin
3. Polycythemia

Sample question

A = 1, 2, 3   B = 1, 3   C = 2, 4   D = 4 only   E = all are correct

1. A 24-year-old male is undergoing an exploratory laparotomy and partial hepatectomy following a motor vehicle accident. General anesthesia is maintained with oxygen, isoflurane, and vecuronium. His vital signs are: blood pressure 100/65 mmHg, temperature 34.7° C, Hb 8.6 gm/dL. His oxygen saturation is 80% by pulse oximetry, but is 98% by blood gas analysis. Possible explanations for this discrepancy include
   1. Hypothermia
   2. Anemia
   3. Hypoperfusion
   4. Interference by ambient light

Answer: 1. B

Chapter 135

Capnography

Function: Provides a continuous visual display of exhaled CO_2 waveform

Provides information regarding

1. Adequacy of ventilation
2. Presence of airway obstruction (based on waveform characteristics)
3. Adequacy of perfusion (low perfusion = low delivery of CO_2 to alveoli)
4. Equipment malfunction (based on waveform characteristics)
5. Positioning of double-lumen tubes (attach separate capnometer to each lumen; if correctly positioned, each lung will exhibit a normal wave)

Accuracy of ETCO$_2$ relies on the assumptions

1. All CO_2 is a product of tissue metabolism, AND:
2. $PaCO_2$ is 5–10 mmHg $> P_ACO_2 \approx ETCO_2$

The typical capnogram has four phases

Phase 1: Gas exhaled from anatomic dead space, devoid of CO_2
Phase 2: CO_2-rich alveolar gas mixes with deadspace gas, creating sharp increase in exhaled CO_2 concentration
Phase 3: After initial sharp rise, steady concentration of CO_2 is exhaled from all lung regions, creating the "alveolar plateau"
Phase 4: The true "end-tidal" CO_2, measured at the very end of exhalation

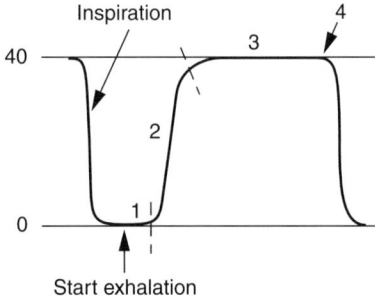

Figure 135–1.

Abnormal waveforms you might see and their differential diagnoses

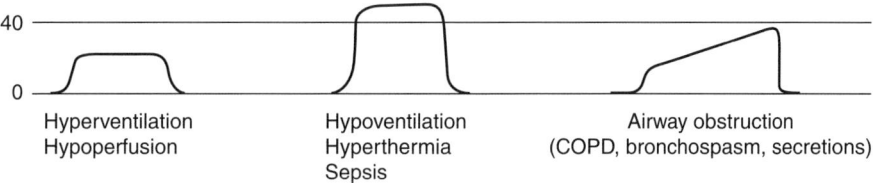

Hyperventilation
Hypoperfusion

Hypoventilation
Hyperthermia
Sepsis

Airway obstruction
(COPD, bronchospasm, secretions)

Figure 135–2.

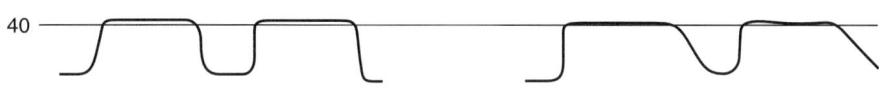

Rebreathing (normal ETCO$_2$, but doesn't return to baseline). Causes include:
Incompetent expiratory valve
Incompetent inspiratory valve
Exhausted CO$_2$ absorbant
Inadequate Mapleson fresh gas flows

Rebreathing (a variant)
This is another way an incompetent inspiratory valve can present. Presence of CO$_2$ in inspired gases prevents the usual sharp drop in CO$_2$ seen during inhalation.

Figure 135–3.

Causes of low ETCO$_2$

1. Increased deadspace ventilation (same thing as hypoperfusion . . . if the CO$_2$ isn't delivered to the alveoli, then the ETCO$_2$ will be lower than the arterial CO$_2$)
2. Embolic phenomena (air, clot, etc . . . tends to cause rapid, progressive decline, but not usually totally absent CO$_2$)
3. Dilution of exhaled CO$_2$ by proximally located fresh gas source (as in Mapleson D and Bain circuits)
4. Sampling flow rate exceeds expired flow rate (entrains fresh gas and dilutes sample)

> **CAVEAT:** Shunting doesn't usually affect ETCO$_2$ because it's so highly diffusible; even if a diminished number of alveoli are perfused, the lung can still eliminate all the CO$_2$.

Causes of high ETCO$_2$

1. Increased CO$_2$ production (sepsis, hyperthermia)
2. Exogenous source of CO$_2$ (abdominal CO$_2$ insufflation, rebreathing, HCO$_3^-$ administration)
3. Release of tourniquet or aortic crossclamp (transcient effect)
4. Condensation in sampling tube

Sample questions

Single best answer

1. A 20-year-old, 80-kg male sustains a pelvic fracture and ruptured spleen in a motor vehicle accident. His vital signs prior to rapid-sequence induction with 350 mg thiopental and 150 mg succinylcholine were: BP

115/68 mmHg, pulse 110/min. Sixty seconds after the institution of mechanical ventilation, the capnograph shows the following waveform

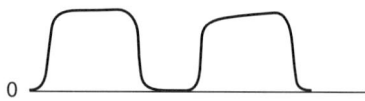

Figure 135–4.

The most likely explanation for this is
1. Incorrect calibration of the capnograph
2. Esophageal intubation
3. Incompetent exhalation valve
4. Sampling rate is too low
5. Hypotension

A = 1, 2, 3   B = 1, 3   C = 2, 4   D = 4 only   E = all are correct

2. During a general anesthetic with mechanical ventilation for appendectomy, the capnograph exhibits the following waveform.

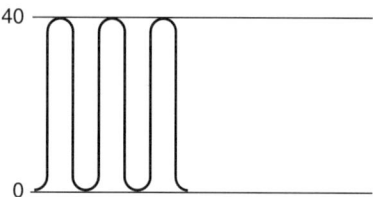

Figure 135–5.

Possible explanations for this include
1. Patient is disconnected from breathing circuit
2. Esophageal intubation
3. Total obstruction of endotracheal tube with secretions
4. Pulmonary embolus

3. Same patient as last question. Fifteen minutes after resolution of first abnormal capnograph, you see the following trace:

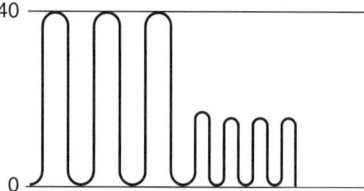

Figure 135–6.

Possible explanations for this include
1. Ruptured endotracheal balloon cuff
2. Partial obstruction of endotracheal tube with secretions
3. Patient is partially disconnected from breathing circuit
4. Reduced minute ventilation

4. Okay, this guy's getting to be a pain in the butt . . . you fixed him the first two times, and now he does this:

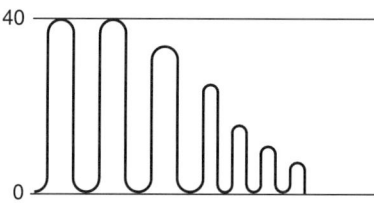

Figure 135–7.

Possible explanations include
1. The surgeon transected the aorta by mistake
2. Pulmonary embolus
3. Massive myocardial infarction
4. Inadequate minute ventilation

Answers: 1. 5   2. A   3. A   4. A

CHAPTER 136

Electrical Confusion in the Operating Room

First, some definitions

Direct current (DC): electrons always flow in the same direction through the circuit

Alternating current (AC): direction of electron flow reverses at regular intervals. (In the United States, the power company delivers 120 volts of AC at 60 Hz, meaning the direction of flow reverses 60 times/sec.)

Impedence: the cumulative effect of all forces oppposing electron flow in a circuit. (For current to flow, there must be a closed loop and a voltage difference across the impedance of the circuit.)

Capacitance: the measure of the ability of a device to store charge

Ground: an object outside the electrical circuit with zero voltage that acts as a huge electron "sink" (typically Earth). If YOU touch the hot wire of a circuit, YOU become part of the circuit by creating a low-impedance pathway for electrons to dump into the earth.

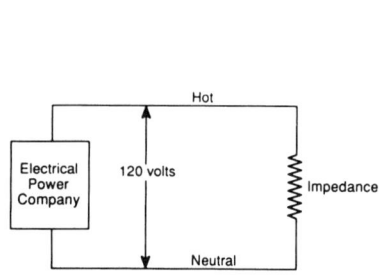

Figure 136–1. Generic Electrical Circuit. From Barash PG, Cullen BF, Stoelting RK. Clinical Anesthesia, ed 2. Philadelphia: Lippincott, 1992, p. 185. Reprinted with permission.

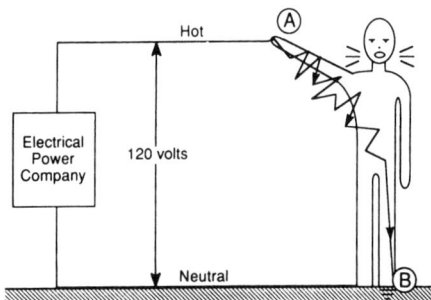

Figure 136–2. You, Acting as Part of the Circuit. From Barash PG, Cullen BF, Stoelting RK. Clinical Anesthesia, ed 2. Philadelphia: Lippincott, 1992, p. 185. Reprinted with permission.

Electrical isolation

The power to the operating room is ungrounded (i.e., it is *isolated* from ground potential). This ungrounded power is created through the use of an isolation transformer (see Figure 136–3).

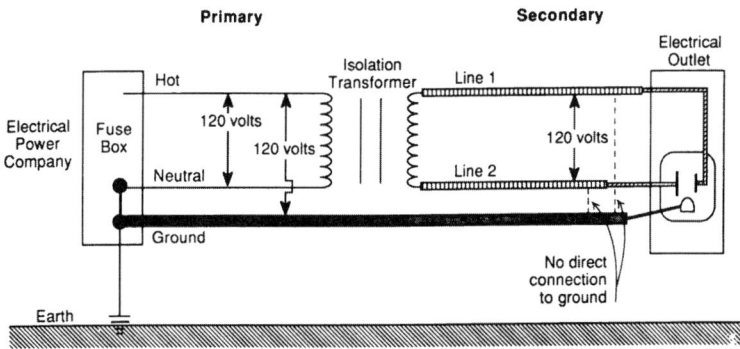

Figure 136–3. From Barash PG, Cullen BF, Stoelting RK. Clinical Anesthesia, ed 2. Philadelphia: Lippincott, 1992, p. 192. Reprinted with permission.

The rapid movement of electrons in the primary coil creates current within the secondary coil, but THERE IS NO DIRECT ELECTRICAL CONNECTION between the two coils. Therefore, the power in the second coil is *isolated* from ground. Note that the 120-V potential difference exists only between the two wires of the isolated circuit and that neither of them is "hot" or "neutral" with respect to ground. This means that you would have to make contact with this circuit in TWO places to complete the circuit and get shocked. (It's SAFER!)

Line isolation monitor

Function is to monitor how well the circuit is isolated from ground. **Warns you of:**

1. **Faulty equipment,** which converts the circuit to a conventional grounded system. (This means that if you plug in a SECOND faulty piece of equipment or contact the circuit in ONE place, you'll get shocked.)
2. **Excess leakage current:** All AC equipment has capacitance (the ability to store charge or current), and this current can "leak" out, reducing the integrity (isolation from ground) of the circuit. The line isolation monitor indicates the amount of leakage current. Bear in mind that the reading on the monitor IS NOT ACTUALLY MEASURING CURRENT, but is indicating how much current will flow at the first fault. **Alarms when 2 milli Amps of leakage current is reached.**

Macroshock

1. Large voltage shock delivered remote from the heart (at skin)
2. Induces ventricular fibrillation at 100 *milli*Amps

Microshock

1. Small-voltage shock delivered directly to heart (via central line)
2. Induces ventricular fibrillation at 100 *micro*Amps

NOTE: that line isolation monitor (which only alarms at ≥ 2 milliAmps) does not warn against microshock!!!

Electrosurgery units

Delivers high-frequency current through a concentrated tip, creating heat that cuts and coagulates tissue.

1. **Unipolar:** current returns to the unit through a large heat-dispersing electrode on the patient (incorrectly called the grounding pad!).
2. **Bipolar:** tip is actually a forcep, and current only travels between the two prongs of the forcep, rather than through the patient as the unipolar does. For use in pacemaker patients, neurosurgery, and opthalmologic surgery.

Prevention of burns from electrosurgical units

1. Return plate must have adequate gel and maintain adequate contact with patient
2. Place pad as close to surgical site as possible
3. EKG pads should be placed as far from surgical site as possible
4. Use lowest possible setting
5. Isolate the ESU from ground

Sample questions

A = 1, 2, 3   B = 1, 3   C = 2, 4   D = 4 only   E = all are correct

1. True statements about a line isolation monitor alarming and a meter reading of 2 mA include
   1. There is a short circuit with 10 mA of current flow in the system
   2. The system is no longer grounded
   3. This protects against the risk of microshock
   4. There is 2 mA worth of leakage current

2. In the operating room
   1. The equipment is grounded
   2. The patient is grounded
   3. The power is ungrounded
   4. Placement of the electrocautery pad grounds the patient

Single best answer

3. Factors that protect against microshock include
   1. Nonconductive shoe covers
   2. The line isolation monitor
   3. Three-wire grounding sytems
   4. Alternating current
   5. None of the above

Answers: 1. D   2. B   3. 5

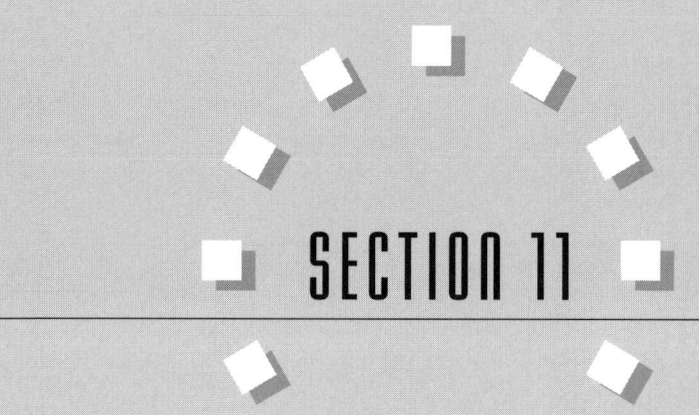

SECTION 11

Airway Management

CHAPTER 137

The Infant Airway versus the Adult Airway

The following table describes the anatomic structures of the infant airway compared to the adult airway.

• **Table 137–1**

Structure	Infant Airway	Clinical Significance
Tongue	Larger in relation to size of oral cavity	Airway obstructs more easily
Larynx	More cephalad (C3-4 vs. C4-5)	Tongue sits closer to roof of mouth: encourages obstruction
		Angle between glottic opening and base of tongue is more acute: visualization is more difficult
Epiglottis	More narrow	Harder to lift with laryngoscope
	Angle not parallel to trachea	
Vocal cords	Anterior attachment is lower	Endotracheal tube can get "hung up" on anterior commissure
Subglottic area	Narrowest part is cricoid cartilage vs. vocal cords in adults	Endotracheal tube may pass easily through nares or cords, but not past cricoid

Key points

1. Because of their relatively large occiput, supine children are already in somewhat of a "sniff" position. THEREFORE: extension of the neck may produce airway obstruction.
2. Because of the acute angulation of the airway, a straight laryngoscope blade is best BUT: all anatomic structures assume adult configuration by ~10–12 years of age.

Sample questions

Single best answer

1. Which of the following structures determines the corrrect-size endotracheal tube in the infant airway?
   1. Glottis
   2. Nares
   3. Vocal cords

4. Cricoid cartilage
5. Thyroid cartilage

A = 1, 2, 3   B = 1, 3   C = 2, 4   D = 4 only   E = all are correct

2. Possible causes of an inability to pass the correct-size endotracheal tube in an infant include
   1. Laryngospasm
   2. Tube is caught in anterior commissure
   3. Excessive degree of neck extension
   4. Endotracheal tube is too large

Answers: 1. 4   2. A

CHAPTER 138

Functional Innervation of the Airway

General innervation

- Table 138–1

Area	Innervation
Nares and nasopharynx	Trigeminal nerve
Tongue and oropharynx	Glossopharyngeal nerve
Larynx and periglottis	Vagus nerve

The larynx consists of three types of muscles

1. Abductors
    A. Posterior cricoarytenoids: abductors **(only abductors of true cords)**
    B. Interarytenoids: close posterior commissure by abduction
2. Adductors
    A. Thyroarytenoids and lateral cricoarytenoids: adduct false cords
    B. Arytenoepiglottis and oblique arytenoids: adduct arytenoepiglottic folds
    C. Cricothyroids: adduct and tense true cords
3. Tensors: cricothyroids: tense true cords (in addition to adduction)

All laryngeal innervation is supplied by two branches of the vagus: the superior laryngeal nerve and the recurrrent laryngeal nerve. Summary of airway innervation and function are in Table 138–2:

- Table 138–2

Nerve	Sensory	Motor
Glossopharyngeal	Posterior $1/3$ of tongue Oropharynx Tonsillar area Gag reflex	None
Superior laryngeal (internal branch)	Base of tongue Epiglottis Supraglottic mucosa Thyroepiglottic joint Cricothyroid joint	None
Superior laryngeal (external branch)	Anterior subglottic mucosa	Cricothyroid Inferior pharyngeal constrictors
Recurrent laryngeal	Subglottic mucosa Muscle spindles	(All other intrinsic laryngeal muscles) Thyroarytenoid Lateral cricoarytenoid Interarytenoid Posterior cricoarytenoid

Effects of specific nerve lesions

1. *Recurrent laryngeal (unilateral lesion):* vocal cord on injured side assumes paramedian position 2° to unopposed adduction by ipsilateral cricothyroid muscle, mild hoarseness, negligible airway obstruction, or aspiration risk
2. *Recurrent laryngeal (bilateral lesion):* stridor or complete airway obstruction, may require tracheotomy
3. *Superior laryngeal external branch (combined with recurrent laryngeal injury):* vocal cord is more medial, less tense, patient is hoarse and at increased risk of aspiration

● Table 138–3

Procedure for Superior Laryngeal Nerve Block	Procedure for Recurrent Laryngeal Nerve Block
Patient supine, head extended	Patient supine, head extended
Laterally displace hyoid bone toward side to be blocked	Palpate ipsilateral lesser cornu of thyroid cartilage in tracheoesophageal groove
Walk needle inferiorly off greater cornu of hyoid, advance ~3 mm	Insert needle perpendicular to patient, directed medially until lesser cornu thyroid cartilage contacted
Note slight loss of resistance as needle passes through thyrohyoid membrane	Withdraw slightly, inject 3 cc local anesthetic
3 cc local anesthetic superficial and deep to membrane	

NOTE: Maintenance of selected functions (sensory, motor) is possible with local anesthesia. All laryngeal functions are depressed in a dose-dependent manner under general anesthesia. Thiopental maintains airway reflexes better than propofol following an induction dose.

Sample questions

A = 1, 2, 3   B = 1, 3   C = 2, 4   D = 4 only   E = all are correct

1. Sensory loss leading to increased risk of aspiration is seen with
    1. Unilateral stellate ganglion block
    2. Bilateral stellate ganglion block
    3. Hypoglossal nerve block
    4. Superior laryngeal nerve block

2. Immediately after extubation following subtotal thyroidectomy for a nontoxic goiter, your patient develops severe respiratory distress and airway obstruction. Fiberoptic examination of the airway reveals both vocal cords in a paramedian position, and they do not abduct when the patient attempts to speak. Possible causes for this include
    1. Hypocalcemia
    2. Bilateral superior laryngeal nerve injury
    3. Hematoma
    4. Bilateral recurrent laryngeal neve injury

3. Nerves that provide motor innervation to the larynx include
    1. Recurrent laryngeal nerve
    2. Superior laryngeal nerve, internal branch
    3. Superior laryngeal nerve, external branch
    4. Glossopharyngeal nerve

Answers 1. C   2. D   3. A

Chapter 139

Management of the Difficult Airway

Anesthesia for "awake" intubations

Direct laryncoscopy, blind, fiberoptic. **Adjuvant medications required:**

1. Some sedation usually needed (fentanyl or midazolam preferred, effects can be reversed if necessary)
2. Give anticholinergics (drying secretions will improve effectiveness of topical techniques)

Anesthesia can be achieved by topical techniques, specific nerve blocks or combination of the two:

1. **Topical anesthesia techniques:**
   A. Nares/nasopharynx:
      1. Use mixture of 1 mL 1% phenylephrine and 4 mL viscous lidocaine
      2. Apply with cotton-tipped applicators, squirting into nare, or smear on the outside of nasal trumpets, placing progressively larger trumpets to dilate nare
   B. Tongue/oropharynx: spray liberally with 10% lidocaine, gargle with viscous lidocaine, or have patient breathe 3–4 mL nebulized 2% lidocaine
2. **Specific nerve blocks**
   A. Glossopharyngeal nerve:
      1. Tissue innervated: pressure sensation at the base of the tongue
      2. Technique: inject 1–2 mL 1% lidocaine in glossopharyngeal arch
   B. Superior laryngeal nerve: see Chapter 138, Functional Innervation of the Airway.

Cricothyroidotomy and transtracheal jet ventilation

1. **Technique**
   A. Insert 12- to 16-gauge angiocath through cricothyroid membrane into trachea.
   B. Confirm intraluminal position by free aspiration of air.
   C. A three-way stopcock connected to the angiocath communicates with the machine's common fresh gas outlet via standard oxygen tubing and an endotracheal tube adapter inserted into the outlet.
   D. Actuate delivery of frequent, short bursts of oxygen by pushing the oxygen flush button on machine.

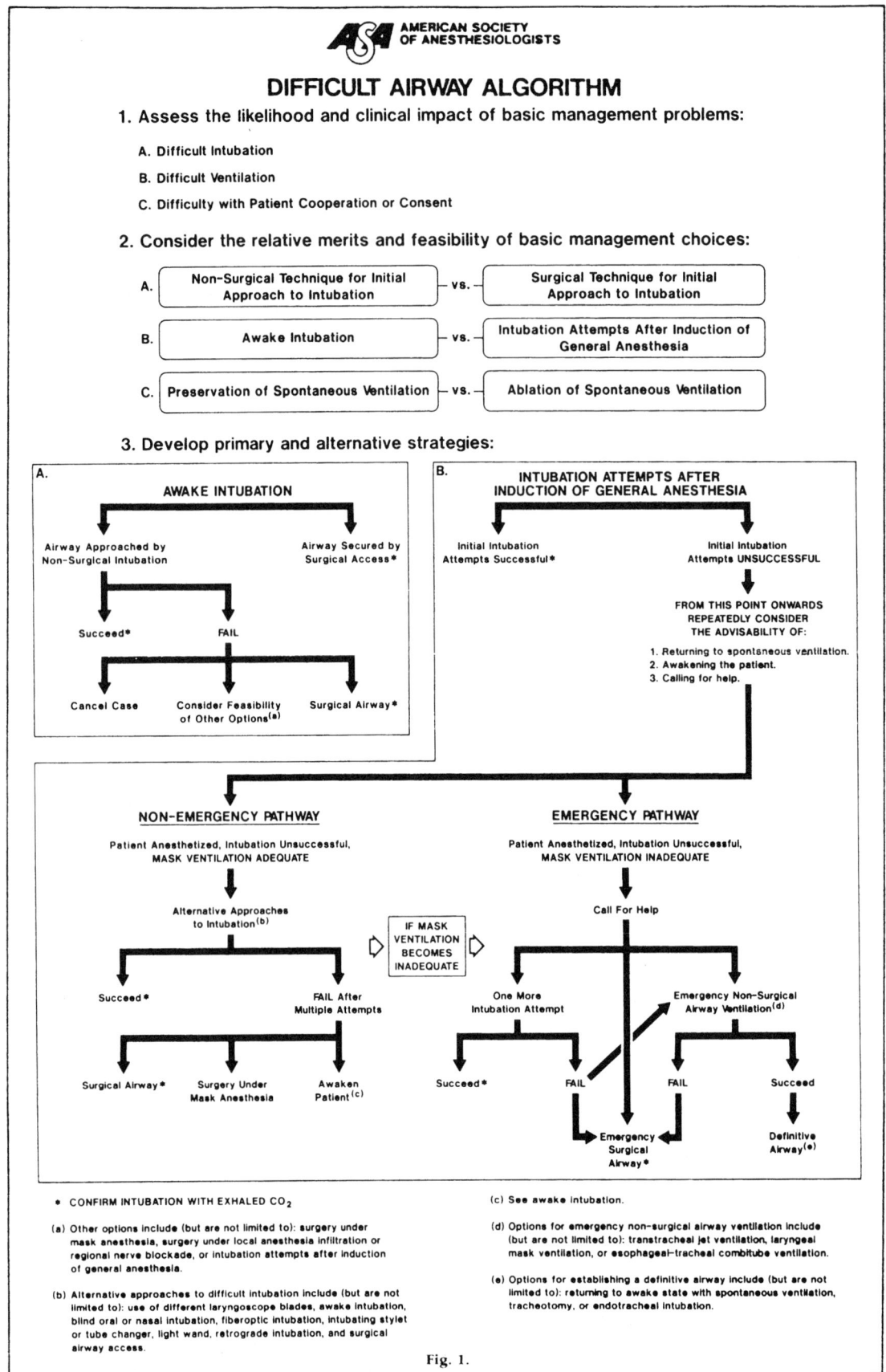

Figure 139–1. From The ASA Task Force on Management of the Difficult Airway. Guidelines for the Management of the Difficult Airway. Anesthesiology 1993; 78: 597–602. Reprinted by permission.

E. Alternatively, ventilation can be performed with a self-inflating ressuscitation bag
2. **Technical limitations**
   A. Limited egress of gas leads to hypercarbia and hyperinflation (risk of barotrauma).
   B. Narrow angiocath lumen necessitates high driving pressures (risk of barotrauma, and self-inflating bag may not provide adequate driving pressure).
   C. Not an option for tracheal injuries (high pressures force gas into surrounding tissues).
   D. Definitive airway still required.
3. **Complications**
   A. Barotrauma (pneumothorax, pneumomediastinum)
   B. Cardiovascular compromise (high intrathoracic pressures due to hyperinflation)
   C. Failure to acquire airway
   D. Subglottic stenosis
   E. Hoarseness

Intubation after cervical spine injury

1. Full stomach
2. Spinal cord injury
3. Head injury (↑ ICP)
4. Airway injury
5. Hypovolemia/hypotension

Techniques for intubation after cervical spine injury

1. **Blind nasal**
   A. Advantages:
      1. Manipulation of C-spine not required
      2. Maintains spontaneous ventilation
   B. Disadvantages:
      1. Risk entering cranial vault if basilar skull fracture present
      2. If topical anesthesia inadequate, patient may retch, vomit, or move head (aspirate, ↑ ICP, or injure spinal cord)
   C. Complications of nasotracheal intubation:
      1. Bleeding
      2. Sinusitis (late)
      3. Erosion of nasal alae (late)
      4. Penetration of brain matter
2. **Awake fiberoptic intubation:** advantages and disadvantages same as blind nasal, but prevents entering cranial vault
3. **Rapid-sequence oral intubation:**
   A. Advantages:
      1. Cricoid pressure ↓ risk of aspiration
      2. Prevents patient from moving
   B. Disadvantages: C-spine immobilization is required (risk of spinal cord injury)
   C. Complications of cricoid pressure:
      1. Degree of pressure during cricoid maneuver may displace cervical fractures
      2. Only prevents passive regurgitation . . . if active retching occurs, release pressure or you risk esophageal rupture

4. **Surgical airway** (cricothyroidotomy, tracheotomy)
   A. Advantages: provides definitive airway
   B. Disadvantages: technically difficult to perform in emergency setting, often not in OR

With all techniques, beware of endobronchial intubation, intraoperative signs of which include

1. Wheezing
2. Unilateral breath sounds
3. Unilateral chest excursion
4. Hypoxemia
5. High peak inspiratory pressures
6. Pressures > 40 cmH$_2$O needed to create "leak" around tube

If patient exhibits hoarseness postextubation, consider the following possible causes

1. Vocal cord paralysis (usually 2° to overinflated cuff exerting pressure on superior laryngeal nerve)
2. Arytenoid dislocation
3. Ulcerated glottic mucosa
4. Vocal cord hematoma

Sample questions: NONE . . . if you're gonna play a doctor in real life, you have to know at least this!

CHAPTER 140

Laryngospasm

Risk factors

1. Light anesthesia
2. Secretions/foreign objects in airway
3. Recent URI (especially children)
4. Airway surgery/pathology

Physiology

Stimulate superior laryngeal nerve → true cord adduction causes partial or complete obstruction of gas entry → concurrent stimulation of recurrent laryngeal nerve → false cords tense, create ball-valve effect in glottic opening → increased obstruction during inspiration

Management

1. Remove irritating factor
2. Anterior displacement of jaw
3. Deepen anesthesia
4. Apply gentle continuous positive pressure (~10–20 cmH$_2$O) with F$_i$O$_2$ 1.0. If spasm doesn't resolve within ~30 sec or if desaturation occurs, administer small dose of succinylcholine (~20 mg IV is usually enough)

Consequences

1. Hypoxemia (can ultimately lead to cardiac arrest, cerebral injury, death)
2. Negative pressure pulmonary edema (transudate due to ↑ negative intrathoracic and transpulmonary pressure)

Sample question

Single best answer

1. A 4-year-old, 25-kg child with a recent history of rhinorrhea undergoes inhalational induction of general anesthesia with nitrous oxide, oxygen, and halothane for tonsillectomy. While you are atttempting placement of the IV, his breathing becomes stertorous. The pulse oximeter reading begins to slowly decline, no paradoxical movements of the chest and abdomen are noted, his respiratory rate increases from 15/min to 30/min

and his gaze is disconjugate. The most appropriate management at this time is
1. Insert an oral airway
2. Apply continuous positive pressure by mask with F_iO_2 1.0
3. Succinylcholine 25 mg IM
4. Anterior displacement of the mandible and increase the delivered concentration of halothane
5. Suction the airway for secretions

Answer: 1. 4

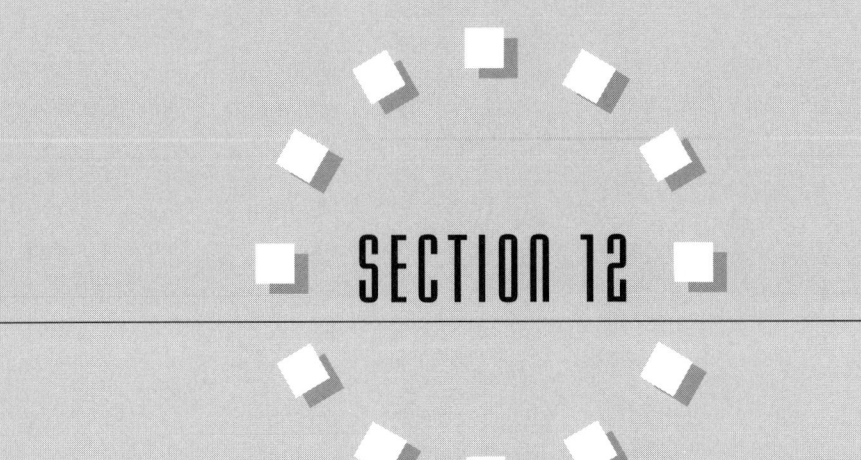

SECTION 12

Complications

Chapter 141

Airway Fire

Procedure: Laser surgery of the airway

Substance burned

1. Endotracheal tube
2. Endotracheal cuff
3. Cotton pledgets or throat packs

Combustion supported by

1. Oxygen
2. Nitrous oxide

Combustion deterred by

1. Low F_iO_2
2. Halothane (mechanism not described)
3. Helium (has high thermal conductivity and may delay ignition of ETT)

Types of lasers capable of inducing airway fire

CO_2 > Nd-YAG, but both can.

Products of combustion

Depends on the endotracheal tube composition:

1. Red rubber ETT produces carbon monoxide when burned.
2. Polyvinyl chloride ETT (what we usually use) produces hydrogen chloride (a pulmonary toxin).
3. Silicone ETT produces silica ash.

Flammability of tubes

Polyvinyl chloride > silicone > red rubber

Measures to prevent fire

1. $F_iO_2 \leq 0.3$.
2. Consider air/O_2 or helium/O_2 mixture.
3. Wrap tube in reflective metal tape (not absolute protection, and doesn't protect cuff).

4. Use specially produced metal tubes (again, not absolute).
5. Double-cuffed tube (protects against inability to ventilate if one is accidentally perforated).
6. Fill cuff with colored saline (allows immediate recognition of perforation, is noncombustible, and possibly will quench a flame).
7. Perform intermittent extubation and laser only during apnea or avoid conventional intubation altogether, instead performing jet ventilation via a ventilating bronchoscope.

Management of an airway fire

1. Stop ventilation.
2. Disconnect patient from breathing circuit.
3. Discontinue oxygen.
4. Remove endotracheal tube.
5. Water or saline to surgical field to extinguish any burning remnants left in airway.
6. Mask-ventilate with F_iO_2 1.0.
7. Reintubate with endotracheal tube or rigid bronchoscope.
8. Perform bronchoscopy to assess airway damage and remove any remaining fragments of tube.

Sample questions

Single best answer

1. During laser surgery of the airway, the gas mixture that is least likely to support combustion is
   1. 73% N_2O, 25% O_2, and 2% halothane
   2. 25% O_2, 73% air, and 2% halothane
   3. 25% O_2, 73% air, and 2% isoflurane
   4. Air and halothane
   5. 25% O_2, 73% helium, and 2% halothane

2. In the event of a fire during laser surgery of the airway, all of the following are indicated except
   1. Discontinue oxygen flow
   2. Airway examination to evaluate the extent of damage
   3. Steroids to prevent airway edema
   4. Reintubation
   5. Disconnect the patient from the anesthesia circuit

Answers: **1.** 5   **2.** 3

CHAPTER 142

Pulmonary Aspiration of Gastric Contents

Predisposing factors

1. Pregnancy
2. Morbid obesity
3. Emergency surgery
4. Decreased level of conciousness
5. Hiatal hernia
6. Scleroderma
7. Presence of a nasogastric tube
8. Diabetic gastroparesis
9. Uremia

Characteristics of the fluid

1. pH is most critical aspect (pH < 2.5 causes immediate severe chemical reaction)
2. Volume is less important (> 25 cc of gastric contents is firmly entrenched in the literature as the point at which you are at risk for aspiration, but this value is not supported by recent research)
3. Solid vs. liquid aspirate—solids are worse than liquids

What substance causes the most damage?

Acid food particles > nonacid food particles > acid liquid > nonacid liquid

Signs/ symptoms

1. Hypoxia—**earliest and most reliable sign** for all types of aspirate material
2. Pulmonary hypertension—all types of aspirate
3. Hypercarbia and acidosis—solids, but not liquids as a rule
4. Wheezing ⎫
5. Coughing ⎬ Bronchospasm
6. Cyanosis ⎭
7. Pulmonary edema
8. Shock
9. Chest X-ray: bilateral perihilar or basal atelectasis/infiltrates, but often see no changes

373

Measures to decrease risk of aspiration

1. NPO for clear liquids at least 2 hr preop (pregnant and emergent surgery still 8 hr), NPO 8 hr for solids
2. Clear, nonparticulate antacids
3. H$_2$-blockers (cimetidine, ranitidine) ⎫
4. Metoclopramide ⎬ Both have problems, see below
5. Sitting or semi-Fowler's position
6. Rapid-sequence induction with cricoid pressure (prevents aspiration from passive regurgitation *and* vomiting)
7. Intubation with a cuffed endotracheal tube

Methods of diagnosis

1. Pulse oximetry or arterial blood gas to detect hypoxia—**most reliable**
2. Chest X-ray can be falsely normal
3. Measurement of pH of fluid in trachea—of no value

Management

1. Supplemental O$_2$
2. Early and aggressive CPAP (mask or ETT) with rapid weaning of F$_i$O$_2$
3. Maintain intravascular fluid status (they can third space large volumes into lungs)

Therapeutic measures that are *not* routinely indicated

1. Steroids
2. Antibiotics—ONLY IF: clinical signs of infection are present OR if the patient is known to have aspirated fecal matter
3. Bronchoscopy—unless solid matter is causing airway obstruction
4. Pulmonary lavage—unless there are large food particles or inspissated secretions

Interesting fact

Did you know that pulmonary lavage with normal saline can cause the same degree of hypoxia as aspirating gastric contents? (Would I lie to you ?)

Drugs we use to (hopefully) reduce risk of aspiration

Metaclopramide

1. **Pharmacodynamics:**
   A. Central action: dopamine antagonist
   B. Peripheral action: stimulates acetylcholine release
2. **Effects:**
   A. Gastric and small intestine motility
   B. ↑ lower esophageal sphincter tone
   C. Relaxation of pylorus and duodenum
3. **Side effects:**
   A. Drug-induced Parkinson's
   B. Tardive dyskinesia

Cimetidine and Ranitidine

1. **Mechanisms by which H_2-blockers alter drug metabolism:**
   A. Inhibition of cytochrome P450 system
   B. Interfere with GI absorption by altering gastric pH
   C. Compete for renal excretion
   D. Alter plasma protein binding
   E. Decrease liver blood flow
2. **Cimetidine pharmacology**
   A. Blocks secretion of hydrochloric acid (must be given ~ 90 min preop to have an effect)
   B. Decreases gastric acidity (but doesn't alter pH of fluid already present in stomach)
   C. Decreases gastric fluid volume
3. **Drug interactions (these apply *only* to cimetidine unless otherwise indicated)**
   A. **Theophylline**—decreased clearance (easily become toxic) ⎱ Both cimetidine *and* ranitidine
   B. **Warfarin**—decreased clearance ⎰
   C. Local anesthetics—↑ serum level of IV lidocaine, bupivicaine (no studies on regionals)
   D. Succinylcholine—no interaction
   E. Beta-blockers (propanalol)—decreased clearance
   F. Phenytoin—increased plasma levels
   G. Calcium channel blockers (nifedipine)—increased plasma levels
   H. Benzodiazepines—altered pharmacokinetics

> **PEARL:** Rapid IV administration of cimetidine can cause bradycardia, hypotension, and cardiac arrest.

Sample questions

A = 1, 2, 3   B = 1, 3   C = 2, 4   D = 4 only   E = all are correct

1. Administration of cimetidine may result in toxic levels of
   1. Theophylline
   2. IV lidocaine
   3. Warfarin
   4. Epidural bupivicaine

2. Pharmacologic effects seen with both cimetidine and metaclopramide include
   1. Increased lower esophageal sphincter tone
   2. Decreased gastric fluid acidity
   3. Increased gastric motility
   4. Decreased gastric fluid volume

3. Following aspiration of gastric contents, routine management would include
   1. Hydrocortisone
   2. Bronchoscopy
   3. Prophylactic antibiotics
   4. Oxygen therapy

Single best answer

4. The greatest reduction in gastric fluid volume is seen with
   1. Sodium citrate
   2. Cimetidine
   3. Metaclopramide
   4. Atropine
   5. Glycopyrolate

5. Which finding is most reliably seen on physical exam following aspiration of gastric contents?
   1. Wheezing
   2. Cyanosis
   3. Perihilar infiltrate on chest X-ray
   4. Hypoxia
   5. Rales

Answers: 1. A   2. D   3. D   4. 3   5. 4

Chapter 143

Methylmethacrylate

Physiologic perturbations following cementing have been attributed to

1. The methylmethacrylate monomer itself
2. Embolization of monomer, fat, bone, air, and clot during insertion of the prosthesis (which forces debris into exposed marrow venous sinuses)

Physiologic changes tend to occur within 1 min of prosthetic placement and include

1. Hypotension (the monomer is a direct vasodilator)
2. Decreased PaO_2
3. Pulmonary hypertension
4. Cardiovascular collapse

Presumed due to emboli, as demonstrated by echogenic material following prosthetic insertion

Prior to cementing, you should

1. Increase intravascular volume
2. Lighten the plane of anesthesia
3. Ensure adequate ventilation and oxygenation

Sample question

Single best answer

1. A 70-year-old, 65-kg female is undergoing total hip replacement under general anesthesia and is 2 hr into the procedure. Estimated blood loss is 1000 cc and she has received 2 L of crystalloid and 1000 cc of colloid. Vital signs are: BP = 110/65, pulse = 88, SaO_2 = 99%. Approximately 2 min after the surgeon inserts the prosthesis into the femoral shaft, her vital signs are: BP = 75/45, pulse = 110, SaO_2 = 99%. The most likely reason for the change is:
   1. Pulmonary embolus
   2. Acute blood loss
   3. Allergic reaction to the methylmethacrylate
   4. Inadequate replacement of blood loss
   5. Direct vasodilation by the methylmethacrylate

Answer: 1. 5

Tourniquet Troubles

Immediate effect of inflation of limb tourniquet

Limb exsanquination → central venous blood volume expansion → ↑ CVP, MAP, and PAP (effect greater during general vs. regional anesthesia)

Physiologic effect on muscle

Cellular hypoxia → anaerobic metabolism within 10 min → cellular acidosis → release of myoglobin, K+, thromboxane → tissue edema and cooling of extremity

Physiologic effect on neurologic function

Hypoxia and direct neural compression → loss of somatosensory evoked potentials within 30 min → pain and hypertension within 1 hr

Effects of tourniquet release

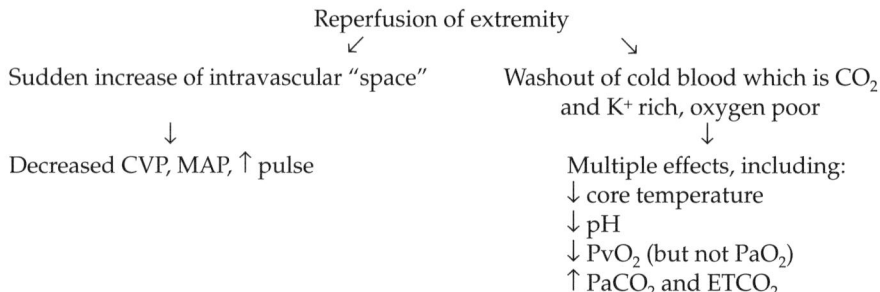

Figure 144–1.

Characteristics and treatment of tourniquet pain

1. Occurs ~45 min after inflation
2. Is thought to be transmitted by A delta and C fibers, mainly C fibers, but still controversial
3. May be prevented by regional block *if* block is dense enough
4. Narcotics and induction of general anesthesia are both unreliable means of treating the pain
5. Most reliable treatment is CUFF DEFLATION

Sample questions

A = 1, 2, 3   B = 1, 3   C = 2, 4   D = 4 only   E = all are correct

1. Risk of nerve injury secondary to the use of a limb tourniquet is
   1. Increased if high inflating pressure are used
   2. Decreased if the cuff is deflated every 90 min
   3. Increased if left inflated longer than 2 hr
   4. Increased with regional anesthesia

2. Physiologic changes following deflation of an extremity tourniquet that was inflated for 75 min include
   1. Decreased systemic vascular resistance
   2. Arterial hypoxemia
   3. Increased end-tidal carbon dioxide levels
   4. Increased hematocrit

Answers: 1. A   2. B

CHAPTER 145

Deep Venous Thrombosis

Physiologic events leading to DVT

1. Venous stasis (intraoperatively due to hypotension, hypovolemia, position)
2. Alterations in the vessel wall
3. Altered coagulation (introperatively due to drugs, circulating factors, hypothermia)

Risk factors for DVT

1. Obesity[1]
2. Age > 40 yr[2]
3. Genitourinary/gynecologic procedures
4. Total hip or knee replacement
5. Laparoscopy
6. Prolonged immobilization[3]
7. Heart failure, myocardial infarction[4]

May reduce risk of DVT with

1. Sequential compression hose
2. Warfarin
3. Low-dose heparin
4. Hydroxychloroquin[5]
5. Regional anesthesia

Sample question

Single best answer

1. A 50-year-old, 105-kg female is scheduled for laparoscopic cholecystectomy. She has a history of hypertension, congestive heart failure, and atrial fibrillation. Her daily medications include baby aspirin, digoxin, and coumadin. Management decisions that may reduce her risk of developing deep venous thrombosis include all of the following EXCEPT:
    1. Continue coumadin therapy until the day before surgery
    2. Continue baby aspirin throughout the perioperative course
    3. Abandon laparoscopic approach in favor of an open cholecystectomy

4. Intraoperative sequential compression hose
5. Addition of low-dose heparin

Answer: 1. 2

References

1. Kakker VV, Howe CT, Nicolaides AN, et al. Deep venous thrombosis of the leg: is there a "high-risk" group? Am J Surg 120: 527, 1970.
2. Ibid.
3. Heatley RV, Hughes LE, Morgan A, et al. Preoperative deep-vein thrombosis. Lancet, 1: 437, 1976.
4. Simmons AV, Sheppard MA, Cox AF. Deep venous thrombosis after myocardial infarction: predisposing factors. Br Heart J 35: 623, 1973.
5. Wu T, Tsapogas M, Jordan R. Prophylaxis of deep venous thrombosis by hydroxychloroquine sulfate and heparin. Surg Gynecol Obstet 145: 714, 1977.

Chapter 146

Anaphylaxis

Clinical manifestations of anaphylaxis under general anesthesia

1. Skin: flushing, erythema
2. Pulmonary: bronchospasm (wheezing, hypoxia, high peak airway pressures), laryngeal edema
3. Cardiovascular: tachycardia, dysrythmias, profound hypotension

Substances producing anaphylaxis of particular interest to anesthesiologists

1. Latex
2. Penicillin (most common drug class causing allergic reactions in OR)
3. Imipenem (a carbapenem) ⎫
4. Aztreonam (a monobactam) ⎬ All cross-react in penicillin-allergic patients
5. Cephalosporins ⎭
6. Sulfonamides
7. Vancomycin (profound histamine release and vasodilation)
8. Muscle relaxants (all have been implicated; those known to release histamine are the most suspect)
9. Ester local anesthetics (also methylparaben, a preservative in multidose vials of amide anesthetics)
10. Thiobarbiturates
11. Narcotics (histamine releasers are worst offenders)

Regarding latex allergy, there are certain high-risk types of patients

1. Patients with spina bifida or genitourinary abnormalities (h/o multiple procedures, frequent bladder catheterization)[1]
2. Patients with a history of atopy[2]
3. Occupational exposure to latex (healthcare workers, rubber industry workers)[3]

Anesthetic implications of latex allergy

1. Identify high-risk patients
2. Pretreatment with steroids and antihistamines may be indicated
3. Minimize introperative exposure (use nonlatex equipment, first case of the day to cut down on airborne latex particles or glove dust)

Management of intraoperative allergic reaction

1. **Immediate treatment**
   A. Discontinue all anesthetic agents
   B. Ventilate with F_iO_2 1.0
   C. Rapid intravascular volume expansion (offsets hypotension)
   D. Epinephrine ~5 µg/kg IV, infusion @ 1–5 µg/kg/min

   If latex reaction suspected, you should also: (1) Have surgeons change gloves; (2) Obtain AlaSTAT and RAST assays

2. **Secondary treatment:**
   A. Hydrocortisone 5 mg/kg IV or methyl prednisolone 1 mg/kg IV
   B. Diphenhydramine 1 mg/kg IV
   C. Aminophylline load with 5 mg/kg, then infuse @ ~0.5 mg/kg/hr
   D. Inhaled β_2-agonists
   E. $NaHCO_3$ PRN for acidosis

Sample questions

Single best answer

1. A 3-year-old patient with a history of extrophy of the bladder presents for revision of her original bladder repair. She has no history of latex allergy and undergoes bladder catheterization three times daily. Thirty min after administration of thiopental and atracurium for induction of general anesthesia, her peak inspiratory pressures are noted to be 50 cmH_2O, pulse oximeter is 94% on F_iO_2 3.0, pulse 95/min, blood pressure 85/50 mmHg. The most likely cause of these findings is
   1. Early anaphylactic reaction to latex IV tubing
   2. Allergic reaction to thiopental
   3. Allergic reaction to atracurium
   4. Endobronchial intubation
   5. Bronchospasm

2. A 40-year-old, 95-kg paraplegic with a history of meningomyelocele repair is undergoing an appendectomy under general anesthesia. Rapid-sequence induction is achieved with thiopental and succinylcholine. Twenty min after incision, he develops multifocal premature ventricular beats on EKG, blood pressure is 65/35 mmHg, pulse 105/min, SaO_2 90% on f_iO_2 0.4 , $ETCO_2$ 44 mmHg, peak inspiratory pressures are ~50 cmH_2O and breath sound are diminished bilaterally. The most likely cause of these findings is
   1. Endobronchial intubation
   2. Allergic reaction to latex
   3. Pulmonary embolus
   4. Pulmonary aspiration of gastric contents
   5. Acute myocardial infarction

Answers: **1. 4   2. 2**

References

1. FDA medical alert. Allergic reactions to latex-containing medical devices. Am Soc Anesthesiol Newsletter 55: 1, 1991.
2. Nguyen DH, Burns MW, Shapiro GG, et al. Intraoperative cardiovascular collapse secondary to latex allergy. J Urol 146: 571–574, 1991.
3. Parisian S. Latex allergies causing more anesthesia problems. Anesthesia Patient Safety Foundation Newsletter 7: 1, 3, 1992.

CHAPTER 147

Intraoperative Hypothermia

Mechanisms of heat conservation in adults

1. Vasoconstriction (impaired under general and regional anesthesia)
2. Shivering (impaired under general anesthesia)

Mechanisms of intraoperative heat loss

1. Radiation **(#1 cause of heat loss)**
2. Convection **(second banana)**
3. Conduction
4. Evaporation (has greater effect on premies, who have thin skin)

Rate of development of hypothermia

1. Initial rapid heat loss phase: (1–1½°C during first hour). Caused by
   A. Anesthesia-induced vasodilation causing *redistribution* of core heat to peripheral tissues. (Caveat: although core temperature decreases, mean temperature doesn't.)
   B. Increased cutaneous heat loss ⎫ Minor contributors to heat loss at
   C. Decreased heat production ⎭ this stage
2. Slow heat loss phase: (additional 1–3°C lost over next ~3 hr). Cause: heat loss exceeds heat production
3. Plateau phase: heat loss = heat production (patients with regional anesthesia may never plateau, because of loss of vasoconstrictive ability)

Effects of moderate hypothermia

1. *The good things*
   A. ↓ basal metabolic rate (protects against hypoxia and ischemia)
   B. ↓ ability to trigger malignant hyperthermia
2. *The bad things*
   A. ↓ drug metabolism
   B. ↓ platelet aggregation (impaired coagulation)

Effects of deliberate, profound hypothermia

1. ↓ total body metabolic rate (thus, ↓ O_2 consumption and CO_2 production . . . beware of inadvertant respiratory alkalosis if you don't decrease minute ventilation in cold patients)
2. Vasoconstriction-induced changes in regional blood flow
   A. Cerebral vasoconstriction→ ↓ CBF (SSEP is temp-dependent, but unaffected if T > 33°C)

B. Renal vasoconstriction → ↓ RBF → ↓ HCO_3^- resorption, ↑ Na^+, K^+, Cl^-, H_2O excretion
C. Decreased hepatic blood flow (↓ metabolism of drugs)
3. Hemodynamic effects: ↑ SVR, SV, and contractility/↓ HR, BP, CO/dysrythmias if < 28°C
4. Acid–base changes: ↑ pH, shift of oxyhemoglobin curve to the left

Prevention and treatment of hypothermia

1. Room temperature to at least 23°C (It's hard for a turkey to get cold in a warm oven.)
2. Cover the patient (reduces convection)
3. Use warm-air blankets (Bair Hugger™)
4. Warm and humidify inhaled gases
5. Warm intravenous fluids

Postoperative shivering

1. Thought to be caused by:
   A. Normal thermoregulatory response to cold **(most likely)**
   B. Increased spinal reflex activity (suspected, but not proven)
2. Treatment:
   A. Meperidine 25 mg IV
   B. Heat lamps directed at face, chest

Sample questions

A = 1, 2, 3   B = 1, 3   C = 2, 4   D = 4 only   E = all are correct

1. Devices that can actively and efficiently increase a patient's body temperature include
   1. Warm air blankets
   2. A warming mattress
   3. Radiant heat lamps
   4. A humidi-vent type humidifier in the patient breathing circuit

2. During isoflurane general anesthesia at steady-state concentrations, a change in body temperature from 37°C to 34°C will cause a decrease in
   1. Carbon dioxide production
   2. Minimum alveolar concentration
   3. Oxygen consumption
   4. Blood–gas partition coefficient of isoflurane

Single best answer

3. The most effective way to maintain adult body temperature during closed reduction and external fixation of a fractured humerus is
   1. Heat the room to 21°C
   2. Warming mattress under the patient
   3. Cover the patient with insulated wrap
   4. Avoid neuromuscular blockade
   5. Avoid regional anesthesia

Answers: **1. B** (tricky . . . warming mattresses are very inefficient, since they only make contact with ⅓ of patients' body surface area. Humidi-vents don't *increase* temperature, they just prevent heat loss.)   **2. A**   **3. 1** (temperature is suboptimal, but still the best choice)

CHAPTER 148

Perioperative Nerve Injury

Mechanisms of injury

1. Compression
2. Stretching } Most common mechanisms, usually due to malpositioning
3. Surgical cutting, cautery, crushing

Which nerve is injured is usually a function of the patient position. Symptoms usually resolve spontaneously and are short-lived.

Nerves injured in supine position

1. Brachial plexus (if arm abducted > 90°)
2. Ulnar (direct compression from armboard or by BP cuff)
3. Radial (from BP cuff)

Nerves injured in lateral decubitus position

1. Suprascapular
2. Long thoracic (causes winging of scapula)
3. Peroneal (on down-side leg)

Nerves injured in prone position

1. Brachial plexus (stretching)
2. Facial
3. Trigeminal } From direct compression on face

Nerves injured in lithotomy position

1. Common peroneal nerve (inadvertant pressure on stirrup edge)
2. Lateral femoral cutaneous
3. Femoral } Kinked during hip flexion
4. Sciatic (stretching)

Nerves injured during vaginal or forceps delivery

Any and all branches of lumbosacral trunk (compressed by fetal head as it passes through birth canal)

Sample questions

Single best answer

1. After vaginal delivery of a 3500-g term infant without analgesia, a 25-year-old female receives a saddle block with 50 mg hyperbaric lidocaine in dextrose for repair of a fourth-degree vaginal tear. Five hours later she has loss of dorsiflexion ability and decreased temperature and pinprick sensation on the dorsum of her right foot. The most likely cause of this is
   1. Injection of lidocaine into the spinal cord
   2. Common peroneal nerve compression from the stirrups
   3. Lumbosacral trunk compression by the fetal head
   4. Anterior spinal artery thrombosis
   5. Epidural abscess

2. True statements regarding ulnar neuropathy include **(k-type question)**
   1. Incidence is lessened in the supine position by laterally rotating arm out of anatomic position
   2. Usually is accompanied by radial neuropathy
   3. May be caused by compression by blood pressure cuff
   4. Relief of symptoms is best managed by local anesthetic nerve block

Answers: 1. 2 2. 2

Venous Air Embolism

Clinical settings

1. Craniotomy in the sitting position: **most common**
2. Orthopedic procedures with bone reaming
3. Ventriculoatrial shunt
4. Vaginal delivery with placenta previa

Precipitated by

Large open veins and intravenous pressure less than atmospheric pressure

Pathophysiology

Embolism of small bubbles or slowly entrained ⇒ dissolve in blood or absorbed in lungs without consequence

Embolism of large bubble or quickly entrained ⇒ occlusion of pulmonary vasculature

Increased pulmonary deadspace	Increased pulmonary artery pressure
⇓	⇓
Increased arterial: end-tidal CO_2 gradient and arterial hypoxemia	Right ventricular airlock, no forward flow
	⇓
	Acute drop in cardiac output

Figure 149–1.

Summary of cardiopulmonary changes

1. *Cardiac*
   A. Cardiac output decreases
   B. Systemic arterial pressure decreases
   C. Pulmonary artery pressure increases
   D. Right atrial pressure increases
2. *Pulmonary*
   A. Increased deadspace
   B. Arterial hypoxia
   C. Arterial hypercarbia
   D. Alveolar hypocarbia

Methods for monitoring for venous air embolus

1. Transthoracic doppler: **most sensitive,** audible signal lets you tend to other duties, yields no information about size of embolus, must be placed in 3rd–6th intercostal space at right sternal border

2. Transesophageal ECHO: extremely sensitive, but nonspecific (can't distinguish air from fat emboli), requires continuous visual attention
3. End-tidal nitrogen: precedes the drop in $ETCO_2$, more sensitive than $ETCO_2$ if embolus is large
4. End-tidal CO_2: will decrease before blood pressure and cardiac output
5. Esophageal stethescope: "mill wheel" murmur heard only with large air embolus
6. Central venous catheter: is more for treatment of VAE rather than monitoring, must be multi-orifice, tip should be at superior vena cava–atrial junction. If placement is EKG directed, you will see a large negative p-wave when at the caval-atrial junction. (mid-atrial placement yields large, biphasic p waves)
7. Arterial line: for beat-to-beat assessment of blood pressure, zero and place transducer at level of head

Management of air embolus

1. Ventilate with 100% oxygen, discontinue N_2O.
2. Aspirate right heart catheter.
3. Stop further air entrainment by:
   A. Packing wound or flooding field
   B. Raising venous pressure via lowering head, applying pressure to jugular vein, adding PEEP (which can actually worsen existing hypotension)
4. CPR and vasopressors as needed.
5. Place patient in left lateral position (supposedly lets air float away from pulmonary outflow tract, but difficult to do chest compressions in this position).

Other complications associated with the sitting position

1. Paradoxical air embolus via patent foramen ovale (rare)
2. Tension pneumocephalus (consider if patient is slow to awaken)
3. Impaired venous drainage from head with resultant massive head/neck/airway edema
4. Peripheral nerve injury (sciatic stretch is a unique risk)
5. Quadriplegia (due to diminished cervical spinal cord perfusion pressure, might be prevented by zeroing arterial line at the level of the head)
6. Kinking of the endotracheal tube due to head flexion

Sample questions

Single best answer

1. During positioning of a 45-year-old male for a sitting craniotomy, the pulse oximeter decreases to 85% and the end-tidal carbon dioxide decreases to zero. The most likely cause of this is
   1. The endotracheal tube is in the esophagus
   2. Venous air embolus
   3. Acute endotracheal tube occlusion
   4. Diminished cardiac output
   5. Disconnection of the anesthesia circuit

2. A 52-year-old female is undergoing posterior fossa craniotomy in the sitting position. Monitoring includes a transthoracic doppler, CVP, and arterial blood pressure. Prior to dural incision, the patient receives a man-

nitol infusion for cerebral decompression. Five minutes after initiating the mannitol, the mean arterial pressure acutely falls from 75 mmHg to 50 mmHg, the arterial wave form dampens, the end-tidal CO_2 decreases by 10 mmHg and the CVP decreases from 6 mmHg to 4 mmHg. The most appropriate action at this time is

1. Position the patient head down, left side down and aspirate the CVP catheter.
2. Slow down the mannitol infusion.
3. Ask the neurosurgeon to flood the field with irrigant.
4. Flush the arterial catheter.
5. Increase the minute ventilation.

Answers: 1. 1   2. 2

Chapter 150

Fat Embolism

Clinic settings

1. Long-bone fracture: most common
2. Chronic steroid therapy
3. Severe burns
4. Pancreatitis

Presentation

Symptoms appear ~24 hr after the embolus occurs

1. Respiratory effects: range from hypoxia to ARDS, with increased A-aDO$_2$
2. Cardiovascular effects: tachycardia, ST segment depression
3. Central nervous system effects: range from disorientation to seizures to coma
4. Hematologic effects:
   A. Petechiae on axilla/thorax/conjunctiva
   B. Thrombocytpenia
   C. Elevated PT/PTT and fibrin split products
   D. Elevated serum lipase
5. Metabolic effects: fever

Therapy

Provide respiratory support as needed and stabilize the fracture

Sample question

A = 1, 2, 3   B = 1, 3   C = 2, 4   D = 4 only   E = all are correct

1. Early signs of fat embolism include
   1. Hypoxia
   2. Fever
   3. Tachycardia
   4. Truncal petechiae

Answer: 1. A

SECTION 13

Pharmacology

CHAPTER 151

Clonidine

(Trade names: Catapres, Yohimbine)

Mechanism of action

1. Central and peripheral presynaptic α_2-agonist, inhibits norepinephrine release
2. Minimal α_1-agonist (may cause paradoxical hypertension)
3. Decreases plasma renin levels

Routes of administration

Transcutaneous, rectal, or PO

Dosage

1. For hypertension: 0.2 mg PR or PO
2. For sedation: 3–5µg/kg PO

Bonus effects

1. Regional anesthesia: prolongs subarachnoid motor block, improves analgesia with spinals and epidurals, intrinsic subarachnoid analgesic effect
2. Decreases IV opioid requirement
3. Decreases MAC
4. Decreases intraocular pressure
5. Decreases cerebral blood flow

Clinical uses

1. Sedation
2. Induced hypotension
3. Management of preeclampsia
4. Treatment of RSD
5. Treatment of post-op shivering

Side effects

1. Sedation
2. Dry mouth
3. Impotence

4. Rebound hypertension after abrupt cessation of treatment:
   A. Occurs ~18 hr after clonidine is discontinued
   B. Develop HTN, tachycardia, headache, flushing
   C. Can be confused with postop emergence delirium/pain
   D. Can be precipitated with naloxone

Sample question

A = 1, 2, 3   B = 1, 3   C = 2, 4   D = 4 only   E = all are correct

1. A 45-year-old, 70-kg male is scheduled for herniorrhaphy for an incarcerated inguinal hernia. He takes clonidine 0.2 mg PO every morning for essential hypertension. He received 25 mg diphenhydramine PO, 1.25 mg droperidol IV, and 1 mg midazolam IV preoperatively. Upon arrival to the operating room, the patient is somewhat sedated. Medications that may be contributing to his drowsiness include
   1. Midazolam
   2. Diphenhydramine
   3. Droperidol
   4. Clonidine

Answer: 1. E

Digitalis Toxicity

Mechanisms of action

1. Inhibits $Na^+ \cdot K^+$ pump, increasing intracellular Na^+. Exchange Ca^{++} for Na^+, increasing intracellular Ca^{++} and thus, myocardial contractility.
2. Decreases conduction through AV node.
3. Increases vagal tone.

Chief clinical uses

1. Treatment of congestive heart failure
2. Control of ventricular rate in patients with atrial fibrillation

Toxic effects

1. Loss of myocardial K^+
2. AV block (often accompanied by atrial tachydysrythmias)
3. Ventricular dysrythmias, bradycardia
4. Nausea/vomiting

Factors increasing risk of digitalis toxicity

1. Hypokalemia due to:
    A. Metabolic acidosis and total body K^+ depletion
    B. Respiratory alkalosis and shifting of K^+ into cells
    C. Insulin infusion and shifting K^+ into cells
2. Hypomagnesemia
3. Hypothyroidism
4. Hypercalcemia
5. Hypoxemia
6. Nifedipine, verapamil, amiodarone

Management of acute intraoperative digitalis toxicity

Which can occur with NORMAL digoxin levels:
1. K^+ infusion to high normal levels
2. Maintain normocarbia
3. Atrial dysrythmias:
    A. Phenytoin 1.25 mg/kg IV load (maximim 15 mg/kg)
    B. Low voltage synchronized cardioversion (pretreatment with lidocaine decreases risk of secondary ventricular dysrythmia)

4. Ventricular dysrythmias:
      A. Phenytoin 1.25 mg/kg IV load
      B. Lidocaine 1 mg/kg IV load (maximum 3 mg/kg)
      C. Low-voltage synchronized cardioversion
   5. Beta-blockers: if AV block ensues, might need transvenous pacer.

BEWARE: Cardioversion can precipitate refractory V FIB!!

Sample question

Single best answer

1. A 65-kg diabetic male under general anesthesia is being mechanically ventilated with rate 10/min and tidal volume 1000 mL. He has a history of atrial fibrillation and congestive heart failure, treated with digoxin and furosemide. Shortly after incision, he develops supraventricular tachycardia. You should immediately
   1. Administer 50 mL dextrose 5% solution and 10 units regular insulin
   2. Reduce the tidal volume to 650 mL
   3. Administer adenosine
   4. Administer potassium chloride 1 mEq/min IV until resolution of the rythym
   5. Perform synchronized cardioversion at 200 joules

Answer: 1. 2

CHAPTER 153

Sodium Nitroprusside

I guarantee they will ask about this.

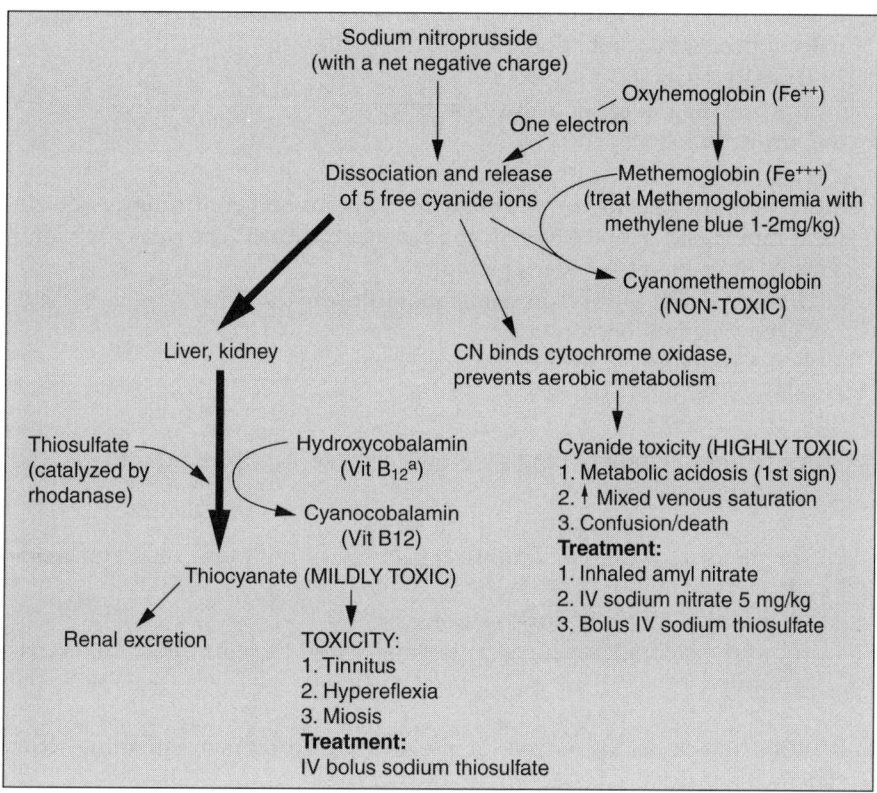

Figure 153–1.

The key features of nitroprusside metabolism are

1. Cyanide removed by: binding with methemoglobin, hydroxycobalamin or **thiosulfate**
2. Thiocyanate: production catalyzed by rhodanase, receives thiol group from body stores of thiosulfate, less toxic than cyanide
3. Cyanide not otherwise removed binds cytochrome oxidase, **extremely toxic,** metabolic acidosis first sign of toxicity
4. Increased risk of cyanide toxicity if patient has liver or renal disease, pernicious anemia

Complications of nitroprusside therapy

1. Rebound hypertension when therapy is discontinued
2. Inhibition of platelet function
3. Intrapulmonary shunting (inhibits hypoxic pulmonary vasoconstriction)
4. Hypothyroidism (prevents iodine uptake by thyroid)
5. Increased intracranial pressure

Sample questions

A = 1, 2, 3   B = 1, 3   C = 2, 4   D = 4 only   E = all are correct

1. A patient with a 30-pack-year smoking history is undergoing clipping of an intracranial aneurysm in the supine position with his head turned to the right. Preoperative pulmonary function tests are normal except for a carboxyhemoglobin level of 4%. Mean arterial pressure is decreased to 55 mmHg with IV nitroprusside 2 µg/kg/min and trimethephan 2 mg/min after the dura is opened. Ten minutes later, the pulse oximeter decreases to 85% and wheezing is noted on auscultation. Possible causes include:
   1. Endobronchial intubation
   2. Trimethephan
   3. Mucous plug in the endotracheal tube
   4. Nitroprusside

2. Same patient. After discontinuing trimethephan and confirming endotracheal tube position and patency, the wheezing clears. The pulse oximeter remains 85%. Possible causes include:
   1. Dilution of the pulse oximeter signal by ambient light
   2. Carboxyhemoglobinemia
   3. Intrapulmonary shunting due to nitroprusside
   4. Methemoglobinemia

3. Same patient. Findings that would suggest nitroprusside to be the causative factor include
   1. The presence of thiocyanate in the urine
   2. The measured arterial saturation is equal to the pulse oximeter reading
   3. An elevated mixed venous saturation
   4. The pulse oximeter returns to normal when the nitroprusside is discontinued

4. If nitroprusside is the source of the low pulse oximeter reading, true statements include:
   1. Methylene blue will improve oxygenation
   2. Amyl nitrite will improve oxygenation
   3. Sodium thiosulfate will improve oxygenation
   4. A lesser degree of desaturation would be seen if his preoperative pulmonary function tests showed moderate to severe obstruction

5. Same patient (are you sick of him yet?). Findings that would suggest carboxyhemoglobinemia as the causative agent include:
   1. An elevated mixed venous saturation
   2. Polycythemia
   3. A P_{50} value of 29 mmHg
   4. The measured arterial saturation is less than the pulse oximeter reading

Single best answer

6. Patients with renal dyfunction are unlikely to develop cyanide toxicity during nitroprusside therapy because
   1. Anemia prevents the production of methemoglobin.
   2. Thiocyanate is produced in the liver.
   3. They have a larger volume of distribution.
   4. Renal excretion of thiosulfate is decreased.
   5. Absorption of cyanocobalamin depends on intrinsic factor.

Answers: 1. A 2. A 3. C 4. D 5. D 6. 2

CHAPTER 154

Deliberate Hypotension

Clinical uses

1. Minimize blood loss while maintaining organ perfusion
2. Facilitation of cerebral aneurysm clipping

Systemic effects of hypotension

1. **CNS:** risk of ischemia if:
    A. MAP < 50 mmHg in normotensive patients (lower limit of autoregulation)
    B. MAP > ~25% below baseline blood pressure
    C. ICP is elevated

    BUT IN GENERAL: no deleterious effects of hypotension > 40 mmHg induced with isoflurane, nitroprusside, or trimethephan

2. **CVS:** risk of ischemia if:
    A. Hypotension causes reflex tachycardia, even in "healthy" patients
    B. Coronary artery disease impairs ability to maintain flow via vasodilation

    SO IN GENERAL: avoid deliberate hypotension in patients with CAD

3. **Pulmonary**
    A. Deadspace increases if concommitant drop in cardiac output occurs
    B. Shunt increases when vasodilators inhibit hypoxic pulmonary vasoconstriction

4. **Renal**
    A. Autoregulation fails if MAP < 75 mmHg
    B. Transcient oliguria occurs, but no permanent sequelae

    SO IN GENERAL: decreased urine output during deliberate hypotension is okay

Possible complications of deliberate hypotension (in addition to above)

1. Visual changes: blurring, retinal thrombosis, blindness (rare)
2. Postoperative bleeding at surgical site (impaired vasoconstriction)
3. Hypoxemia (due to inhibition of hypoxic pulmonary vasoconstriction)
4. Prolonged emergence, cerebral thrombosis

Drugs used to induce hypotension

These are the ones they always ask about.

• Table 154–1

Parameter Measured	Nitroprusside	Nitroglycerin	Trimethephan	Isoflurane
Vasodilation	Arterial > venous	Venous > arterial	Arterial = venous	Venous > arterial
Preload	↓	↓↓	↓	↓
Afterload	↓↓	—	↓	—
Cardiac output	—(↓ if hypovolemic)	—	—	—
Coronary perfusion	↓	↑		
Coronary steal	Yes	No		
Reflex tachycardia	Yes (young > old)	Yes	No effect	
Hypoxic pulmonary vasoconstriction	Inhibits most	Inhibits	No effect	Inhibits least except for trimethephan
CBF and ICP	↑ (maintains autoregulation)	↑	↑ (lose autoregulation)	↑

Specific characteristics of each of the drugs

• Table 154–2

Nitroprusside	Nitroglycerin	Trimethephan	Isoflurane
Renin-angiotensin activated, prevented with captopril Reflex tachycardia blocked by propanolol Tissue PO_2 < arterial Highly toxic	Maintains coronary flow the best	Nonspecific ganglionic blocker Tachyphylaxis Histamine release Hydrolyzed by pseudocholinesterase Potentiates succinylcholine effect	Better preservation of $CMRO_2$ than the other three drugs

Characteristics of drugs less commonly used for deliberate hypotension

1. Hydralazine: smooth-muscle relaxant/↓ SVR/no Δ cardiac output/↑ ICP
2. Phentolamine: α-blocker/↓ SVR/no Δ ICP
3. Esmolol: β-blocker/↓ cardiac output/↑ SVR /↓ renin-angiotension system
4. Labetolol: $α_1$-, $β_1$-, $β_2$-blocker/↓ cardiac output/↓ SVR/no Δ ICP/long duration
5. Adenosine: Arterial dilation/↑ cardiac output/coronary vasodilator but causes "steal"/↑ ICP

Sample questions

A = 1, 2, 3   B = 1, 3   C = 2, 4   D = 4 only   E = all are correct

1. Compared to nitroprusside, trimethephan
   1. Causes less intrapulmonary shunting
   2. Preserves coronary artery flow better
   3. Causes more bronchospasm
   4. Increases cerebral blood flow more

2. Shortly after induction of general anesthesia for clipping of an intracranial aneurysm, the blood pressure of a normotensive patient is lowered to 50 mmHg with IV trimethephan 2 mg/min and nitroprusside 2 µg/kg/min. During emergence, the patient's pupils are noted to be markedly dilated. Possible explanations for this include
   1. Decreased cerebral perfusion pressure prior to opening the dura
   2. Cyanide toxicity
   3. Expected effect of trimethephan
   4. Thiocyanate toxicity

3. Compared to nitroprusside, nitroglycerin
   1. Decreases tone in capacitance vessels more
   2. Is less toxic
   3. Maintains coronary artery flow better
   4. Causes less intrapulmonary shunting

4. Inducing deliberate hypotension to a mean arterial pressure of 55 mmHg with nitroprusside causes
   1. Increased mixed venous saturation
   2. Decreased ventilation/perfusion ratio
   3. Decreased physiologic deadspace
   4. Decreased PaO_2

Answers: 1. B   2. B   3. E   4. E

CHAPTER 155

Furosemide versus Mannitol

● Table 155–1

	Furosemide	Mannitol
Drug classification:	Loop diuretic	Osmotic diuretic
Mechanism of action	Inhibits active resorption of Cl^- at ascending thick loop accompanied by Na^+, Ca^{++}, large Na^+ load to distal tubule causes K^+ and H^+ loss in exchange for Na^+	Filtered at glomerulus and not resorbed by tubules, causes osmotic diuresis. Increased flow through nephrons impairs Na^+ resorption
Pharmacodynamics	↑ renal blood flow ↑ renin production ? protects against ischemic renal failure Systemic vasodilation and lowered LV filling pressures (seen before diuresis occurs) Normal serum osmolality ↓ ICP by diuresis and reduces CSF production	↑ renal blood flow ↓ renin production ? protects against ischemic renal failure Transcient ↑ extracellular volume, may precipitate CHF ↑ serum osmolality ↓ ICP by diuresis, ↓ CSF production
Side effects	Hypotension Vasodilation Potentiates curare (see Chapter 167, Neuromuscular Relaxants) Hyponatremia Hypochloremic metabolic alkalosis ↓ K^+, Ca^{++}, Mg^{++} Hyperglycemia Hyperuricemia (prerenal) Ototoxicity Nephrotoxicity	Hypotension Vasodilation No effect on curare Hyponatremia CHF, pulmonary edema Histamine release

Sample questions

A = 1, 2, 3   B = 1, 3   C = 2, 4   D = 4 only   E = all are correct

1. Electrolyte and metabolic effects of both mannitol and furosemide include
   1. Hyponatremia
   2. Hypokalemia
   3. Decreased production of CSF
   4. Hyperglycemia

2. A 67-kg diabetic patient under goes a 3-hr craniotomy during which he receives mannitol 65 g and lactated Ringer's 2000 mL. His urine output was 800 mL intraoperatively and is 1000 mL after 45 min in the recovery room. Possible causes include:
   1. Hyperglycemia
   2. Excessive fluid administration intraoperatively
   3. Mannitol-induced osmotic diuresis
   4. Nephrogenic diabetes insipidus

3. Effects of mannitol during cerebral aneurysm clipping include
   1. Transcient rise in ICP
   2. Increased production of cerebrospinal fluid
   3. Transcient increase in intravascular volume
   4. Increased renin levels

Single best answer

4. Furosemide causes diuresis by
   1. Aldosterone inhibition
   2. Altered distribution of renal blood flow
   3. Potentiation of carbonic anhydrase
   4. Antagonism of antidiuretic hormone
   5. Altered tubular reabsorption

Answers: 1. B   2. B   3. B   4. 5

CHAPTER 156

Thiopental

Class: Barbiturate

Mechanism of action

Binds GABA receptor, decreases dissociation of GABA from receptor

Systemic effects

CNS: ↓ CBF, ICP, and $CMRO_2$, may ↑ CPP if drop in ICP exceeds drop in MAP.
SSEP: ↑ latency and ↓ amplitude
CVS: ↓ MAP, SVR, CVP, CO, and myocardial contractility, ↑ HR
Respiratory: ↓ VT, minute ventilation and causes right shift of CO_2 response curve
Renal: RBF changes correlate with changes on cardiac output
Endocrine: ↑ antidiuretic hormone, no adrenal supression
Analgesia: antianalgesic effect

Clinical effect terminated by

1. **For single bolus:** redistribution
2. **For repeat doses/infusions:**
    A. Hepatic metabolism (slow 2° to high protein binding)
    B. Uptake by adipose tissue (which is slow, but becomes important as hepatic enzymes get saturated and lean tissue concentration equilibrates with blood levels)

Metabolism

Hepatic (liver disease decreases protein binding of thiopental): **slow,** because hepatic extraction ratio is low (0.15) and % protein binding is high (85%)

Excretion

Renal (renal disease decreases protein binding of thiopental)

Side effects

Histamine release

Contraindications

1. Acute intermittent porphyria
2. H/o asthma or anaphylaxis (relative contraindication)

Sample questions

A = 1, 2, 3   B = 1, 3   C = 2, 4   D = 4 only   E = all are correct

1. Repetitive doses of thiopental will result in delayed emergence because
   1. It is taken up by adipose tissue and released very slowly
   2. Hepatic metabolism of thiopental is slow
   3. The capacity of lean tissues to dilute the thiopental is reduced
   4. The hepatic extraction ratio decreases

2. Clinical effects of thiopental include
   1. Renal vasodilation
   2. Increased water reabsorption by the kidney
   3. Decreased cerebrospinal fluid production
   4. Heightened sensitivity to pain

Answers: 1. A   2. C

Chapter 157

Comparison of Thiopental and Methohexital

They like to ask about these, since they're the most commonly used barbiturates.

Mechanism of action

Bind GABA receptors, preventing GABA dissociation. Also increase Cl- conduction, hyperpolarizing the neuron and preventing firing.

Pharmacokinetic profiles

• Table 157–1

	pK	% Ionized at pH 7.4	Lipid Solubility	Potency	% Protein Bound	Volume of Distribution (L/kg)	Clearance	t½β (hr)	Hepatic Extraction Ratio	Single Bolus Effect Ends by
Thiopental	7.5	40	High	1	~85	~2	~3	~8	0.1	Redistribution
Methohexital	7.9	25	High	2.5	~85	~2	~10	~3	0.5	Redistribution

The take-home message

1. They have roughly the same degree of ionization, lipid solubility, and protein binding; *therefore,* onset time of clinical effect is the same.
2. They have roughly the same volume of distribution and protein binding; *therefore,* the much shorter half-life of methohexital is due to its very high rate of clearance.
3. They both depend on redistribution to terminate the effect of a single bolus, *but* methohexital is less likely to accumulate with repeated doses due to its high rate of clearance.

Complications/contraindications

Both: are contraindicated in acute intermittent porphyria
Methohexital causes more: excitation and pain on injection, but no histamine release, arterial spasm or skin sloughing from infiltrated IV
Thiopental causes more: venous thrombosis, histamine release, skin sloughing if IV is infiltrated, and arterial spasm if injected into artery

Management of arterial injection of thiopental

Spasm → pain → ischemia → gangrene → loss of tissue

1. Relieve spasm:
   A. Brachial plexus/stellate ganglion block (improves blood flow)
   B. Papaverine/lidocaine/procaine (vasodilation)
2. Dilute the drug: saline flush
3. Prevent thrombosis: give IV heparin

Factors that decrease barbiturate dose requirements

1. Burns ⎫
2. Malnutrition ⎪
3. Malignancy ⎬ ↓ protein binding
4. Uremia ⎪
5. Cirrhosis ⎭
6. Shock
7. Hypothermia (↓ $CMRO_2$)
8. Acute intoxication (sober alcoholics need more)
9. Anemia
10. Acidosis (↑ nonionized drug, so more crosses the blood–brain barrier)

For systemic effects of barbiturates, read Chapter 156, Thiopental, and Chapter 161, Comparison of Physiologic Effects and Pharmacokinetics of Thiopental, Propofol, Etomidate, and Ketamine. Methohexital exerts the same effects as thiopental, except it produces even more tachycardia and less vasodilation.

Chapter 158

Propofol

Class: Hindered phenol

Mechanism of action

Enhances GABA transmission

Systemic effects

CNS: ↓ CBF, ICP, CMRO$_2$, CPP (CPP drops due to drop in MAP).
SSEP: ↑ latency, ↓ amplitude
CVS: ↓ MAP, SVR, CVP, CO, myocardial contractility and HR (changes are more profound than those seen with thiopental)
Respiratory: ↓ VT, minute ventilation and right shift of CO$_2$ response curve
Renal: RBF changes correlate to changes in cardiac output
Endocrine: ↑ antidiuretic hormone, no adrenal supression
Analgesia: none

Clinical effect terminated by

1. **For single bolus:** redistribution and rapid hepatic metabolism
2. **For infusion:** hepatic metabolism, following return from deep compartment to central compartment

Metabolism

1. Hepatic: very fast (hepatic disease not reported to alter pharmacokinetics)
2. Extra-hepatic (mechanism unknown)
3. Protein binding: 98%
4. Clearance: exceeds hepatic blood flow

Excretion

Renal (renal disease not reported to alter pharmacokinetics)

Side effects

1. Histamine release
2. Myoclonus
3. Pain on injection

Contraindications

No absolute contraindications, but beware of hypovolemia and patients who can't tolerate profound hypotension

Sample questions

A = 1, 2, 3   B = 1, 3   C = 2, 4   D = 4 only   E = all are correct

1. A 50-year-old, 65-kg man with stable angina undergoing exploratory laparotomy for small-bowel obstruction has a blood pressure of 105/63 mmHg, pulse 99/min, and temperature 38°C. Rapid-sequence induction is performed with propofol 130 mg IV and succinylcholine. True statements regarding his expected cardiovascular responses include
   1. He will be more hypotensive than if he had been induced with thiopental 260 mg IV
   2. Reflex tachycardia is likely
   3. Myocardial ischemia is more likely than with thiopental
   4. Allergic reaction to propofol is more likely than with thiopental

2. The rapid recovery from a single bolus of propofol is due to
   1. Urinary excretion of conjugated metabolites
   2. Hepatic conjugation to glucuronide
   3. The lack of hypnotic activity of metabolites
   4. Redistribution to lean tissues

Answer: 1. B   2. C

CHAPTER 159

Etomidate

Class: Imidazole

Mechanism of action

Increased GABA transmission

Systemic effects

CNS: ↓ CBF, ICP, $CMRO_2$, may ↑ CPP since MAP is maintained.
  SSEP: ↑ latency and amplitude
CVS: no change in MAP, SVR, CVP, CO, myocardial contractility, or HR
Respiratory: ↓ VT, minute ventilation, and right shift of CO_2 response curve
Renal: RBF changes correlate to any changes in cardiac output
Endocrine: ↑ antidiuretic hormone, causes adrenal suppression
Eyes: ↑ intraocular pressure
Analgesia: none

Clinical effect terminated by

1. **For single bolus:** redistribution and rapid hepatic metabolism
2. **For infusion:** hepatic metabolism

Metabolism

1. Hepatic: fast (but hepatic disease may increase volume of distribution)
2. Hepatic extraction ratio high (0.5)
3. Protein binding high (75%)

Excretion

Renal (renal disease may increase volume of distribution)

Side effects

1. Myoclonus/epileptogenesis
2. Pain on injection
3. Adrenal suppression
4. High incidence of nausea/vomiting

Contraindications

1. Acute intermittent porphyria
2. Patients with seizure disorders

Sample question

A = 1, 2, 3   B = 1, 3   C = 2, 4   D = 4 only   E = all are correct

1. Possible side effects of prolonged infusion of etomidate include
   1. Hyponatremia
   2. Elevated ACTH
   3. Hyperkalemia
   4. Hypotension not responsive to ephedrine

Answer: 1. E (inhibition of 11 β-hydroxylase blocks production of cortisol and aldosterone)

Chapter 160

Ketamine

Class: Arylcyclohexylamine (related to phencylidine . . . PCP)

Mechanism of action

Dissociation between thalamocortical and limbic systems, interacts with CNS acetylcholine and spinal opiate receptors

Systemic effects

CNS: ↑ CBF, ICP, CMRO$_2$, may ↓ CPP since ICP is increased. SSEP: no change in latency, ↑ amplitude
CVS: ↑ MAP, SVR, and HR, no change in CVP, CO. Myocardial contractility can be decreased if catecholamines are depleted
Respiratory: ↓ VT, minute ventilation, right shift of CO$_2$ response curve, bronchodilation, maintain airway reflexes
Renal: RBF changes correlate to any changes in cardiac output
Endocrine: no increase in antidiuretic hormone, no adrenal supression
Analgesia: good analgesic effect

Clinical effect terminated by

1. **For single bolus:** redistribution
2. **For infusion:** hepatic metabolism

Metabolism

1. Hepatic: fast (alterations in hepatic blood flow will affect clearance)
2. Hepatic extraction ratio is high
3. Protein binding 12% (high percent of free drug aids metabolism)

Excretion

Renal

Side effects

1. Histamine release
2. Myoclonus (doubtful if it's truly epileptogenic)
3. Dysphoria/hallucinations

Contraindications

Intracranial hypertension

Sample question

A = 1, 2, 3   B = 1, 3   C = 2, 4   D = 4 only   E = all are correct

1. A patient with a history of daily cocaine abuse, abdominal pain, and vomiting for the last 3 days is undergoing an emergent appendectomy. Rapid-sequence induction is performed with ketamine and succinylcholine. After induction, his blood pressure is 88/54 mmHg, pulse 99/min, and he remains so even after incision. Possible causes include
   1. Myocardial depression by ketamine
   2. Ventricular dysfunction due to unrecognized prior myocardial infarction
   3. Depleted stores of endogenous catecholamines
   4. Relative hypovolemia

Answer: 1. E

Chapter 161

Comparison of Physiologic Effects and Pharmacokinetics of Thiopental, Propofol, Etomidate, and Ketamine

Central nervous system effects

• Table 161–1

Drug	CBF	ICP	CMRO$_2$	CPP	SSEP
Thiopental	↓	↓	↓	↑ or no change	↑ latency ↓ amplitude
Propofol	↓	↓	↓	↓ or no change	↑ latency ↓ amplitude
Etomidate	↓	↓	↓	↑	↑ latency and amplitude
Ketamine	⇑	⇑	⇑	⇓	No difference in latency, ↑ amplitude

Cardiovascular effects

• Table 161–2

Drug	MAP	SVR	CVP (venodilation)	Cardiac Output	Contractility	HR
Thiopental	↓	↓	↓	↓	↓	⇑
Propofol	↓↓	↓↓	↓↓	↓↓	↓↓	↓↓
Etomidate	No change	No change	No change	No change	No change	No change
Ketamine	↑	↑	No change	No change	No change or ↓ if catechols are depleted	↑

Pharmacokinetic profiles

- Table 161-3

Drug	Volume of Distribution (L)	Hepatic Extraction Ratio	Protein Binding (%)	Elimination Half-life ($t_{1/2}\beta$) (hr)
Thiopental	100–200	0.15	85	10
Propofol	200–500	~1	98	1.5
Etomidate	200–500	0.9	75	2.5
Ketamine	200	~1	12	2.5

Sample questions

A = 1, 2, 3   B = 1, 3   C = 2, 4   D = 4 only   E = all are correct

1. Administration of halothane will increase the elimination half-life of
   1. Ketamine
   2. Propofol
   3. Etomidate
   4. Thiopental

2. The short elimination half-life of propofol is due to
   1. Rapid hepatic conjugation
   2. The high degree of protein binding
   3. Extrahepatic mechanisms
   4. Renal excretion

3. A decrease in hepatic blood flow will prolong elimination of
   1. Thiopental
   2. Ketamine
   3. Propofol
   4. Etomidate

4. Myoclonus is a side effect of
   1. Ketamine
   2. Propofol
   3. Etomidate
   4. Thiopental

Single best answer

5. The difference in elimination half-life between thiopental and propofol is primarily due a difference in
   1. The degree of protein binding
   2. The rate of renal excretion
   3. The rate of hepatic metabolism
   4. The volume of distribution
   5. Redistribution to vessel-poor groups

Answers: 1. A   2. B   3. C   4. A   5. 3

Chapter 162

Benzodiazepines

Featuring their favorite three: midazolam, diazepam, and lorazepam.

Mechanism of action: Enhance GABA transmission and mimic glycine (both are inhibitory neurotransmitters).

Pharmacokinetic characteristics

• Table 162–1

	% Protein Binding	Distribution Half-life (min)	Elimination Half-life (hr)	Volume of Distribution (L/kg)	Clearance (mg/kg/min)	Relative Potency	Lipid Solubility
Lorazepam	90	3	15	1	1	5	Least (Lorazepam)
Midazolam	94	15	3	2	7	3	Most (Midazolam)
Diazepam	98	30	20–50!!!	1	0.2	1	

Take-home message

1. Protein binding and volume of distribution all roughly the same.
2. Clearances vary greatly and are predictive of elimination half-life.
3. Termination of clinical effect of single bolus is by redistribution.

Systemic effects of benzodiazepines

CNS: all three cause ↓ CBF, $CMRO_2$, reduction in MAC and no Δ ICP. Central muscular relaxation
CVS: all three cause mild ↓ SVR, MAP, and slight reflex tachycardia
Respiratory: decreased minute ventilation response for any given $PaCO_2$

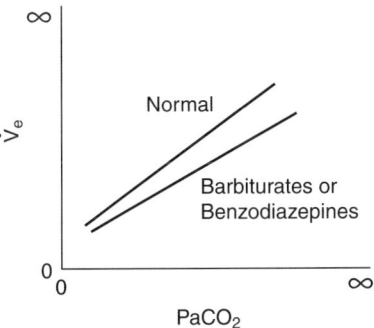

Figure 162–1.

Metabolism

1. All three undergo hepatic metabolism.
2. Only diazepam has clinically significant active metabolites.
3. $t_{1/2}\ \beta$ of metabolite > parent diazepam, so repeated doses leads to accumulation of both.

Special considerations

1. There is ↑ volume of distribution and ↓ elimination in elderly and cirrhotic patients.
2. Cimetidine decreases the clearance of diazepam.

Sample question

A = 1, 2, 3   B = 1, 3   C = 2, 4   D = 4 only   E = all are correct

1. The dose of diazepam should be reduced in patients
   1. With hepatic insufficiency
   2. Who are elderly
   3. Also taking cimetidine
   4. Also taking tricyclic antidepressants

Answer: 1. A

Chapter 163

Flumazenil

Class: Benzodiazepine antagonist (an imidazobenzodiazepine derivative)

Mechanism of action

Binds specifically to benzodiazepine receptor and antagonizes all clinical effects: Hypnosis, muscle relaxation, amnesia, sedation, anticonvulsant effect, anxiolysis

Dosing

1. The more potent the benzodiazepine, the higher the required dose of flumazenil. Potency: lorazepam > midazolam > diazepam
2. Dose required for reversal of clinical effects varies: hypnosis (smallest dose) > muscle relaxation > amnesia > sedation > anticonvulsant > anxiolysis (biggest dose of flumazenil)

Systemic effects

No significant effects on any system except **CNS**: weak intrinsic anticonvulsant activity transient reversal of hepatic encephalopathy no change in CBF or ICP.

Metabolism

Hepatic (no active metabolites)

Excretion

Renal (90%), fecal (10%)

Pharmacokinetics

- Table 163–1

Onset (min)	Elimination Half-life (min)	Duration of Effect (hr)	% Protein Binding	Hepatic Extraction Ratio
5	60	1–3.5	50	0.6

Complications/warnings

1. Precipitates withdrawal in benzodiazepine-dependent patients
2. Resedation occurs if used with long-acting benzodiazepine (diazepam)

Sample questions

A = 1, 2, 3   B = 1, 3   C = 2, 4   D = 4 only   E = all are correct

1. Flumazenil will reverse the effects of
   1. Methohexital
   2. Ethyl alcohol
   3. Morphine
   4. Oxazepam

2. The brief duration of benzodiazepine antagonism by flumazenil is due to its
   1. Low protein binding
   2. High degree of renal excretion
   3. High hepatic extraction ratio
   4. High degree of ionization at pH 7.4

Answers: 1. D   2. B

CHAPTER 164

Opioids

Opioids have specific receptors, which are most heavily concentrated in

1. The periaqueductal gray area of the brain
2. The substantia gelatinosa of the spinal cord

Opioid receptors and the effects they mediate

mu_1	mu_2	kappa	sigma
Supraspinal analgesia	Respiratory depression	Spinal analgesia	Dysphoria
	↓ GI motility	Respiratory depression	Hallucinations
	Cardiovascular effects	Sedation	
		Miosis	

Systemic effects of opioids

CNS:
1. Analgesia, mood alteration, cough supression, nausea/vomiting
2. Myoclonus/myotonic activity without EEG changes. Exception: meperidine metabolite normeperidine is truly epileptogenic
3. Muscle rigidity: specifically, rigidity of chest wall and laryngeal/pharyngeal muscles. Note: it's a centrally mediated rigidity, but neuromuscular blockers will attenuate the effect.

CVS:
1. Dose-dependent bradycardia (mediated by vagus, attenuated by atropine). Exception: meperidine, which is structurally similar to atropine, produces tachycardia
2. Arterial and venous vasodilation
   A. Morphine, meperidine: dilation due to histamine release, morphine reduction of blood pressure greater than with fentanyl, sufentanil or alfentanil
   B. Fentanyl, sufentanil, alfentanil: dilation due to direct effect or neurogenic action
3. Myocardial contractility is maintained. Exception: meperidine decreases contractility at clinically used doses
4. Prolonged AV conduction and decreased SA node activity (minimal)

Respiratory:
1. Respiratory depression (at equianalgesic doses, all opioids produce same amount)
2. Low doses ↓ respiratory rate, higher doses ↓ V_T too
3. CO_2 response shifts to right (a higher CO_2 is required to stimulate breathing, but once stimulated, the response is equal to nonmedicated patient)

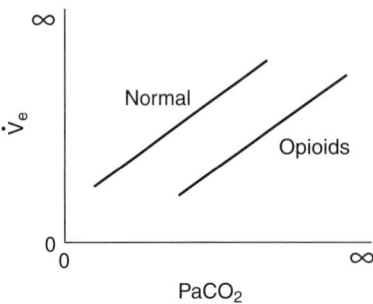

Figure 164–1.

4. In the asleep/medicated patient, the response will be flattened, as well as shifted right
5. Response to hypoxia is also blunted

GI:
1. Opioids produce smooth-muscle spasm, leading to:
   A. Intestinal hypertonus, but decreased peristalsis (delayed gastric emptying)
   B. Sphincter of Oddi spasm. Degree of sphincter spasm: fentanyl > morphine > meperidine > codeine > butorphanol. Reversal of spasm can be achieved with: (1) naloxone; (2) glucagon; (3) nitroglycerin; (4) atropine

Renal/GU:
1. Ureteral spasm (despite alleviating pain due to kidney stones)
2. Increased tone of bladder detrusor and urinary sphincter (get urinary retention)

Endocrine:
1. Inhibition of GnRH, CRF, cortisol release
2. Increased levels of prolaction, growth hormone

Pregnancy: Nonteratogenic, but risk of fetal addiction

Metabolism

1. Hepatic
2. Active metabolites with:
   A. Morphine: morphine 6-glucuronide, analgesic effect > parent compound
   B. Meperidine: normeperidine, half the analgesic effect of parent compound, but very powerful convulsant effect

Excretion

1. Renal
2. Percentage of drug excreted unchanged in urine (most affected by renal insufficiency):

   morphine > meperidine > fentanyl > sufentanil ≈ alfentanil

Pharmacokinetic characteristics

- Table 164–1

Drug	$t_{1/2} \alpha$ (min)	$t_{1/2} \beta$ (hr)	Vdss (L/kg)	Clearance (mg/kg/min)	Hepatic Extraction Ratio	Octanol/H_2O Partition Coefficient (lipid sol.)	% Protein Binding	% Ionized at pH 7.4	pKa
Morphine	1.5	4	3.5	15	.7	1.5	35	75	7.9
Meperidine	5	4	3	15	.5	40	65	95	8.5
Fentanyl	12	5	4	12	.6	850	80	90	8.5
Sufentanil	18	2.5	1.5	13	.7	1800	90	80	8
Alfentanil	12	1.5	0.8	6.5	.6	150	90	10	6.5

Take-home message

1. Morphine's clinical effects do not parallel its pharmacokinetics because its low lipid solubility delays entry into CNS.
2. Although alfentanil has a much slower hepatic clearance than fentanyl, its total body clearance is much greater due to a very small volume of distribution as well as a lower lipid solubilty, which keeps more of the drug in the blood and available for metabolism.
3. Although the clinical effects of fentanyl are much shorter than morphine, fentanyl has a longer elimination half-life due to its large volume of distribution.
4. All have high hepatic extraction ratios (are dependent on hepatic blood flow for clearance).

Highlights of specific agents

1. **Morphine:**
   A. Least lipid soluble
   B. **Most likely** opioid to accumulate active metabolites in the presence of renal disease
   C. Plasma concentration achieved after IM injection > IV, because IV dose is rapidly distributed to steady-state volume
2. **Meperidine:** active metabolite accumulates if renal disease present, produces seizures

Side effects (as occur at equianalgesic doses)

1. Nausea/vomiting: all opioids produce same amount
2. Respiratory depression: all opioids produce same amount
3. Histamine release: meperidine > morphine. The others don't release histamine.

Drug interactions

1. MAO inhibitors: LIFE-THREATENING hyperpyrexia/excitation reaction with meperidine
2. Propanolol: decreased first-pass effect of fentanyl by lungs
3. Amphetamines, clonidine: increase analgesic effects of opioids
4. Cimetidine: prolongs elimination half-life of fentanyl
5. MAOI, TCA, phenopthiazines: exaggerate/prolong depressant effect of all opioids

Sample questions

A = 1, 2, 3   B = 1, 3   C = 2, 4   D = 4 only   E = all are correct

1. Intramuscular premedication with morphine
   1. Produces higher serum concentrations than IV injection with the same dose
   2. Alters the response to carbon dioxide for 10 hr
   3. Produces sphincter of Oddi spasm
   4. Is contraindicated in patients with asthma

2. In patients with congestive heart failure, morphine is preferred over fentanyl because
   1. Fentanyl has no vasodilating properties
   2. Morphine produces bradycardia
   3. Fentanyl causes coronary artery "steal"
   4. Morphine lowers systemic vascualar resistance

3. The slow onset of analgesia by morphine is due to
   1. Low lipid solubility and delayed entry into the CNS
   2. A short elimination half-life
   3. A high degree of ionization at pH 7.4
   4. A large volume of distribution

4. Decreased hepatic blood flow will significantly increase the elimination half-life of
   1. Morphine
   2. Meperidine
   3. Fentanyl
   4. Sufentanil

5. Opioids whose metabolites possess analgesic activity include
   1. Morphine
   2. Fentanyl
   3. Meperidine
   4. Alfentanil

6. A 72-year-old, 65-kg man undergoes induction of general anesthesia with thiopental 300 mg, succinylcholine 130 mg, and fentanyl 150 µg. He is ventilated with N_2O/O_2 (70/30) prior to intubation. During laryngoscopy, his jaw is difficult to open. Possible causes include
   1. Fentanyl
   2. Early stage malignant hyperthermia
   3. Nitrous oxide synergism of opioid- induced muscle rigidity
   4. Succinylcholine-induced masseter spasm

7. A patient with a history of cholecystitis and angina complains of substernal chest pain, nausea, and shortness of breath. The EKG is normal. The diagnosis of biliary colic can be made by
   1. Cholangiogram
   2. Worsening of symptoms following administration of meperidine
   3. Relief of symptoms following administration of glucagon
   4. Relief of symptoms following administration of nitroglycerin

Single best answer

8. Meperidine has a faster onset of analgesia than morphine because its
   1. Lipid solubility is higher
   2. Volume of distribution is smaller
   3. Redistribution to vessel-rich groups is slower
   4. Protein binding is higher
   5. Ionization at pH 7.4 is higher

9. Despite having a longer elimination half-life than morphine, fentanyl has a shorter duration of action due to
   1. A higher hepatic extraction ratio
   2. Redistribution
   3. Lower protein binding
   4. Less ionization at pH 7.4
   5. Rapid renal excretion

Answers: 1. E 2. D 3. B 4. E 5. B 6. E 7. A 8. 1 9. 2

CHAPTER 165

Mixed Narcotic Agonists/Antagonists

Definitions
1. **Competitive antagonist:** binds mu-receptor only, has no intrinsic activity but blocks opioid effects
2. **Partial agonist:** binds mu-receptor only, exerts limited effect
3. **Agonist/antagonist:** all drugs in this class are mu-antagonists with agonist activity at kappa sigma (predominantly kappa). **Exceptions:**
   A. Nalbuphine: mu activity is partial agonist
   B. Nalorphine: kappa activity is partial agonist

Which drugs are which?
1. Competitive antagonist: naloxone, naltrexone
2. Partial agonist: buprenorphine (by binding receptor, it effectively "antagonizes" opioids)
3. Agonist/antagonist: butorphanol, pentazocine, nalbuphine, nalorphine

Review of opioid receptors and the effects they mediate

Mu	Analgesia	Respiratory depression	Euphoria (mu-phoria)	Addiction
Kappa	Analgesia	Respiratory depression	Sedation	
Delta			Dysphoria	

Strength of mu-receptor antagonism

Naloxone > buprenorphine > nalorphine > nalbuphine > pentazocine > butorphanol

Strength of analgesic effect compared to morphine

Buprenorphine > butorphanol > nalbuphine, nalorphine > pentazocine

Comparison of the narcotic agonists/antagonists

● Table 165–1

Drug	Analgesic Potency (morphine = 1)	Produces Respiratory Depression	Induces Withdrawal in Opioid Addicts	Abuse Potential	Incidence of Dysphoria	Cardiovascular Effects
Buprenorphine	25	+++	No		Low	None
Butorphanol	5	+	No	Low	High	↑ PAP, ↓ MAP and HR
Pentazocine	¼	+	Yes	High	High	↑ PAP, MAP, HR
Nalbupine	1	+	Yes	High	Low	None
Nalorphine	1	+	Yes	Low	High	None

NOTES:
1. Unlike narcotics, the mixed agonists/antagonists have a "ceiling" to their analgesic and respiratory depressant effects. Higher doses don't provide more analgesia or respiratory depression.
2. While they do all reduce MAC, the effect is less than with narcotics.
3. Buprenorphine is noteworthy for withdrawal symptoms upon discontinuation of chronic use.

Naloxone

1. Receptors antagonized: mu, kappa, sigma **(predominantly mu)**
2. Onset time (min): 1–2
3. Elimination half-life (min): 60 (less than morphine, meperidine and fentanyl)
4. Duration of effect (hr): 1–4 (depends on dose of narcotic)
5. Drugs it can reverse: All narcotics and mixed agonists/antagonists (buprenorphine requires very large doses)

Side effects/complications

1. All narcotic effects are reversed in parallel (respiratory depression goes away, but so does analgesia)
2. Hypertension, dysrythmias (? catechol release due to pain)
3. Pulmonary edema
4. Death
5. Withdrawal in opioid-dependent patients

Sample questions

A = 1, 2, 3   B = 1, 3   C = 2, 4   D = 4 only   E = all are correct

1. Premedication with buprenorphine
    1. Produces respiratory depression that can be prevented by prior administration of naloxone
    2. Precipitates withdrawal symptoms in opiod-dependent patients
    3. Reduces the analgesic effect of subsequent doses of fentanyl
    4. Produces respiratory depression that it easily reversed with naloxone

2. 2 mg of butorphanol given IV
   1. Produces the same amount of respiratory depression as 10 mg IV morphine
   2. Will increase pulmonary artery pressure
   3. Is equianalgesic to 10 mg IV morphine
   4. Produces a withdrawal syndrome in opioid-dependent patients

Single best answer

3. A 68-year-old, 70-kg female has just completed a 5-hr total hip arthroplasty. Preoperative EKG shows lateral T-wave inversion. Preoperative medications include NPH insulin and propanolol. General anesthesia includes morphine 20 mg, thiopental 350 mg, vecuronium, nitrous oxide, and oxygen. Train-of-four stimulation is $1/4$, and atropine 1 mg and neostigmine 5 mg are given IV. Five minutes later, spontaneous tidal volume is 500 mL, respiratory rate 10/min, pupils are midline and 2 mm in size, pulse 140/min, blood pressure 180/95 mmHg, and the patient is diaphoretic. Despite no measurable end-tidal volatile agent, she is unarousable. The most appropriate action at this time is
   1. Administer naloxone 0.1 mg IV
   2. Administer esmolol 10 mg IV
   3. Administer 25 mL of 5% dextrose IV
   4. Extubate the patient
   5. Administer neostigmine 2 mg IV

Answers: 1. B   2. A   3. 3

CHAPTER 166

Ketorolac

Class: Nonsteroidal antiinflammatory

Mechanism of action

Reduces prostaglandin synthesis by inhibiting cyclooxygenase, the enzyme necessary for converting arachidonic acid to prostaglandins

Route of administration

PO, IV, IM

Clinical effects

1. Analgesic: potency of 10–30 mg IM ketorolac = 12 mg IM MSO_4 analgesia when combined with opioid > analgesia ketorolac only
2. Antipyretic
3. Inhibition of platelet function

Advantages over opioids

Less nausea, sedation, respiratory depression and no addictive element

Use with caution if

1. Hepatic disease present (undergoes hepatic metabolism)
2. Renal disease present (undergoes renal excretion, can also precipitate acute renal insufficiency, hyperkalemia, and fluid overload)
3. Prolonged bleeding poses risk of adverse outcome (e.g., tonsillectomy, craniotomy)

Contraindications

1. Nasal polyps
2. h/o bronchospastic reaction to aspirin or other NSAIDs
3. h/o angioedema

Side effects

1. Somnolence
2. GI upset
3. Platelet inhibition
4. Elevated LFTs
5. Peptic ulceration/GI bleeding
6. Acute renal insufficiency

Sample questions

A = 1, 2, 3   B = 1, 3   C = 2, 4   D = 4 only   E = all are correct

1. Compared to meperidine, ketorolac
   1. Causes less somnolence
   2. Is approximately half as potent for treating moderate pain
   3. Produces less respiratory depression
   4. Has equal affinity for mu-receptors

Single best answer

2. A 24-year-old female is having endoscopic sinus surgery and removal of nasal polyps. She complains of shortness of breath with exertion, which is relieved with over-the-counter sympathomimetics. Postoperative analgesia should be achieved with
   1. Ketorolac
   2. Morphine
   3. Fentanyl
   4. Acetominophen with codiene
   5. Naproxen

Answers: 1. A   2. 3

CHAPTER 167

Neuromuscular Relaxants

(Only the ones commonly used in the United States)

There are 2 main classes

1. Depolarizers: succinylcholine
2. Nondepolarizers: all the rest

Mechanisms of action (pharmacodynamics)

1. Depolarizers: bind postsynaptic nicotinic receptors, induce depolarization and flaccid paralysis
2. Nondepolarizers: bind one of the two alpha subunits of the postsynaptic nicotinic receptor and competitively antagonize ACH, but lack intrinsic activity
3. Both classes also block, by two mechanisms, the ion channels used for repolarization/depolarization
   A. Open channel blockade: all the relaxants are charged molecules and are electrochemically attracted to Na^+, Ca^{++}, and K^+ channels. They enter and bind channels, blocking ingress/egress of ions and ability to repolarize. This is noncompetitive blockade and can be accentuated by ACH or anticholinesterases.
   B. Closed channel blockade: relaxants prevent channels from ever opening (this is how aminoglycosides act)

Characteristics of nondepolarizing blockade

1. Train of four: fade
2. Tetanus: fade
3. Posttetanic stimulation: yes

Clinical significance of the pharmacokinetics of nondepolarizers

• Table 167–1

Drug	Elimination Pathway	Duration in Renal Disease	Duration in Hepatic Disease	Duration in Elderly	Duration in Neonates	Duration in Pseudocholinesterase Deficiency
d-Tubocurarine	Renal = biliary	↑	↑	↑	↑	No change
Pancuronium	Renal	↑	No change	↑	↑	No change
Vecuronium	**Biliary (unchanged)**, renal excretion of metabolites	↑ (slight)	↑	↑	↑	No change
Atracurium	**Ester hydrolysis**, Hoffman degradation	No change	No change	No change	No change	Possibly increased
Mivacurium	Plasma cholinesterase hydrolysis	No change	No change	No change	No change	Increased

Factors causing residual blockade despite adequate doses of reversal

1. Hypothermia
2. Intense block prior to reversal
3. Disease states that prolong elimination
4. Duration of antagonist vs. relaxant
5. Residual volatile agent
6. Respiratory *acidosis* and metabolic *alkalosis*

Special notes about each drug

d-Tubocurarine: causes the most histamine release, ganglionic blockade, hypotension, bradycardia

Pancuronium: causes tachycardia and hypertension due to muscarinic activity and prevention of catecholamine reuptake, may need higher doses in liver disease due to increased volume of distribution

Vecuronium: devoid of side effects, renally excreted active metabolite can accumulate in renal disease and prolong clinical effect

Atracurium: causes histamine release.

Metabolism:
1. Ester hydrolysis (main pathway)
2. Hoffman degradation: impaired by *hypothermia*, acidosis.
3. Active metabolite: laudanosine which undergoes renal excretion, causes cerebral excitation/seizures, increases MAC
4. Note: possible prolonged effect in pseudocholinesterase deficiency

Mivacurium:
1. Causes histamine release
2. Onset: 3.5 minutes (slower than sux)
3. Metabolism: hydrolyzed by pseudocholinesterase and hepatic esterases. Rate of hydrolysis 70% that of sux
4. Reversal: effect of anticholinesterases is additive to spontaneous hydrolysis (i.e., it reverses faster than other nondepolarizers)
5. Note: prolonged effect in pseudocholinesterase deficiency

Differential muscle sensitivity to neuromuscular relaxants

1. Speed of onset of blockade: larynx > diaphragm > obicularis oculi > adductor pollicis

2. Speed of recovery: larynx > obicularis oculi = diaphragm > adductor pollicis
3. Sensitivity to blockade: adductor pollicis > larynx = diaphragm = obicularis oculi
4. "Take home message": obicularis is a better indicator of laryngeal blockade than adductor pollicis. Monitoring obicularis for induction allows early intubation. Monitoring adductor for reversal insures laryngeal reflexes are already recovered.

Factors that cause resistance to nondepolarizers

See Chapter 168, Succinylcholine.

1. Drugs: xanthine derivatives (theophylline, aminophylline), phenytoin, carbamazepine, steroids
2. Extrajunctional receptor proliferation (burns, crush injuries, deafferentation states like upper and lower motor neuron disorders)

Factors that increase sensitivity to nondepolarizers

See Chapter 168, Succinylcholine.

1. Electrolyte disorders: low K^+ and Ca^{++}, high Na^+ and Mg^+
2. Drugs: beta-blockers, local anesthetics, volatile agents, steroids, aminoglycosides, dantrolene, furosemide (furosemide inhibits cAMP → decreased breakdown of ATP → decreased release of ACH)
3. Neuromuscular disease: muscular dystrophy, myasthenia gravis
4. Extreme young age (neonates) . . . note that neonates have an increased volume of distribution (expect higher dose requirements) but are also more sensitive (expect lower dose requirements). The two cancel out, and the dose requirements are the same as for adults. Duration is still greater than adults, though, because the high volume of distribution outweighs their increased clearance rates.

Sample questions

A = 1, 2, 3   B = 1, 3   C = 2, 4   D = 4 only   E = all are correct

1. Nondepolarizing neuromuscular blockers are potentiated by
    1. Halothane 1%
    2. Fentanyl 4 µg/kg
    3. Isoflurane 1.5%
    4. Morphine 2 mg/kg

2. The steady-state volume of distribution of pancuronium is
    1. Increased in cirrhosis
    2. Roughly equivalent to that for d-tubocurarine
    3. Larger than for vecuronium
    4. Equal to that for thiopental

3. Compared to adults, neonates have
    1. Increased sensitivity to vecuronium
    2. Higher clearance rates of vecuronium
    3. Prolonged blockade with equipotent doses of vecuronium
    4. Similar elimination half-lifes of atracurium

4. Nondepolarizing relaxants with active metabolites include
   1. Vecuronium
   2. Atracurium
   3. Pancuronium
   4. Mivacurium

Single best answer

5. The effects of vecuronium are potentiated by
   1. Hypermagnesemia, hypernatremia, hypokalemia
   2. Hypokalemia, hypocalcemia, hyponatremia
   3. Hypokalemia, hypocalcemia, hypomagnesemia
   4. Hypokalemia, hypercalcemia, hypermagnesemia
   5. Hyperkalemia, hypocalcemia, hypermagnesemia

6. The nondepolarizing agent most dependent on biliary excretion is
   1. Pancuronium
   2. d-tubocurarine
   3. Atracurium
   4. Vecuronium
   5. Mivacurium

Answers: 1. B   2. A   3. E   4. A   5. 1   6. 4

Reversal of Neuromuscular Blockade

(acetylcholinesterase inhibitors)

Pharmacodynamics (mechanism of action) of acetylcholinesterase inhibitors

1. Inhibition of acetylcholinesterase increases length of time ACh can spend at motor endplate (Ach can't displace relaxant . . . relaxant dissociates from receptor, then Ach can bind open receptor)
2. Increased release of Ach via K^+ channel blockade (if K^+ can't exit cell to terminate depolarization, then Ca^{++} influx continues to cause release of Ach)

> **NOTES:** 1. *These effects are seen at both nicotinic and muscarinic receptors.*
> 2. *Physostigmine, another acetylcholinesterase inhibitor, is rarely used because of its ability to cross the blood–brain barrier and produce central cholinergic effects.*
> 3. *Renal failure reduces clearance of reversal agents more than the clearance of relaxants; therefore, there's little risk of "recurarization."*

Characteristics of the common acetylcholinesterase inhibitors

● Table 168–1

Agent	Onset of Action (min)	Duration (min)	Max Dose	Effect of Renal Disease on $t^1/_2$	Cross Blood–Brain Barrier?	Anticholinergic of Choice
Edrophonium	1	60	1 mg/kg	↑	No	Atropine
Neostigmine	7	60	70 µg/kg	↑	No	Glycopyrolate
Pyridostigmine	12	115	300 µg/kg	↑	No	Glycopyrolate

Factors that influence ability to reverse

1. Factors that potentiate blockade make it harder to reverse (see Chapter 167, Neuromuscular Relaxants)

2. Choice of antagonist: if block is moderate, edrophonium is fastest/if block intense, neostigmine is fastest
3. Dose of antagonist: once maximum effect is achieved (~10 min), recovery from profound blockade is dependent on clearance of relaxant. Thus, recovery from long-acting drug is slower)
4. Intensity of blockade: the deeper the block, the slower the recovery
5. Half-life of relaxant: low clearance = slow recovery

Side effects of acetylcholinesterase inhibitors

Think: cholinergic crisis

Table 168-2

Muscarinic	Nicotinic	Central Nervous System (only w/physostigmine)
Bradycardia (the only one commonly encountered)	Muscle weakness	Confusion/delirium
Bronchospasm	Tachycardia	Seizures
Increased bronchial secretions		Loss of conciousness
Vomiting (↑ gut motility)		Respiratory depression
Miosis		

Since (1) we require the nicotinic stimulation to reverse neuromuscular blockade and (2) we don't use reversal agents that cross the blood–brain barrier, the only side effects we need to prevent are the muscarinic effects. This is done by concurrent administration of anticholinergics.

Characteristics and side effects of anticholinergics

• **Table 168-3**

Characteristic	Atropine	Glycopyrolate
Onset	1 min	2 min
Crosses blood–brain barrier	Yes	No
CNS effects	Excitation/delirium/ hyperpyrexia ("central anticholinergic syndrome")	None
Cardiovascular effects	Tachycardia, flushing	Much less than atropine
Respiratory effects	↓ bronchial secretions Bronchodilation (↑ anatomic and physiologic deadspace)	Much less than atropine
Gastrointestinal effects	Antisialogogue ↓ motility ↑ pH if halothane used	More than atropine for all GI effects
Eye	↑ IOP (OK in wide angle glaucoma)	

Treatment of central anticholinergic syndrome

Physostigmine (so it's actually good for something).
So after all this, what's the best way to decide if your patient is ready for extubation? No single test is adequate, but here are some favorites:

- **Table 168–4**

Estimated % Receptors Occupied When Normal Response Achieved	Test	Advantage/Disadvantage
50	Head lift for 5 sec	Requires cooperation
50	Inspiratory force > –35 cmH$_2$O	Cooperation not necessary
50	Sustained tetanus @ 100 Hz	Painful
70	Double-burst stimulation	More sensitive than TOF
75	TOF ratio 0.7	

Sample questions

A = 1, 2, 3   B = 1, 3   C = 2, 4   D = 4 only   E = all are correct

1. A 20-year-old, 70-kg patient with a history of fever and vomiting for 2 days undergoes emergency surgery for a rupture appendix. Ninety minutes after 6 mg pancuronium, administration of 3.5 mg neostigmine does not reverse neuromuscular blockade. Possible causes include
   1. Hypercarbia
   2. Hypochloremia
   3. Hypokalemia
   4. Metabolic acidosis

2. A 70-year-old 60-kg patient with open angle glaucoma is to have cataract removal. Premedication with 0.6 mg atropine will
   1. Cause respiratory depression
   2. Aggravate the glaucoma
   3. Produce miosis
   4. Increase physiologic deadspace

3. Neostigmine antagonizes nondepolarizing blockade by all of the following except
   1. Decreasing the breakdown of acetylcholine at the motor endplate
   2. Preventing potassium efflux from the cell
   3. Increasing the release of acetylacholine at the motor endplate
   4. Depolarization of the motor endplate

Single best answer

4. In the recovery room, a 65-kg intubated patient with three twitches on train-of-four stimulation receives 3 mg neostigmine for reversal of pancuronium-induced blockade. Extubation is uneventful, and he complains of surgical pain. Ten minutes after receiving 5 mg morphine, his respirations are shallow and his oxygen saturation is falling. Train of four reveals one twitch. The most appropriate action is
   1. Administer naloxone
   2. Administer neostigmine 2 mg
   3. Reintubate and institute positive pressure ventilation
   4. Administer atropine 0.6 mg
   5. Administer edrophonium 65 mg

5. Which of the following tests reflects the greatest degree of recovery from pancuronium-induced neuromuscular blockade?
   1. Train of four
   2. Head lift for 5 sec

3. Sustained tetanus for 5 sec at 100 Hz
4. Negative inspiratory force of −35 cmH$_2$O
5. Double-burst stimulation

6. Following emergency laparotomy for a ruptured appendix, a 60-kg patient receives neostigmine 4 mg and atropine 1.2 mg to reverse vecuronium-induced block. Extubation is uneventful. In the recovery room, the patient keeps pulling off his oxygen mask and trying to climb out of bed. Respiratory rate is 20/min, temperature is 39°C, pulse is 115/min, SaO$_2$ is 98%. The most appropriate course of action is
   1. Apply four-point restraints
   2. Administer physostigmine
   3. Administer morphine 5 mg
   4. Sedate and intubate the patient
   5. Increase the F$_i$O$_2$

Answers: 1. B   2. D   3. D   4. 1   5. 2   6. 2

Succinylcholine

Pharmacodynamics: Noncompetitively binds cardiac muscarinic receptors as wells as sympathetic and parasympathetic nicotinic receptors, produces depolarization at all receptors.

Phases of blockade and characteristics of each

- Table 169–1

	Tetanic Stimulation	Posttetanic Facilitation	Train-of-Four Response	Effect of Anticholinesterases
Phase I	No fade	No	~No fade	Potentiate block
Phase II	Fade	Yes	Fade	Reverse block

Pharmacokinetics

1. Onset: ~30 sec.
2. Duration: ~5 min.
3. Metabolism: rapid hydroysis *in plasma* by pseudocholinesterase (thus, very little of IV dose ever reaches the motor endplate)
4. Termination of effect: *diffusion* away from motor endplate (no pseudocholinesterase at the motor endplate . . . diffusion explains why even pseudocholinesterase-deficient patients eventually recover from sux blockade)

Factors causing prolonged blockade

1. Atypical pseudocholinesterase (see Chapter 170, Pseudocholinesterase Deficiency)
2. Liver disease (dilutional effect, as well as reduced production of enzyme)
3. Pregnancy (dilutional effect)
4. Organophosphate poisoning (irreversible cholinesterase inhibitors)
5. Echothiophate (an organophosphate, used to treat glaucoma)
6. Anticholinesterases (because they block pseudocholinesterase, too)
7. Metaclopramide
8. Lithium
9. Magnesium (reduces ACH release)

Side effects

1. Dysrythmias: sinus bradycardia: most common, due to muscarinic stimulation; increased risk if second dose of sux given; prevented and/or treated with atropine/glycopyrolate

2. Hyperkalemia: proliferation of extrajunctional receptors increases risk (burns, trauma, neuromuscular disease). Renal patients at risk because of baseline hyperkalemia
3. Malignant hyperthermia: especially in patients already at risk for MH (see Chapter 22)
4. Masseter spasm: a harbinger of MH
5. ↑ intracranial pressure
6. ↑ intragastric pressure: due to fasciculations, pretreatment with small dose of nondepolarizer prevents
7. ↑ intraocular pressure: pretreatment with nodepolarizer prevents
8. Myalgias: due to fasciculations, prevention with nondepolarizer unreliable, lower incidence in children due to relative lack of fasciculations

Contraindications

1. MH-susceptible patients
2. Pseudocholinesterase deficiency/inhibition (for any reason)
3. ↑ ICP (relative to need to secure airway)
4. Open-eye injury
5. Extrajunctional receptor proliferation (burns, trauma, spinal cord transection, etc.)

When is it safe to give succinylcholine to these patients?

1. Burns: injury <24 hr old or >6 months
2. Spinal cord transection: <24 hr old; after that, it's probably never safe

Sample questions

A = 1, 2, 3   B = 1, 3   C = 2, 4   D = 4 only   E = all are correct

1. A 70-kg patient on magnesium for pre-eclampsia develops fetal distress and requires emergency C-section. Thrombocytopenia necessitates general anesthesia. Rapid-sequence induction is performed with thiopental 200 mg and succinylcholine 140 mg. All of the following are true except
   1. She has reduced activity of pseudocholinesterase
   2. Magnesium lowers the required dose of thiopental
   3. She has a dibucaine number of 40
   4. Magnesium potentiates the phase I block of succinylcholine

2. After reversing neuromuscular relaxation with neostigmine and atropine, the surgeon announces that he needs 15 more minutes of relaxation to retrieve a sponge. You administer succinylcholine and expect
   1. Delayed onset of phase I block
   2. Increased risk of phase II block
   3. Decreased risk of hyperkalemia
   4. Prolonged phase I block

Single best answer

3. Following an intubating dose of succinylcholine, the intragastric pressure of a neonate will
   1. Increase due to abdominal muscle fasciculations
   2. Increase due to pyloric fasciculations
   3. Increase due to muscarinic effects on the lower esophageal sphincter
   4. Not change
   5. Increase to peak levels within 90 sec and resolve over 5 min

4. A 60-kg man is intubated with succinylcholine 120 mg and then placed on a succinylcholine infusion for the removal of arch bars. He underwent an uneventful general anesthetic 2 months ago with succinylcholine at induction and vecuronium for maintenance relaxation. The case lasts 20 min. With no detectable end-tidal volatile agent and no narcotics on board, the patient remains apneic. Train-of-four stimulation reveals fade and posttetanic facilitation. True statements about this patient include
   1. His dibucaine number is 40
   2. He has low levels of succinylmonocholine
   3. The previous exposure to succinylcholine depleted his pseudocholinesterase stores
   4. Edrophonium will antagonize the neuromuscular block

Answers: 1. D   2. D   3. 4   4. 4

CHAPTER 170

Pseudocholinesterase Deficiency

Pseudocholinesterase action: Hydrolysis of succinylcholine → succinylmonocholine → succinic acid and choline

Location in body

Plasma only (not at motor endplate)

Defect in deficient patients

Genetic variant resulting in atypical enzyme lacking normal activity

Phenotypes

1. Homozygous normal: normal enzyme ativity
2. Heterozygous atypical: mildly reduced enzyme activity
3. Homozygous atypical: profoundly reduced enzyme activity

Diagnostic tests

Dibucaine number: dibucaine, an amide local anesthetic, inhibits 80% of the activity of normal pseudocholinesterase. It also inhibits atypical enzyme, but not nearly as much.

- Table 170–1

	Normal Enzyme	Heterozygous Atypical	Homozygous Atypical
% inhibition	80	40	20
Dibucaine number	80	40	20

Drugs that have prolonged effect in pseudocholinesterase-deficient patients

1. Succinylcholine
2. Mivacurium
3. Atracurium (possibly)
4. Ester local anesthetics (possibly)
5. Trimethephan

Sample questions

Single best answer

1. A 60-kg patient with homozygous atypical pseudocholinesterase receives succinylcholine 100 mg. You expect him to have increased
   1. Circulating succinylmonocholine
   2. Risk of malignant hyperthermia
   3. Inhibition of pseudocholinesterase by dibucaine
   4. Dose requirement of succinylcholine
   5. Duration of phase I block

2. 75-kg female presents for dilation and evacuation for retained placenta. She has had uneventful general anesthesia with succinylcholine in the past. An intubating dose of 130 mg succinylcholine is given IV. You expect

	Cholinesterase activity	Dibucaine number
1.	Low	20
2.	Normal	80
3.	Normal	45
4.	Low	80
5.	Normal	20

Answers: 1. 5   2. 2

CHAPTER 171

Droperidol

Trade names: Inapsin, Innovar (combination with fentanyl)

Mechanism of action

1. Binds postsynaptic GABA receptors, causes buildup of dopamine in synaptic cleft
2. Occupies central dopamine receptors (competitive antagonism)
3. Minimal α_1 blockade

Drug class

Butyrophenone

Routes of administration

IV, IM

Dose

1. For sedation: 0.1 mg/kg (may cause dysphoria when given alone)
2. For antiemesis: 0.6–1.25 mg/70-kg adult

Uses

1. Neuroleptic
2. Antiemetic

Systemic effects

1. CBF, $CMRO_2$: never studied by itself, slight decrease when combined with fentanyl
2. Respiratory: no significant depression
3. Cardiovascular: antiarrythmic properties, α-blockade causes vasodilation, slight hypotension

Side effects

1. Extrapyramidal symptoms (acute dystonic reactions, treat with diphenhydramine)
2. Hypotension (especially in patients already on vasodilators or hypovolemic)
3. Neuroleptic malignant syndrome
    A. Presents with fever, muscle rigidity, autonomic instability (looks like MH)
    B. Treat with dantrolene and/or bromocriptine

Contraindications

1. Parkinson's disease
2. Monoamine oxidase inhibitor therapy

Sample questions

Single best answer

1. All of the following drugs are contraindicated in the patient with Parkinson's disease **except**
    1. Metaclopramide
    2. Chlorpromazine
    3. Hydroxyzine
    4. Droperidol
    5. Promethazine

A = 1, 2, 3   B = 1, 3   C = 2, 4   D = 4 only   E = all are correct

2. The pharmacologic actions of droperidol include
    1. Antidopaminergic activity
    2. Analgesia
    3. Inhibition of the chemoreceptive trigger zone
    4. Respiratory depression

Answers: 1. 3   2. B

CHAPTER 172

Monoamine Oxidase Inhibitors

Mechanism of action: Increased CNS levels of epinephrine, norepinephrine, dopamine, and serotonin by blocking their breakdown by the enzyme monoamine oxidase

Common agents

1. Phenelzine (Nardil)
2. Tranylcypromine (Parnate)
3. Isocarboxazid (Marplan)

Clinical use

Atypical depression, not responsive to tricyclic antidepressants

Side effects

1. Altered metabolism of endogenous/exogenous catecholamines, leads to:
    A. Intraoperative autonomic instability
    B. Orthostatic hypotension
    C. Hypertensive crisis, which is:
        1. Precipitated by indirect-acting sympathomimetics (ephedrine) or food containing tyramine (an indirect sympathomimetic)
        2. Treated with IV phentolamine (an α-blocker)
2. Inhibition of hepatic microsomal enzymes (leads to impaired breakdown of opioids, barbiturates, ETOH . . . see below)

Drug interactions

1. Meperidine (all other opioids safe): causes hyperpyrexia, seizures, excitation. Less commonly, causes hypotension and respiratory depression.
2. Barbiturates, ETOH: exaggerated respiratory depression, prolonged sedation
3. Halothane: hyperthermia, muscle rigidity (mimics MH).
4. Potentiates action of following drugs, leading to hypertensive crisis:
    A. Guanethedine (which promotes norepinephrine release)
    B. Reserpine (which blocks reuptake of norepinephrine)
    C. L-Dopa (eventually converted to catechols)
    D. Ephedrine, metaraminol (indirect-acting sympathomimetics)
    E. Cocaine (which blocks reuptake of norepinephrine)

Anesthetic considerations

1. Consider stopping MAOI's 2 to 3 weeks before elective cases (weigh against risk of suicide in depressed patients)
2. If discontinuation not an option:
   A. Avoid indirect-acting sympathomimetics
   B. Avoid meperidine (all other opioids have been used safely)
   C. Avoid halothane

Sample question

A = 1, 2, 3   B = 1, 3   C = 2, 4   D = 4 only   E = all are correct

1. A 34-year-old male scheduled for emergency appendectomy has a history of cocaine abuse and depression treated with phenelzine. Premedication is with 25 mg IV meperidine, followed by induction of general anesthesia. During surgical prepping, his blood pressure is 75/45 mmHg, treated with 5 mg ephedrine IV. Shortly after incision, his blood pressure is 200/110 mmHg, pulse 105/min, and T° = 38.5°C. Possible causes include
   1. Meperidine
   2. Cocaine
   3. Ephedrine
   4. Inadequate depth of anesthesia

Answer: 1. A

CHAPTER 173

Cyclosporine Toxicity

Class: Immunosupressant

Mechanism of action

1. Inhibits production of interleukin-1
2. Blocks secretion of interleukin-2
3. Blocks activation of CD-4 cells

Toxicity

CNS: seizures
CVS: hypertension (possibly by renin activation)
Renal: How ironic . . . the drug that prevents rejection can kill the organ!
1. Produces interstitial renal fibrosis and tubular atrophy
2. Occurs with acute and chronic administration
3. Result is increased BUN and creatinine
Hepatic: hepatocellular injury with increased SGOT, SGPT
Miscellaneous: gingival hyperplasia

Sample question

A = 1, 2, 3   B = 1, 3   C = 2, 4   D = 4 only   E = all are correct

1. A 45-year-old sickle cell patient received a cadaveric renal transplant 72 hr ago. Current medications include phenytoin for a seizure disorder as well as prednisone, azathioprine, and cyclosporine. Despite normal renal function for the first 48 hr, laboratory studies now reveal: BUN 48, creatinine 3.2, SGOT 88, SGPT 72. Possible explanations include:
   1. Rejection of the transplanted kidney
   2. Phenytoin toxicity
   3. Acute sickle crisis
   4. Cyclosporine toxicity

Answer: 1. D

KEYWORDS

Note: *Keywords are followed by a comma, test years by a semicolon, and by first page of chapter in which keyword is used.*

A-aDO$_2$: causes of increased, 1996, 1998; 17
AAA mgmt: aortic declamping, 1995; 234
Abdominal surgery: PFT's after, 1993, 1994, 1998; 26
Abdominal surgery: gas exchange after, 1993, 1998; 26
ABG interpretation during hypothermia, 1994, 1998; 211
ABG's during CPR: mgmt, 1994; 253
Acetylcholinesterase: pharmacodynamics, 1995, 1996; 437
Acetylcholinesterase inhibitors: side effects, 1995; 53, 437
Acetylcholinesterase inhibitors: muscarinic effects, 1994; 53, 437
ACLS: priorities for therapy, 1995; 253
ACT: uses and limitations, 1994, 1995; 237
Acute hypocarbia and arrhythmias, 1993; 346
Acute tubular necrosis: diagnostic criteria, 1994, 1996; 83
Aging: effect on PFTs, 1993; 26
Airway fire: management, 1993, 1994, 1995, 1996, 1998; 371
Airway: infant vs. adult, 1993, 1996, 1998; 359
Alfentanil vs. Fentanyl: kinetics, 1993; 423
Alfentinil: pharmacodynamics/pharmacokinetics, 1993, 1995; 423
Allergic transfusion reaction: management, 1994, 1998; 265
Anaphylactoid reaction: antibiotics, 1993; 382
Anaphylaxis: management, 1995, 1996; 382
Anesthesia for awake intubation, 1994, 1996 × 2; 363
Anesthesia for upper arm vascular surgery, 1995; 189
Anesthesia ventilator: function, 1993, 1994; 337
Anesthesia ventilator: implications of bellows hole, 1994; 337
Anesthesia ventilator: malfunction, 1995; 337
Anesthesia ventilator: mechanics, 1993; 337
Ankle block: anatomy, 1993 × 2, 1995 × 2, 1996, 1998; 193
Antegrade flow with chest compression, 1994; 253
Anticholinergic side effects: treatment, 1993, 1995, 1996; 437
Antiemetics: pharmacology of, 1995; 446
Antihypertensives: rebound hypertension, 1994, 1998; 395
Aortic cross-clamp and myocardial ischemia, 1996; 234
Aortic cross-clamping and renal preservation, 1994; 234
Aortic dissection: hypotensive treatment, 1994, 1996; 234
Aortic insufficiency: hemodynamics, 1995, 1998; 230
Aortic regurgitation: management of acute, 1996; 230
Aortic stenosis: anesthetic considerations, 1993; 228
Aortic stenosis and acute ischemia: management, 1995, 1996; 228
Aortic stenosis and spinal anesthesia, 1996; 228
Aortic valve replacement: anesthetic management, 1993; 228
Aortocaval compression: management, 1995, 1996; 133
ARDS: CO$_2$ retention, 1995; 34
ARDS: mechanical ventilation, 1993, 1995; 34
ARDS: pathophysiology and treatment, 1995; 34
Arterial catheterization, 1993; 209
Arterial pressure monitoring: artifacts, 1993, 1995; 209
Aspiration: perioperative, diagnosis of, 1996, 1998; 373
Aspiration: perioperative, management of, 1993, 1994, 1998; 373
Aspiration prophylaxis: side effects, 1994; 373
Asthma: anesthetic considerations, 1994; 37
Asthma: intraoperative signs, 1995; 37
Asthma: management, 1996; 37
Atracurium: factors affecting metabolism, 1994; 433

Atracurium: metabolism, 1995; 433
Atracurium and laudanosine, 1993; 433
Atropine and hyperthermia, 1993; 437
Atropine toxicity, 1993; 437
Auditory evoked response: anesthetic implications, 1995; 295
Autonomic hyperreflexia, 1993, 1998; 298
Autonomic hyperreflexia: bradycardia, 1994; 298
Autonomic hyperreflexia: prevention, 1995 × 2; 298
Axillary block: anatomy, 1994, 1998; 189
Axillary block: dx and tx of inadequate block, 1994; 189
Axillary block: factors affecting spread, 1993; 189
Axillary block: median nerve failure, 1995; 189
Axillary brachial plexus: anatomy, 1994; 189

Bain circuit, 1994; 325
Banked blood: characteristics and considerations, 1993, 1996; 261
Banked blood vs. cell saver, 1994; 261
Barbiturate coma: indications, 1995, 1998; 282
Barbiturates and cerebral protection, 1993, 1996; 282, 417
Barbiturates: cerebral effects, 1994, 1996; 417
Barbiturates: kinetics, 1993; 407, 409, 417
Barotrauma: sequelae, 1993; 340
Benzodiazepines: comparative pharmacology, 1993, 1995; 419
Benzodiazepines in the elderly, 1995; 419
Bicarbonate: side effects, 1993; 253
Bicarbonate in cardiac arrest, 1994, 1998; 253
Bleeding parturient: causes, 1995, 1996; 144
Blood compatibility, 1995, 1998; 261
Blood pressure measurement: effect of site, 1993; 209
Blood pressure: viscosity, 1995; 209
Blood transfusion and typing, 1993, 1998; 261
Brachial plexus: anatomy, 1993, 1998; 189
Brachial plexus block: onset characteristics, 1994, 1996; 189
Bradycardia during neurosurgery: causes, 1995; 282
Brain death: criteria, 1994, 1996, 1998; 282
Brain herniation: treatment, 1994; 282
Brain swelling and hypocarbia, 1993; 282
Breech delivery: anesthesia for, 1994; 142
Bronchitis: preoperative assessment, 1993; 31
Bronchospasm: diagnosis of intraoperative, 1993, 1998; 37
Bupivicaine: toxicity, 1993, 1998; 155
Burns and electrocautery units, 1993, 1994, 1998; 354

C-section: anesthesia for and neonatal effects, 1995, 1998; 139
C-section: effects of low dose halothane, 1993; 139
C-section and GA: anesthetic considerations, 1994; 139
CABG: differential diagnosis for hypotension after, 1993; 241
Capnography and airway obstruction, 1994, 1998; 350
Capnography: applications, 1995; 350
Capnography: DDx of abnormal waveforms, 1993, 1996, 1998; 350
Carbon monoxide poisoning, 1993 × 2, 1995, 1996, 1998; 43
Cardiac failure, 1995; 206

Cardiac output: effect of arteriovenous shunt, 1996; 216
Cardiac output and dead space, 1995; 17
Cardiac output thermodilution: valvular regurgitation, 1995; 216
Cardiac tamponade: anesthetic management, 1993, 1998; 222
Cardiac tamponade: diagnosis, 1994, 1998; 222
Cardiopulmonary bypass: ABGs during, 1993; 241
Cardiopulmonary bypass: causes of hypoxemia following bypass, 1995, 1998; 241
Cardiopulmonary bypass: defibrillation after, 1993; 241
Cardiopulmonary bypass: flow & pressure determinants 1994; 241
Cardiopulmonary bypass: venous saturation during, 1995; 241
Cardiovascular derived variables, 1993; 216
Carotid endarterectomy: carotid body denervation, 1996; 291
Carotid endarterectomy: chemoreceptors after, 1993; 291
Carotid endarterectomy: EEG interpretation, 1994; 291
Carotid endarterectomy: neurologic deficit after, 1995; 291
Carotid endarterectomy: physiologic effects of, 1995, 1998; 291
Carotid endarterectomy: ventilatory drive after, 1994, 1996; 291
Causalgia: diagnosis, 1993, 1998; 177
Celiac plexus block: anatomy, 1994, 1996; 188
Celiac plexus block: avoiding complications, 1996; 188
Celiac plexus block: complications, 1995, 1996; 188
Celiac plexus block: indications, 1993, 1994; 188
Celiac plexus block: pancreatic cancer treatment, 1994; 188
Celiac plexus block: physiology, 1994, 1995, 1998; 188
Central anticholinergic syndrome, 1993; 437
Central anticholinergic syndrome: treatment, 1996; 437
Cerebral aneurysm: rupture at induction, 1995; 288
Cerebral aneurysm clipping: anesthetic management, 1994; 288
Cerebral blood flow: autoregulation, 1993 × 2, 1995, 1996, 1998; 279
Cerebral blood flow autoregulation: physiologic inferences, 1994; 279
Cerebral blood flow: perioperative regulation, 1995, 1998; 279
Cerebral ischemia: detection, 1995; 293
Cerebral perfusion and hypocarbia, 1994; 282
Cerebral perfusion pressure: determinants, 1994, 1996, 1998; 279
Cerebral vasospasm: characteristics, 1996; 288
Cerebral vasospasm: treatment, 1993, 1998; 288
Cervical cord injury (acute): anesthesia, 1995; 298
Cervical plexus block: complications, 1996, 1998; 187
Cervical trauma: intubation after, 1993; 363
Cervical trauma: intubation after, 1993; 298
Chemical neurolysis: indications, 1994, 1996; 185
Chronic anemia: compensatory mechanisms, 1995; 21
Cigarette smoking: pulmonary effects, 1994; 42
Circle system: dead space, 1993, 1995; 328
Cirrhosis: cardiovascular abnormalities, 1994; 75
Cirrhosis: pharmacokinetic implications, 1994; 75
Cirrhosis and liver function tests, 1996, 1998; 75
Cirrhosis and muscle relaxants, 1995; 75, 433
Citrate intoxication: predisposition, 1994, 1998; 261
Clonidine: anesthetic implications of preoperative, 1993, 1994, 1998; 395
Clonidine: side effects, 1996, 1998; 395
Closed-circuit anesthesia, 1993; 331
$CMRO_2$ and anesthetics, 1994, 1998; 279
$CMRO_2$ and hypothermia, 1995; 279
CO_2 absorption: byproducts of, 1993, 1995, 1996; 333
CO_2 absorption in a circle system, 1993, 1995; 328
CO_2: causes of inspired, 1994; 350
CO_2 response curve: anesthetic implications, 1994, 1998; 9
CO_2 response curve: drug effect, 1994, 1998; 9
Cocaine: signs of acute intoxication, 1993, 1994; 81
Cocaine: treatment of hypertension after, 1993; 81
Cocaine intoxication: anesthetic implications, 1995; 81
Colloid therapy: viral risks, 1993; 268
Colloid vs. Crystalloid, 1993; 268
Compression volume: clinical implications, 1994; 340
Concentration effect, 1993; 5
Congenital heart disease: effect of intracardiac shunt on uptake, 1993, 1994, 1996; 5
Congestive heart failure and myocardial O_2 consumption, 1994, 1998; 206

COPD: hemodynamic monitoring, 1993; 31
COPD: mechanical ventilation, 1994, 1996, 1998; 31
COPD: preoperative therapy, 1996, 1998; 31
COPD: PFT's in advanced disease, 1996; 24
COPD: spinal anesthesia, 1993; 31
Coronary artery disease: tx of postinduction hypotension, 1993; 203
Coronary blood flow: physiology, 1993, 1996; 293
Coronary steal: pathophysiology, 1995; 293
Coumadin reversal for emergency surgery, 1994, 1995, 1998; 239
CPAP: induced lung changes, 1995; 340
Cricoid pressure: effects, 1994; 363
Cricothyroidotomy: ventilatory implications, 1994; 363
Croup vs. Epiglottitis, 1993, 1995, 1998; 102
CVP: accurate measurement, 1996; 213
CVP: venous waves, 1994; 213
Cyanide toxicity, 1995, 1998; 399
Cyanide toxicity: treatment, 1995; 399
Cyclosporine toxicity, 1993, 1994; 450
Cylinders: pressures of gases, 1993; 307

Dantrolene: pharmacology, 1995, 1998; 58
DDAVP: perioperative indications for, 1995, 1998; 266
DDD pacer function, 1993, 1998; 219
Deep cervical plexus block, 1994, 1998; 187
Deep venous thrombosis: prevention, 1993; 380
Deep venous thrombosis: perioperative, 1995; 380
Defibrillation: and thoracic impedance, 1993; 253
Desflurane: rate of rise of F_A/F_I vs. N_2O, 1996; 5
Desflurane pharmacology, 1995, 1998; 9, 11
Desflurane vaporizer: function, 1995, 1996; 320
Dextran: side effects, 1994; 268
Diabetes insipidus: diagnosis and treatment, 1995, 1996, 1998; 286
Diabetes insipidus vs. Flouride toxicity: DDx, 1993, 1998; 286
Diabetes insipidus: post traumatic, 1994, 1998; 286
Diabetic ketoacidosis, 1995, 1996; 45
Diaphragmatic hernia: management, 1993, 1994, 1995; 104
Dibucaine number: interpretation, 1995, 1998; 444
DIC in obstetric patients, 1994; 144, 146
Differential nerve sensitivity, 1994, 1996; 155
Difficult airway: management, 1995, 1998; 363
Diffusion hypoxia: principle, 1993, 1998; 344
Digitalis toxicity: management of acute, 1994, 1998; 397
Digitalis toxicity: perioperative causes and tx, 1994; 397
Double lumen tube: indications, 1993; 247
Double lumen tubes: malposition, 1996; 247
Double lumen tube: placement, 1993, 1994; 247
Droperidol: pharmacology, 1993; 446
Droperidol: side effects, 1994; 446
Duchenne's: preoperative evaluation, 1995; 64
Duchenne's: succinylcholine effects, 1995; 64, 441
DVI pacer: perioperative inhibition, 1994; 219

ECT: anesthetic considerations, 1994; 302
ECT: duration of seizure, 1996; 302
ECT and hemodynamic management, 1994; 302
ECT: physiologic effects, 1996, 1998; 302
E cylinder: pressure, flow and volume, 1994; 307
EEG: anesthetic effects on, 1993, 1996; 293
EKG: pacemaker, 1994; 219
EEG burst suppression: causes, 1995, 1998; 293
Electrical safety in the OR, 1994; 354
EMD: causes, 1996; 253
EMD: CPR, 1993; 253
Emphysema: chest X-ray, 1993; 31
Endobronchial intubation: signs of, 1995, 1998; 363
Epidural anesthesia: cardiorespiratory effects, 1993 × 2; 166
Epidural anesthesia: complications, 1993 × 2, 1998 × 2; 166
Epidural anesthesia: duration, 1994; 166
Epidural anesthesia: effects of T8 level, 1994; 166
Epidural: management of retained catheter, 1994; 166

Epidural morphine: pharmacodynamics/pharmacokinetics, 1993; 173
Epidural narcotics: respiratory depression, 1993; 173
Epidural opioids: rostral migration, 1994; 173
Epidural opioids: site of action, 1993; 173
Epidural opioids: spread, 1993; 173
Epidural space: anatomy, 1996, 1998; 166
Epidural steroids: indications, 1994, 1995, 1998; 175
Epidural steroid: low back pain, 1995; 175
Epidural: test dose failure, 1993, 1998; 166
$ETCO_2$ and neurosurgery, 1994, 1998; 388
$ETCO_2$/arterial CO_2: causes of increased gradient, 1993, 1994, 1995, 1996, 1998; 350
$ETCO_2$: causes of low, 1993; 350
$ETCO_2$: equipment causes of high values, 1994; 350
$ETCO_2$: factors affecting, 1995, 1998; 350
ETOH: anesthetic implications of acute intoxication, 1993, 1995, 1996, 1998; 80
Etomidate: adrenal suppression, 1993, 1996; 413
Etomidate: comparative pharmacology, 1994; 417
Etomidate: side effects, 1994; 413
Extrapyramidal drug effects: treatment, 1995, 1998; 373
Eye surgery: bradycardia during, 1995; 69
Eye surgery: regional vs. general, 1994, 1998; 69

Failsafe device in anesthesia machine, 1993; 322
Fat embolism: signs, 1994, 1998; 391
Femoral nerve block, 1995; 193
Fentanyl: effect on heart rate, 1996, 423
Fentanyl: pharmacokinetics, 1993, 1996; 423
Fetal adaptation at birth, 1993, 1998; 115, 123
Fetal distress: diagnosis, 1994, 1998; 129
Fetal heart rate decelerations: causes, 1994; 129
Fetal heart rate: drug effects, 1993, 1996; 129
Fetal heart rate: monitoring, 1993, 1996, 1998; 129
Fetal hemoglobin, 1995; 21
Fetal hemoglobin vs. adult, 1993, 1995; 21
Fetal monitoring, 1993; 129
FFP: indications, 1993, 1994; 266
First trimester: anesthesia for, 1994, 1995, 1998; 151
Flowmeter sequence, 1993; 312
Flow proportioning system, 1996; 322
Flow-volume loops in COPD, 1996; 24, 31
Fluid resuscitation: distribution characteristics, 1994, 1998; ???
Flumazenil: duration, 1996; 421
Flumazenil: pharmacology, 1994; 421
Fluoride toxicity, 1993; 83, 286
Frank Starling relationships, 1993, 1996, 1998; 206
FRC and general anesthesia, 1994, 1998; 26
FRC: factors reducing, 1996, 1998; 26
FRC: positional effects, 1994, 1998; 26
Furosemide: metabolic effects, 1995; 405

Gastric pH and emptying: drugs for, 1996; 373
Gastroschisis repair: anesthetic implications, 1994; 106
General anesthesia and heat loss: mechanisms, 1995, 1996, 1998; 384
General anesthesia and pulmonary gas exchange, 1995; 9
Giant A waves: significance, 1993, 1998; 213
Glasgow coma scale: criteria, 1994; 282
Glasgow coma scale: use and limits, 1994; 282
Glaucoma: anesthetic considerations in closed angle, 1996; 69
Glaucoma: drug interactions, 1995, 1998; 69
Glycopyrolate: effects, 1995; 437

H_2 blockers: drug interactions, 1993; 373
Halothane: cardiovascular effects, 1993, 1995; 11
Halothane: ventilatory response to hypoxia, 1993; 11
Head trauma: anesthetic management, 1993, 1998; 282
Heat loss in exposure: mechanisms, 1994, 1998; 384
Hemiparesis: nondepolarizing muscle relaxants, 1994; 433

Hemolytic transfusion reaction: tests for, 1993, 1998; 265
Hemolytic transfusion reaction: treatment, 1994, 1998; 265
Hemophilia A and emergency surgery, 1995; 273
Heparin: effects of preoperative administration, 1993, 1998; 237
Heparin: factors affecting duration, 1993; 237
Heparin induced thrombocytopenia, 1993, 1996; 237
Heparin resistance, 1995; 237
Heparin resistance: management, 1996; 237
Hepatic blood flow: intraop determinants, 1994; 75
Hepatic dysfunction: postoperative, 1995, 1996, 1998; 75
Hepatitis B: immediate tx after exposure, 1994; 79
Hepatitis B testing: interpretation, 1995; 79
Hetastarch: pharmacology, 1993; 268
HIV: inactivation of, 1994; 86
HIV: management of contamination, 1993; 86
Hoarseness: mechanisms of postoperative, 1994; 47, 363
Hypercarbia: intraoperative effects, 1993, 1996; 346
Hyperglycemia: effects of chronic, 1993; 45
Hyperglycemia: perioperative management, 1995, 1998; 45
Hyperglycemia: preoperative management, 1993; 45
Hyperthyroidism: beta blockers, 1996; 47
Hyperthyroidism:intraop management, 1994, 1998; 47
Hyperthyroidism: perioperative concerns, 1995, 1998; 47
Hypocarbia: physiologic effects, 1994; 346
Hypoglycemia: signs of acute perioperative, 1994; 45
Hypotensive drugs and ICP, 1994; 282
Hypothermia and gas transport, 1994; 211
Hypothermia: effects of profound, 1995, 1996; 384
Hypothermia: Intraoperative, prevention of, 1993; 384
Hypothermia: perioperative effects of moderate, 1993, 1994, 1996, 1998; 384
Hypothermia: physiology of deliberate, 1993×2, 1994; 384
Hypothyroidism: anesthetic considerations, 1993, 1998; 47
Hypoventilation: effects, 1993; 17
Hypoxia during emergence, 1994, 1998; 344
Hypoxia: early postoperative causes, 1994, 1998; 344
Hypoxia: intraoperative causes, 1993, 1994, 1995, 1996; 344
Hypoxic mechanisms in pregnancy, 1993, 1994, 1995, 1996; 26, 131
Hypoxic pulmonary vasoconstriction: drug effects, 1996; 250
Hypoxic pulmonary vasoconstriction: inhibition, 1996; 250

IABP: hemodynamic effects, 1995, 1998; 243
IABP: limitations, 1993; 243
ICP: intraoperative management of increased, 1995×2, 1996×2; 282
ICP: pharmacologic management of increased, 1993, 1994, 1996; 282
ICP: reduction of following head trauma, 1993; 282
IHSS: drugs worsening, 1994; 232
IHSS: intraoperative management, 1993, 1995; 232
IHSS: management of inhalational anesthesia, 1996; 232
IMV: demand vs. continuous flow, 1994; 340
IMV vs. IPPV, 1994; 340
Indications for platelet transfusion, 1996; 266
Infant airway: anatomy, 1993, 1994, 1996; 359
Infants born to myasthenic women: respiratory failure at delivery, 1993; 114
Inhalational anesthesia: respiratory effects, 1994, 1995; 9
Inhalational induction: child vs. adult, 1995, 1998; 5
Inhalational induction in infants, 1993; 5
Inhaled anesthetics: uptake and distribution of, 1993, 1994, 1998; 5
Innervation of the larynx, 1995, 1996; 361
Inspiratory valve malfunction: consequences, 1994; 328
Inspired anesthetic concentration: determinants, 1994; 5
Interscalene block and phrenic paralysis, 1995; 189
Interscalene block: complications, 1993×2; 189
Interscalene block: landmarks, 1995; 189
Intracranial elastance, 1995; 282
Intraocular pressure: drugs affecting, 1993; 69
Intraoperative hypothermia in infants, 1995, 1998; 117
Intraoperative hypotension: therapeutic intervention, 1993, 1995; 206
Intrathecal neurolytic block: techniques, 1994; 185

Isoflurane effects: CBF and $CMRO_2$, 1993; 11
IV regional anesthesia: effects and duration, 1994; 196
IV regional anesthesia: technique, 1994; 196
IV regional anesthesia: termination of, 1993; 196
IV regional anesthesia: tourniquet management, 1994; 196

Ketamine: adverse effects, 1995; 415
Ketamine: cardiovascular effects, 1994; 415
Ketamine: pharmacology, 1993, 1994, 1996; 415, 417
Ketorolac: contraindications, 1994, 1998; 431
Ketorolac: pharmacology, 1993, 1995; 431
Ketorolac vs. Meperidine, 1993; 431
Knee surgery: nerves that must be blocked, 1993, 1994, 1998; 193
Kyphoscoliosis: respiratory effects, 1995; 26

Labor: analgesia techniques for first stage, 1994, 1998; 137
Labor: dermatomes affected during second stage, 1993, 1996, 1998; 137
Labor: fetal distress and epidural, 1994; 137
Laparoscopy and gas embolism, 1993; 87, 388
Laparoscopy: complications, 1995, 1998; 87
Laparoscopy: pulmonary effects, 1995; 87
Laparoscopy: response to CO_2 insufflation, 1993, 1998; 87
Laryngeal function: local anesthesia & GA, 1994; 361
Laryngospasm: consequences, 1994; 367
Laryngospasm: management, 1995; 367
Laryngospasm: physiology, 1996; 367
Laser airway fire: prevention, 1993, 1995, 1998; 371
Latex allergy: anesthetic implications, 1994, 1995, 1996; 382
Leakage current: recommended level, 1993; 354
Left ventricle failure, acute: management, 1996; 206
Leg tourniquet pain: anesthetic implications, 1994, 1998; 378
Leg tourniquet pain: treatment, 1996; 378
Line isolation monitor: alarm, 1993; 354
Line isolation monitor: function, 1994; 354
Lithotripsy and regional anesthesia: hemodynamic effects, 1994; 73
Lithotripsy: timing, 1994; 73
Liver disease and muscle relaxants, 1993, 1998; 75, 433
Liver disease and Thiopental, 1996; 75, 407
Liver disease: anesthetic implications, 1995, 1998; 75
Liver disease: anesthetic induction, 1993; 75
Liver disease: coagulopathy in, 1995; 75
Liver disease: hypoxemia with severe disease, 1993, 1995; 75
Liver disease: intraoperative hypotension, 1993; 75
Liver disease: preoperative evaluation, 1993; 75
Liver function tests, 1994, 1998; 75
Liver transplant: management, 1994; 80
Liver transplant: venovenous bypass during, 1995; 80
Local anesthetic: alkalinization, 1993; 155
Local anesthetic: cardiotoxicity, 1994, 1995, 1998; 155
Local anesthetics: clinical implications of IV administration, 1994; 155
Local anesthetic: duration, 1993; 155
Local anesthetic: mechanism of action, 1993; 155
Local anesthetic onset: pharmacologic manipulation, 1994; 155
Local anesthetic: PABA allergy, 1995; 155
Local anesthetic: physicochemical properties, 1994; 155
Low back pain: treatment, 1993; 175
Lower esophageal sphincter: drug effects, 1993; 373
Lower extremity blocks: anatomy, 1993, 1994, 1995; 193
Lower extremity nerve injury: causes, 1996, 1998; 386
Lung compliance: anesthetic factors and disease, 1994; 17
Lung resectability: criteria, 1994, 1998; 250
Lung resection and preoperative PFT's, 1993, 1995, 1998; 250

MAC and volatile anesthetic potency, 1994 × 2, 1998; 3
MAC: definition, 1994; 3
MAC: factors affecting, 1994, 1996; 3
Machine check, 1994; 322
Machine: check valves, 1993, 1995; 322

Machine check with no oxygen flow, 1993; 322
Machine design to prevent hypoxia, 1994, 1998; 322
Magnesium: drug interactions, 1994; 146, 433
Magnesium: neuromuscular effects, 1995, 1996; 123, 146, 433
Magnesium: pharmacology, 1996, 1998; 146
Magnesium: side effects, 1993; 146
Magnesium toxicity: neonatal, 1994; 123, 146
Malignant hyperthermia: clinical signs, 1993; 58
Malignant hyperthermia: early diagnosis, 1996; 58
Malignant hyperthermia: testing susceptibility, 1996, 1998; 58
Malignant hyperthermia history: anesthetic management, 1994; 58
Mannitol: nondiuretic effects, 1993; 405
Mannitol: pharmacology, 1995, 1996; 405
Mannitol vs. furosemide: cardiovascular effects, 1994; 405
MAO inhibitors: anesthetic implications, 1993, 1995; 448
Masseter spasm: characteristics, 1996; 58
Massive transfusion and coagulopathy, 1993; 261
Massive transfusion and coagulation, 1994, 1998; 261, 266
Maternal-fetal levels of bupivicaine, 1993, 1994; 135
Maternal-fetal O_2 transport, 1994; 21, 135
Mechanical ventilation and increased VD/VT, 1996; 340
Mechanical ventilation: increased PIP, 1993, 1996; 340
Meconium aspiration: resuscitation after, 1993, 1998; 121
Mediastinoscopy: complications, 1995; 245
Metaclopramide and cimetidine: GI effects, 1995; 373
Metaclopramide: pharmacology, 1993, 1994, 1996; 373
Methyl methacrylate: hemodynamic effects, 1993, 1994; 377
Micro shock: causes, 1996; 354
Midazolam vs. Diazepam, 1993; 419
Midazolam vs. Thiopental: pharmacology, 1993; 419
Mitral regurgitation: hemodynamic management, 1995; 226
Mitral regurgitation: management of acute, 1993, 1996; 226
Mitral stenosis: anesthetic management, 1994; 224
Mitral stenosis: pathophysiology, 1994, 1998; 224
Mitral stenosis: signs and symptoms, 1994; 224
Mitral stenosis: tx of acute intraop atrial fibrillation, 1994; 224
Mitral valve disease and tachycardia, 1995; 224
Mitral valve prolapse: anesthetic implications, 1993, 1998; 226
Mivacurium duration of action: factors affecting, 1996; 443
Mivacurium: pharmacology, 1996; 443
Mixed venous O_2: and high FiO_2, 1996; 218
Mixed venous O_2: factors decreasing/increasing, 1993, 1994, 1996, 1998; 218
Morbid obesity: anesthetic implications, 1993, 1995, 1998; 39
Morbid obesity: cardiovascular implication and complications, 1994, 1998; 39
Morbid obesity: pharmacokinetic considerations, 1994; 39
Morbid obesity: PFTs, 1993, 1994; 26, 39
Morphine: duration in renal disease, 1995, 1998; 423
Morphine: elimination in renal failure, 1994; 83, 423
Morphine: site of action, 1996; 423
Muscle relaxants: liver disease, 1993, 1998; 75, 433
Muscle relaxants in renal failure, 1993, 1994, 1995, 1998; 423, 433
Muscular dystrophy: anesthetic implications, 1994; 64
Myasthenia gravis, 1995; 53
Myasthenia gravis: PFTs, 1993, 1994; 26, 53
Myasthenic crisis vs. cholinergic, 1995; 53
Myasthenic syndrome: characteristics, 1993, 1994, 1995; 56
Myocardial ischemia: detection of intraoperative, 1994, 1998; 203
Myocardial ischemia: treatment of postoperative, 1993, 1998; 203
Myocardial O_2 supply: anesthetic effects, 1994; 203
Myocardial oxygenation: determinants, 1994; 203
Myotonic dystrophy: anesthetic implications, 1995; 64

N_2O and air in closed spaces, 1993, 1996; 13
N_2O: cerebral effects, 1995; 11, 13
N_2O and eye surgery, 1996; 13
N_2O: physical properties, 1994; 13, 307
Nalbuphine: pharmacology, 1995; 428
Naloxone: pharmacology, 1994; 428
Narcotic addict: premedication, 1993; 428
Narcotic agonists/antagonists: analgesia with, 1994; 428

Nasal prongs: FiO$_2$ with, 1993; 310
Nasotracheal intubation: complications, 1993; 363
Necrotizing enterocolitis: perioperative management, 1994; 110
Negative inspiratory force: intraop assessment, 1994; 437
Negative pressure pulmonary edema, 1993; 367
Neonates and postoperative apnea, 1994, 1998; 93, 119
Neonatal fluid management, 1995, 1998; 96
Neonatal HCO$_3^-$ therapy, 1995, 1998; 123
Neonatal hypothermia: effects, 1995, 1998; 117
Neonatal hypoxemia: physiologic causes, 1995, 1998; 93
Neonatal perioperative desaturation: mechanisms, 1994; 93
Neonatal respiratory failure, 1993; 93
Neonatal respiratory physiology, 1996; 93
Neonatal resuscitation, 1995 × 4, 1998; 123
Neonatal resuscitation: maternal addiction, 1994; 123
Neonatal temperature regulation, 1995, 1998; 117
Neonatal ventilation, 1996; 340
Neonatal vs. adult thermoregulation, 1994, 1998; 117
Neostigmine and relaxant metabolism, 1994; 437
Nerve injuries: forceps delivery, 1996; 386
Nerve injuries: vaginal delivery, 1993; 386
Neuroleptic malignant syndrome, 1993; 62
Neurolytic blocks: head and neck cancer, 1994, 1998; 185
Neuromuscular blockade and antibiotics, 1993; 433
Neuromuscular block reversal: clinical influences, 1993, 1994, 1998; 437
Neuromuscular relaxation: differential muscle sensitivity, 1994, 1998; 433
Neuromuscular relaxation: resistance to, 1995; 433
Neuromuscular relaxation reversal: criteria for extubation after, 1994; 437
Neuromuscular relaxation reversal: atropine vs. glycopyrolate, 1994, 1995; 437
Nitroprusside: coronary steal, 1994; 402
Nitroprusside: pharmacology, 1993, 399, 402
Nitroprusside toxicity: signs, 1993, 1994, 1998; 399
Nitroprusside vs. Nitroglycerin: pharmacodynamics, 1994; 402
Nitroprusside vs. Trimethaphan, 1993; 402
Nitroprusside-propanolol interactions, 1994; 402
Nondepolarizing blockade: characteristics, 1993; 433
Nondepolarizing blockade: duration, 1996; 433
Nondepolarizing blockers: dosing with burns, 1996; 433
Nondepolarizing blockers: dosing with diseases, 1993; 433
Nondepolarizing blockers: histamine release, 1996; 433
Nondepolarizing relaxants: pharmacodynamics, 1994; 433

O$_2$ transport, hematocrit and viscosity, 1995; 21
O$_2$ delivery: determinants of, 1995, 1998; 21
Oculocardiac reflex: causes, 1993, 1998; 198
Oculocardiac reflex: clinical implications, 1993, 1994; 69, 198
Oculocardiac reflex: pathways, 1993, 1994, 1998; 198
Oculocardiac reflex: prevention and treatment, 1993, 1998; 198
Oliguria: interpretation of lab data, 1993, 1995, 1998; 83
Oliguria: postoperative causes, 1995; 83
Oliguria: postoperative, diagnostic criteria, 1994, 1998; 83, 106
Omphalocele: fluid therapy, 1996; ???
Omphalocele repair: complications, 1995; 106
One lung ventilation: anatomic considerations, 1994; 250
One lung ventilation: hypoxic pulmonary vasoconstriction during, 1994; 250
One-lung ventilation: management of hypoxia during, 1993, 1995, 1998; 250
One lung ventilation: PaO$_2$, 1994, 1998; 250
Opiate receptor antagonists, 1993; 428
Opioid anesthesia: awareness and, 1995; 423
Opioid side effects: treatment, 1993; 423
Opioids and histamine release, 1996; 423
Opioids and muscle rigidity, 1994, 1995; 423
Opioids: treatment of opioid induced biliary spasm, 1995 × 2; 423
Oxygen analyzer: function in the circuit, 1993, 1996; 328
Oxygen analyzer: malfunction, 1996; 328
Oxygen content: factors affecting, 1994; 21

Oxygen cylinder volume, 1996; 307
Oxygen delivery masks: characteristics, 1994; 310
Oxygen flowmeter leak, 1994; 312
Oxygen flowmeter malfunction: consequences, 1994; 312
Oxygen flush valve function, 1995; 322
Oxygen pressure safety devices, 1994; 322
Oxygen supply and demand: assessment, 1994, 1998; 218
Oxygenation: infant vs. adult, 1993; 93
Oxyhemoglobin shift: causes, 1993, 1995, 1998; 21

p50: altered value and tissue O$_2$ delivery, 1995; 21
Pacemaker: fixed vs. synchronous mode, 1995; 219
Pacemaker: indications for preoperative insertion, 1994, 1996; 219
Pacemaker mode conversion, 1994; 219
PAD:LVEDP: causes of abnormal gradient, 1994; 213
PAOP: factors affecting accuracy, 1996; 213
PAOP: interpretation, 1993, 1996; 213
PAOP and LV volume: pitfalls, 1995; 213
Parkinson's disease: anesthetic implications, 1995, 1996; 67
Parkinson's disease: drug interactions, 1993; 67
Patient positioning: neurologic complications, 1994, 1998; 386
Pediatric caudal anesthesia, 1994; 170
Pediatric caudal anesthesia: complications, 1993; 170
Pediatric circuits: fresh gas flow requirements, 1993, 1994, 1996; 325
Pediatric fluid management, 1993, 199?, 1998; 96
Pediatric postoperative pain management, 1993; 170
PEEP: cardiopulmonary effects, 1994, 1996; 340
PEEP: complications, 1995; 340
PEEP: effect on right ventricle, 1995; 340
Perioperative desaturation in neonates: mechanisms, 1994, 1998; 119
Perioperative nerve injuries: lower extremity positioning, 1994, 1998; 386
Persistent fetal circulation: factors causing, 1993, 1996, 1998; 115
PFTs: flow-volume loop interpretation, 1993, 1995; 24
PFTs: in obstructive and restrictive disease, 1994; 24
Phase II block, 1993, 1995; 441
Phenol vs. alcohol, 1993, 1998; 185
Pheochromocytoma: mgmt of hypotension after resection, 1993, 1995; 50
Pheochromocytoma: preoperative management, 1994; 50
Physics: gas flow, 1993; 312
Pierre-Robin syndrome: anesthetic implications, 1994; 112
Placental abruption: management, 1996; 114
Placental oxygen exchange, 1993; 135
Placental transfer: determinants, 1993, 1995, 1998; 135
Placental transfer: local anesthetics, 1993, 1994; 135
Placental transfer: relaxants, 1996; 135
Plasma cholinesterase genotypes, 1995; 444
Platelet transfusion: thrombocytopenia, 1993; 266
Positioning and peroneal nerve injury, 1995, 1998; 386
Positive pressure ventilation: physiologic effects, 1995, 1996; 340
Postherpetic neuralgia, 1993, 1994, 1995; 183
Preeclampsia and epidural anesthesia, 1996; 146
Preeclampsia: hemodynamic effects, 1994; 146
Preeclampsia: pathophysiology, 1995; 146
Pregnancy and volatile anesthetic induction, 1994, 1996; 139
Pregnancy: hypoxic mechanisms in, 1993; 139
Pregnancy: PFT's during, 1994; 26, 131
Prematurity: anesthetic risks, 1993, 1998; 119
Prerenal azotemia: diagnosis, 1995; 83
Prerenal oliguria, 1993, 1998; 83
Pressors and preload, 1995, 1998; 206
Pressure cycled ventilators, 1993, 1995; 340
Pressure support ventilation, 1993, 1995; 340
Preterm infants: hypothermia, 1993; 117, 119
Prolonged bleeding time: preoperative therapy, 1994; 266
Prolonged PT, 1996; 266
Propofol: cardiovascular effects, 1993; 411, 417
Propofol: pharmacodynamics, 1994; 411, 417
Propofol: pharmacology, 1993; 411, 417
Protamine: cardiovascular effects, 1996; 239

Protamine reaction and management, 1993, 1994, 1995; 239
Pseudocholinesterase deficiency: clinical implications, 1996; 444
Pseudocholinesterase deficiency: diagnosis, 1994; 444
Pseudocholinesterase: pharmacology, 1993; 444
Pulmonary artery blood gas: interpretation, 1994; 218
Pulmonary artery catheter and pulmonary hypertension, 1993; 213
Pulmonary artery catheter: complications, 1994; 213
Pulmonary blood flow: distribution, 1995; 17
Pulmonary fibrosis: anesthetic considerations, 1993; 26
Pulse oximetry: artifacts, 1993, 1996; 348
Pyloric stenosis: preoperative abnormalities, 1993, 1994, 1998; 98

Recurrent laryngeal nerve block: anatomy, 1993; 361
Recurrent laryngeal nerve block: effects, 1995; 361
Recurrent laryngeal nerve paralysis: causes, 1993; 361
Recurrent laryngeal nerve resection: effects, 1995, 1996; 361
Reflex sympathetic dystrophy: characteristics, 1994, 1995, 1998; 177
Reflex sympathetic dystrophy: early and late signs, 1994, 1996 × 2, 1998; 177
Reflex sympathetic dystrophy: management, 1993, 1996, 1998; 117
Relaxant pharmacology: neonate, 1995; 433
Renal failure: electrolyte effects of, 1996; 83
Renal failure: pharmacokinetics, 1993; 83
Residual muscle blockade after GA, 1995; 433
Respiratory distress: postoperative causes, 1994; 344
Respiratory function: adult vs. child, 1993; 93
Restrictive lung disease: pathophysiology, 1995; 26
Retained placenta: anesthesia for, 1993; 144
Retinopathy of prematurity, 1995; 119
Retrobulbar block: apnea and, 1993; 198
Retrobulbar block: complications, 1993, 1994, 1995, 1996, 1998; 198
Retrobulbar block: contraindications, 1995; 198
Retrobulbar block: effects, 1996, 1998; 198
Reversal of fibrinolytics, 1995; 239
Right to left shunt: management during anesthesia, 1993; 100

Scavenging systems: features and types, 1994, 1995; 335
Sciatic nerve: landmarks, 1993; 193
Second gas effect, 1993, 1998; 5
Seizure potential: anesthetic drugs, 1993; 302
Shivering: treatment of postoperative, 1993, 1994; 384
Shoulder block interscalene block: anatomy, 1994, 1998; 189
SIADH: diagnosis, 1996; 286
SIADH: treatment, 1995; 286
Sickle cell anemia: neonatal considerations, 1994, 1998; 274
Sickle cell crisis: management, 1994, 1998; 274
Sinus arrest: anesthetic implications, 1994; 253
Sitting position: complications, 1995, 1998; 388
Smoking cessation: preoperative, 1993, 1998; 42
Soda lime: exhaustion of, 1996; 333
Sodium citrate toxicity, 1995; 261
Spinal cord injury: acute, 1993, 1994, 1996; 298
Spinal cord injury and succinylcholine, 1993; 298
Spinal headache, 1993, 1994, 1996; 161
Spinal opioids and ventilatory depression, 1994; 173
SPO_2: causes of artifactual values, 1995, 1996; 348
SPO_2: causes of decreased, 1994; 348
Spontaneous vs. Control ventilation: effect on CO_2 gradient, 1996; 340
SSEP: anesthetic effects, 1995, 1996, 1998; 295
SSEP: interpretation, 1993, 1998; 295
SSEP: moderating factors, 1995; 295
SSEP: pathways, 1995; 295
SSEP: spinal cord function, 1995; 295
SSEP: uses, 1993; 295
Stellate ganglion block: anatomy, 1995, 1998; 179
Stellate ganglion block: complications, 1993, 1994; 179
Stellate ganglion block: effects, 1993; 179
Stellate ganglion block: signs, 1994; 179
Subarachnoid block: advantages of paramedian, 1993, 1998; 161

Subarachnoid block: cardiovascular collapse with and resuscitation, 1994, 1998; 161
Subarachnoid block: cardiovascular effects, 1993, 1998; 161
Subarachnoid block: causes of failed block, 1995; 161
Subarachnoid block: causes of hypotension during, 1993, 1995, 1998; 161
Subarachnoid block: differential neural sensitivity, 1994; 161
Subarachnoid block: distribution of local anesthetic, 1993, 1995, 1998; 161
Subarachnoid block: duration of local anesthetic, 1994; 161
Subarachnoid block: dyspnea with high level, 1994; 161
Subarachnoid block: effects/signs of high level, 1994, 1995; 161
Subarachnoid block: hypobaric spinal anesthesia, 1995; 161
Subarachnoid block: mechanism of respiratory arrest during, 1994; 161
Subarachnoid block: midline vs paramedian anatomy, 1994; 161
Subarachnoid block: nausea with high level, 1995; 161
Subarachnoid block: physiologic effects of T4 level, 1994; 161
Subarachnoid block: quadriplegia and, 1994; 298
Subarachnoid block: recovery, 1995; 161
Subarachnoid hemorrhage: signs of, 1996; 288
Subendocardial blood flow, 1993; 203
Succinylcholine after neuromuscular reversal, 1995; 441
Succinylcholine and preeclampsia, 1993; 146, 441
Succinylcholine and pseudocholinesterase deficiency, 1993, 1998; 441, 444
Succinylcholine: contraindications, 1994, 1998; 58, 441
Succinylcholine: effects in Duchenne's, 1995; 58, 64, 441
Succinylcholine: hyperkalemia, 1994, 1998 × 2; 58
Succinylcholine: pharmacokinetics, 1993; 58
Succinylcholine: prolonged recovery, 1996; 58
Superficial cervical plexus block: anatomy, 1995; 187
Superior laryngeal nerve, 1993; 361
SVT: management, 1995, 1996; 253

Tamponade: hemodynamic manipulation, 1994, 1998; 222
TE fistula: complications, 1993, 1994; 108
Tetralogy of Fallot: management of cyanosis, 1993, 1994, 1995, 1996, 1998; 100
Tetralogy of Fallot: pathophysiology, 1995; 100
Thermodilution CO: measurement errors, 1993, 1994, 1996, 1998; 216
Thiopental and liver disease, 1996; 75, 407
Thiopental level: maternal-fetal, 1995; 135
Thiopental: redistribution, 1996, 1998; 407
Thiopental: treatment of intra-arterial injection, 1996; 234, 409
Thoracic aneurysm repair: nerve injuries after, 1996; 409
Thoracic aneurysm repair: paraplegia after, 1995; 409
Thyroid surgery: airway obstruction following, 1993, 1995; 47
Thyroid surgery: causes of hoarseness following, 1994, 1996; 47, 361
Thyroid surgery: complications, 1995; 47
Tocolysis: effects and complications, 1993, 1994, 1995; 149
Tocolysis in preterm labor, 1996; 149
Tourniquet release: physiologic effects, 1993, 1994, 1996, 1998; 378
Tracheal trauma: airway management, 1994; 363
Transducers: resonance/dampening effects, 1994; 209
Transducers: zeroing (where to), 1993 × 2, 1998; 209
Transfusion reaction: causes, 1996; 265
Transfusion reaction: diagnosis, 1996; 265
Transtracheal jet ventilation technique, 1993, 1995; 363
Trimethephan: pharmacodynamics, 1994; 402
TURP: causes of agitation following, 1995; 71
TURP: causes of postoperative hypoxia, 1995; 71
TURP: coagulopathy, 1993; 71
TURP: complications, 1994; 71
TURP: differential diagnosis of bladder perforation, 1996; 71
TURP: effect of glycine during, 1993, 1994, 1995, 1996; 71
TURP: hypervolemia, 1993; 71
TURP: proximate nerve anatomy, 1996; 71
TURP syndrome, 1993; 71
TURP: treatment of hyponatremia, 1996; 71
Type and screen, 1994, 1998; 261

Upper airway: innervation, 1993, 1994, 1995; 361
Uterine blood flow: determinants, 1994, 1996; 133
Uterine blood flow during labor, 1995; 133
Uterine contractions: anesthetic effects, 1993; 133
Utero placental blood flow: physiology, 1994, 1996; 133

V/Q mismatch: effects, 1995; 17
V/Q mismatch: factors affecting, 1993, 1998; 17
Vapor concentration: calculation of, 1993; 318
Vapor pressure: determinants, 1994; 315
Vaporizer hazards, 1996; 315
Vaporizer output: determinants, 1993; 315
Vaporizer: tipped, 1993; 315
VD/VT: factors affecting, 1996; 17
Vecuronium pharmacology: neonate, 1996; 433
Venous air embolus: cardiopulmonary changes, 1993; 388
Venous air embolus: diagnosis and treatment, 1993, 1994 × 2, 1996 × 2, 1998; 350, 388

Venous air embolus: end tidal gases, 1993; 350, 388
Ventilation volume: effect of flow rate on, 1996; 340
Ventilators: factors affecting measured Vt, 1993; 340
Ventilators: factors affecting tidal volume, 1995; 340
Ventilatory disconnect: detection, 1996; 337
Ventilatory disconnect: monitoring, 1995; 337
Ventricular tachycardia: management, 1993, 1994, 1996; 253
Volatile agents: cardiopulmonary effects, 1993, 1994, 1995, 1998; 9, 11
Volatile agents and non ischemic heart disease, 1994; 11
Volatile agent uptake: effect of cardiac output, 1993; 5
Von Willebrand's disease: intraop treatment, 1993, 1998; 271
Von Willebrand's disease: preoperative preparation, 1996; 271
Von Willebrand's disease: treatment, 1995; 271

Work of breathing: factors affecting, 1994; 17